Advances in the Treatment of Athletic Injury

Editor

MARK S. MYERSON

FOOT AND ANKLE CLINICS

www.foot.theclinics.com

Consulting Editor
MARK S. MYERSON

March 2021 • Volume 26 • Number 1

ELSEVIER

1600 John F. Kennedy Boulevard ● Suite 1800 ● Philadelphia, Pennsylvania, 19103-2899

http://www.theclinics.com

FOOT AND ANKLE CLINICS Volume 26, Number 1
March 2021 ISSN 1083-7515, ISBN-978-0-323-75591-7

Editor: Lauren Boyle
Developmental Editor: Nicole Congleton

Foot and Ankle Clinics (ISSN 1083-7515) is published quarterly by Elsevier, Inc., 360 Park Avenue South, New York, NY 10010-1710. Months of issue are March, June, September, and December. Periodicals postage paid at New York, NY, and additional mailing offices. Subscription price per year is $344.00 (US individuals), $741.00 (US institutions), $100.00 (US students), $371.00 (Canadian individuals), $778.00 (Canadian institutions), $100.00 (Canadian students), $479.00 (international individuals), $778.00 (international institutions), and $215.00 (international students). To receive student/resident rate, orders must be accompanied by name of affiliated institution, date of term, and the *signature* of program/residency coordinator on institution letterhead. Orders will be billed at individual rate until proof of status is received. Foreign air speed delivery is included in all *Clinics* subscription prices. All prices are subject to change without notice. **POSTMASTER:** Send address changes to *Foot and Ankle Clinics*, Elsevier Health Sciences Division, Subscription Customer Service, 3251 Riverport Lane, Maryland Heights, MO 63043. **Customer Service: 1-800-654-2452 (US and Canada). From outside of the United States and Canada, call 314-447-8871. Fax: 314-447-8029. E-mail: JournalsCustomerService-usa@ elsevier.com (for print support); JournalsOnlineSupport-usa@elsevier.com (for online support).**

Reprints. For copies of 100 or more, of articles in this publication, please contact the Commercial Reprints Department, Elsevier Inc., 360 Park Avenue South, New York, NY 10010-1710. Tel.: 212-633-3874; Fax: 212-633-3820; E-mail: reprints@elsevier.com.

Contributors

CONSULTING EDITOR

MARK S. MYERSON, MD
Visiting Professor, Department of Orthopedics, University of Colorado, Past President, American Orthopedic Foot and Ankle Society, Editor in Chief, *Foot and Ankle Clinics of N. America,* Executive Director and Founder, Steps2Walk, Denver, Colorado, USA

AUTHORS

NORMAN E. WALDROP, III, MD
Foot and Ankle Surgeon, Managing Partner, Andrews Sports Medicine and Orthopaedic Center, Birmingham, Alabama, USA

JORGE I. ACEVEDO, MD
Department of Orthopedics, Southeast Orthopedic Specialists, Director, Foot and Ankle Center, Jacksonville, Florida, USA

TYLER ALLEN, BS
University of Nevada Reno School of Medicine, Reno, Nevada, USA

J. NIENKE ALTINK, BSc
Department of Orthopaedic Surgery, Amsterdam Movement Sciences, Amsterdam UMC, Location AMC, University of Amsterdam, Academic Center for Evidence Based Sports Medicine (ACES), Amsterdam Collaboration for Health and Safety in Sports (ACHSS), AMC/VUmc IOC Research Center, Amsterdam, the Netherlands

DANIEL BAUMFELD, MD, PHD
Adjunct Professor, UFMG - Federal University of Minas Gerais, Brazil

WILLIAM A. DAVIS III, MD
Orthopaedic Sports Medicine and Foot and Ankle Surgeon, DuPage Medical Group, Team Physician – North Central College, Naperville, Illinois, USA

FRED T. FINNEY, MD
Peachtree Orthopedics, Atlanta, Georgia, USA

CHRISTOPHER W. HODGKINS, MD
Attending Orthopedic Surgeon, Miami Orthopedics and Sports Medicine Institute, Miami, Florida, USA

TODD A. IRWIN, MD
OrthoCarolina Foot and Ankle Institute, Associate Professor, Atrium Health Musculoskeletal Institute, Charlotte, North Carolina, USA

MEGHAN KELLY, MD, PhD
Department of Orthopedic Surgery, University of California, Davis, Assistant Professor of Foot and Ankle Surgery, Department of Orthopedic Surgery, Mount Sinai Icahn School of Medicine, New York, New York, USA

GINO M.M.J. KERKHOFFS, MD, PhD
Professor, Department of Orthopaedic Surgery, Amsterdam Movement Sciences, Amsterdam UMC, Location AMC, University of Amsterdam, Academic Center for Evidence Based Sports Medicine (ACES), Amsterdam Collaboration for Health and Safety in Sports (ACHSS), AMC/VUmc IOC Research Center, Amsterdam, the Netherlands

JEFF KLOTT, MD
Department of Orthopedics, Indiana University, Fishers, Indiana, USA

PETER G. MANGONE, MD
Department of Orthopedics, Blue Ridge Division of EmergeOrtho, Foot and Ankle Center, Arden, North Carolina, USA

NACIME SALOMÃO BARBACHAN MANSUR, MD, PhD
Foot and Ankle Sector, Department of Orthopedics and Traumatology, Escola Paulista de Medicina, Federal University of São Paulo, São Paulo, Sao Paulo, Brazil

CAIO NERY, MD, PHD
Associate Professor, UNIFESP - Federal University of São Paulo, São Paulo, Sao Paulo, Brazil

DAVID A. PORTER, MD, PhD
Methodist Sports Medicine/TOS, Volunteer Clinical Faculty, Department of Orthopedics, Indiana University, Indianapolis, Indiana, USA; Consultant, Indianapolis Colts, Indiana University, Purdue University, Wabash College, Indiana, USA

QUINTEN G.H. RIKKEN, BSc
Department of Orthopaedic Surgery, Amsterdam Movement Sciences, Amsterdam UMC, Location AMC, University of Amsterdam, Academic Center for Evidence Based Sports Medicine (ACES), Amsterdam Collaboration for Health and Safety in Sports (ACHSS), AMC/VUmc IOC Research Center, Amsterdam, the Netherlands

ELI SCHMIDT, BS
University of Iowa, Carver College of Medicine, Iowa City, Iowa, USA

JOHN R. SHANK, MD
Department of Orthopedic Surgery, Colorado Center of Orthopaedic Excellence, Colorado Springs, Colorado, USA

CAROLYN M. SOFKA, MD, FACR
Professor of Radiology, Weill Cornell Medicine, Attending Radiologist, Director, Education, Department of Radiology and Imaging, Hospital for Special Surgery, New York, New York, USA

MICHAEL P. SWORDS, DO
Michigan Orthopedic Center, Chair, Department of Orthopedic Surgery, Director of Orthopedic Trauma, Sparrow Hospital, Lansing, Michigan, USA

NICHOLAS A. WESSLING, MD
Attending Orthopedic Surgeon, Lenox Hill Hospital, New York, New York, USA

GAUTAM P. YAGNIK, MD
Sports Medicine Orthopaedic Surgeon, Miami Orthopaedic and Sports Medicine Institute, Clinical Assistant Professor of Orthopaedic Surgery, Florida International University, Herbert Wertheim College of Medicine, Team Physician, NFL Miami Dolphins and NHL Florida Panthers, Baptist Health South Florida, Coral Gables, Florida, USA

Editorial Advisory Board

Contents

Turf toe injuries have been increasing in numbers in recent years. Injury to the plantar restraints of the first metatarsophalangeal joint can lead to significant disability in athletes, affecting their push-off and ability to perform on the athletic field. Most turf toe injuries can be treated conservatively with rest, ice, compression, immobilization if needed, and a dedicated rehabilitation program; however, in some injuries, the plantar restraints are torn and the joint becomes unstable. If necessary, turf toe injury and its many variants can be surgically repaired with the expectation that the athlete will be able to return to play.

Much has changed since Lisfranc described lesions at the tarsometatarsal (TMT) joint in 1815. What was considered an osseous high-energy condition nowadays is understood as myriad possible presentations, occurring in minor and inconspicuous traumas. Advancements in diagnostics of Lisfranc injury allow recognizing many variants of this trauma presentation, most of them with a focus on ligaments. This perception shifted trends in surgical planning, especially for implants and fixation techniques. These revolutions established a new and evolving universe around TMT lesions, different from what was known only a few years ago and still not enough to completely settle the disease scenario.

Proximal fifth metatarsal fractures are common in the athlete and can be a source of significant, temporary disability and missed playing time. The pattern of fracture can vary, and the type of fracture leads to a significantly different prognosis and treatment. Jones fractures of the fifth metatarsal are particularly common and difficult to treat in the athlete, can have recurrence and refracture, and require expertise to heal. Intramedullary screw fixation is currently the preferred method of fixation. Most other (non-Jones fractures and os vesalianum) proximal fifth metatarsal fractures can be treated successfully without surgery.

patients with OLTs because lesion and patient characteristics guide treatment. This current concepts review covers clinical and preclinical evidence on OLT etiology, presentation, diagnosis, and treatment, all based on the Amsterdam perspective.

Primary lateral ankle ligament reconstruction has a high success rate, but failures may lead to recurrent instability. In patients with recurrent lateral ankle instability, it is important to determine the mode of failure. Underlying cavovarus deformity and joint hypermobility must be identified and addressed at the time of revision surgical stabilization. The modified Brostrom-Gould procedure is typically performed for primary lateral ankle ligament reconstruction, but it may be used in revision stabilization procedures utilizing suture-tape augmentation. Revision lateral ankle stabilization surgery can also be addressed with anatomic allograft reconstruction of the ATFL and CFL, and is the authors' preferred technique.

Ankle impingement refers to a chronic painful mechanical limitation of ankle motion caused by soft tissue or osseous abnormality affecting the anterior or posterior tibiotalar joint. Impingement can be associated with a single traumatic event or repetitive microtrauma. These syndromes are a possible etiology of persistent ankle pain. An arthroscopic approach to this pathology, when indicated, is considered as ideal treatment with its high safety and low complication rate. We describe the clinical and potential imaging features, and the arthroscopic/endoscopic management strategies, for the 4 main impingement syndromes of the ankle: anterolateral, anterior, antero-medial, and posterior.

The epidemiology of any given topic sometimes is overlooked. This is true particularly with sports physicians and sports injuries. The identification of sports-specific injury patterns by collection and examination of data can help prevent injuries. Thus, as a physician involved in any sport, it is essential to have this knowledge because understanding it and imparting it may allow a valuable contribution to the health and safety of the athletes and success of the teams.

In athletes, foot injuries present with a variety of mechanisms, severity, and implications for return to play. Although potentially given less attention than knee and shoulder injuries by the team physician, foot injuries are common and thus require knowledgeable consideration. In this article, we review the anatomy, presentation, workup, and management of several of the most common athletic foot injuries, including turf toe, Lisfranc injuries, Jones fractures, and navicular stress fractures. The goal is to provide the team physician with the information necessary to evaluate and manage these injuries on the sideline and in the training room.

Foot and ankle instability can be seen both in acute and chronic settings, and isolating the diagnosis can be difficult. Imaging can contribute to the clinical presentation not only by identifying abnormal morphology of various supporting soft tissue structures but also by providing referring clinicians with a sense of how functionally incompetent those structures are by utilizing weight-bearing images and with comparison to the contralateral side. Loading the affected joint and visualizing changes in alignment provide clinicians with information regarding the severity of the abnormality and, therefore, how it should be managed.

In the past 2 decades, there has been a rapid expansion of clinical studies investigating the safety and efficacy of biological treatment methods for a wide range of diseases. These biological treatment methods increasingly are used in clinical practice based on limited available evidence. This article provides an overview of evidence on biological treatment methods for foot and ankle pathologies, including ankle osteoarthritis, osteochondral lesions of the talus, and Achilles tendinopathy.

FOOT AND ANKLE CLINICS

RELATED SERIES

Clinics in Sports Medicine
Orthopedic Clinics
Physical Medicine and Rehabilitation Clinics

THE CLINICS ARE NOW AVAILABLE ONLINE!
Access your subscription at:
www.theclinics.com

Foreword

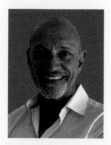

Mark S. Myerson, MD
Consulting Editor

This issue marks the 25th anniversary of *Foot and Ankle Clinics of North America*. When I began as the consulting editor in 1996, I could not have imagined the direction and academic growth that we have enjoyed. We have maintained our goals for high-quality review papers bringing the readership up-to date information on current and controversial topics. In addition to the guest editors who have been such a reliable and generous source of support, I would like to acknowledge the work of the editorial advisory board, including Kent Ellington, Shuyuan Li, Stefan Rammelt, Jeffrey Seybold, and Federico Usuelli.

Each issue is very carefully planned 2 years in advance, and with the support of the incredible Elsevier staff, the process from selection of the guest editor, topics, and contributors, through production and publication has been seamless. It is hard to understand the complexity of producing each issue, and the constant support and dedication of the editorial staff have made my task so much easier. We could not have accomplished this without the author contributors, but also you, the readership, and I encourage all of you to communicate with me directly at mark4feet@gmail.com with any ideas, thoughts, or suggestions for future articles and topics for discussion. I thoroughly enjoy the privilege of being the consulting editor and hope that I can continue to find innovative and thoughtful topics for publication in the years to come.

Mark S. Myerson, MD
Department of Orthopedics
University of Colorado
1635 Aurora Court Anschutz Outpatient
Pavilion, 4th floor
Aurora, CO 80045, USA

E-mail address:
mark4feet@gmail.com

Foot Ankle Clin N Am 26 (2021) xiii
https://doi.org/10.1016/j.fcl.2020.12.002
1083-7515/21/© 2020 Published by Elsevier Inc.

Assessment and Treatment of Sports Injuries to the First Metatarsophalangeal Joint

Norman E. Waldrop III, MD

KEYWORDS

- Turf toe • Hallux • Sports • Metatarsophalangeal joint sprain • Plantar plate

KEY POINTS

- Turf toe injuries have increased in frequency in recent years, leading to significant disability in athletes.
- Injuries to the first metatarsophalangeal joint have many different variants, and understanding these mechanisms and the physical examination signs can help physicians better diagnose and appropriately treat this injury.
- Turf toe injuries are hyperextension injuries of the great toe that lead to compromise of the plantar restraints, leading to difficulty with push-off, affecting the athlete's ability to perform.
- Although uncommon, surgical treatment of turf toe injuries restores stability of the joint and allows successful return to play of the athlete.

Awareness of injuries of the first metatarsophalangeal (MTP) joint has become more heightened over recent years. It is a common injury seen in sports and can significantly affect an athlete's gait and mechanics, and career. Commonly known as turf toe, the injury is typically described as a hyperextension force on the first MTP joint with foot in a flxed position. This hyperextension leads to injury of the plantar plate of the first MTP joint, resulting in an injury to the joint that can significantly compromise the function of the foot. The term turf toe is used to describe the many variants of injury to the first MTP joint, including the isolated hyperextension injury, varus and valgus injuries that also injure the collateral ligaments, as well as associated injury to the sesamoids. Despite more recent awareness of this condition, there still remains some confusion regarding the injury.

The term turf toe was first used to describe injuries to the first MTP joint by Bowers and Martin[1] in 1976. The investigators described a hyperextension injury to the great toe in collegiate football players. They found an average of 5.4 turf toe injuries per year

Andrews Sports Medicine and Orthopaedic Center, 805 St. Vincent's Drive, Suite 100, Birmingham, AL 35205, USA
E-mail address: Norman.waldrop@andrewssm.com
Twitter: @newaldroplII (N.E.W.)

Foot Ankle Clin N Am 26 (2021) 1–12
https://doi.org/10.1016/j.fcl.2020.07.003
1083-7515/21/© 2020 Elsevier Inc. All rights reserved.

in collegiate football players, whereas Coker and colleagues[2] at the University of Arkansas, and Clanton and colleagues[3] at Rice University, found numbers that were comparable.[2,3] Numerous studies have shown the prevalence of the injury at various levels of football, including professional football players in the National Football League, who reported an incidence of 45% in a survey of 80 active players.[4] This injury has also been reported in soccer, wrestling, basketball, and other jumping sports. Much of the increase in incidence of the injury is attributed to changes in shoewear, with athletes wearing more flexible, lightweight shoes that allow greater motion of the forefoot.

ANATOMY

The first MTP joint is an inherently unstable joint that relies on its soft tissue complex to maintain its stability. Only a minor amount of the stability of the joint is afforded from the shape of the joint, with the shallow socket of the proximal phalanx articulating with the convex surface of the metatarsal head. This structure inherently provides the joint with a wide range of motion. Joseph[5] reported that the normal range of the motion in dorsiflexion was nearly 80°. The capsuloligamentous complex provides most of the stability to the joint. There are fan-shaped medial and lateral collateral ligaments that provide stability to varus and valgus forces. These ligaments fan out from the metatarsal head, inserting on the proximal phalanx and the plantar plate. The plantar plate resides on the inferior portion of the joint. It consists of a thickened capsule that extends from the metatarsal head to a stronger, firm attachment on the proximal phalanx. The short flexor tendons contribute to this complex as well. The flexor hallucis brevis becomes confluent with the plantar plate distally as it inserts on the proximal phalanx. As the tendon extends distally from the proximal musculature, it envelops the medial and lateral sesamoids. These bones contribute to the stability of the joint as well as increase the lever arc for strength of push-off for the great toe. This plantar plate is a thick, strong, fibrous pad that encases the plantar aspect of the sesamoids, linking the sesamoids to the base of the proximal phalanx. This portion of the plantar plate has 2 distinct bands as they extend from the sesamoids distally to the proximal phalanx. The tibial and fibular phalangeosesamoid ligaments are the thickened portions of the plantar plate that provide much of this strength and stability (**Fig. 1**). These ligamentous structures attach the sesamoids to the proximal phalanx, whereas the abductor and adductor hallucis tendons do not connect with the sesamoids. The sesamoids themselves are connected through the intersesamoid ligament.

The first MTP joint complex must sustain and support 40% to 60% of the body weight during the normal gait cycle.[6] This force can triple with athletic activities and increase up to 8-fold with a running jump.[7] Because such significant forces must be withstood in athletes, this strong joint complex is essential to an athlete's performance.

MECHANISM OF INJURY

A turf toe injury is classically described as a sprain of the first MTP joint caused by hyperextension of the joint. This injury typically occurs when an axial load is applied to a foot fixed in an equinus position, forcing the great toe into hyperextension. Once the hyperextension forces become too great and the toe is taken outside of its normal ranges of motion, or even extreme ranges of motion, disruption of the capsuloligamentous plantar plate occurs. For example, in football, the injury often occurs when the foot is fixed to the ground with the heel elevated. With the foot in this position, another

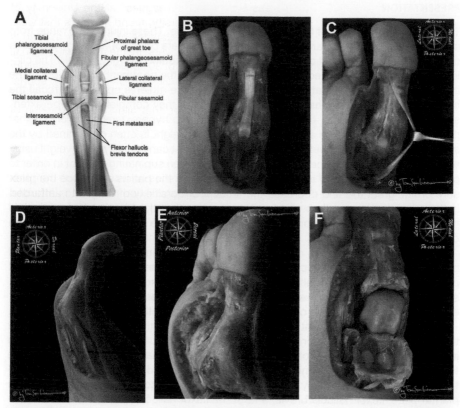

Fig. 1. (A) The plantar plate anatomy of the first MTP joint. (B) Plantar anatomy of the first MTP joint. (C) Plantar plate anatomy with flexor hallucis longus tendon retracted. (D) Side view. (E) Close-up side view of plantar plate anatomy. (F) Plantar view with plantar plate reflected off proximal phalangeal attachment. ([A.] From Clanton TO, Waldrop NE. Athletic Injuries to the soft tissues of the foot and ankle. In: Coughlin MJ, Saltzman CL, Anderson RB, eds. Mann's Surgery of the Foot and Ankle. 9th ed. Philadelphia, PA: Elsevier Saunders; 2014: 1531-1687; with permission. Illustrated by Andy Evansen.)

player lands on the back of the heel, causing extreme hyperextension of the first MTP joint, resulting in injury to the plantar plate.[8]

There are variations of turf toe injuries that can occur. Depending on the forces on the toe, the directed force can have a medial or lateral component, leading to injury of the collateral ligaments and/or the abductor or adductor attachments. This injury can result in a traumatic hallux valgus or varus, resulting in a coronal plane deformity in addition to loss of the plantar restraints.[9]

Another variation of injury that can occur is injury involving the sesamoids. Instead of an isolated soft tissue injury, the sesamoids can be injured. The hyperextension moment of the great toe can lead to fractures of 1 or both of the sesamoids. In many cases, it can be difficult to discern whether the injury is a disruption of the fibrous connection of a bipartite sesamoid or an acute fracture of the sesamoid. Nearly 15% of the population has a bipartite sesamoid; as a result, these turf toe injuries can occur through the dense fibrous tissue connecting the ossification centers of the bipartite sesamoid.[10]

PRESENTATION

The spectrum of severity of turf toe injuries can be wide. These injuries can range from subtle sprains of the plantar ligaments where the athlete does not miss any practices or games, to frank dislocation of the first MTP joint, requiring surgical repair. The clinical presentation and subsequent work-up determine the treatment. The history of the injury can guide the evaluation of the injury. Often the athletes specifically recall the injury, describing the mechanism of injury. Typically, they complain of a hyperextension injury, often recalling the toe getting forced into hyperextension when another player fell on the foot. The athlete's ability to bear weight is often determined by the severity of the injury. In lower-grade injuries, the patient can typically bear weight using an antalgic gait, favoring the side of the injury and often supinating the foot in order to off-load the medial side of the foot. Doing this allows the patient to reduce the pressure on the great toe and decrease the amount of dorsiflexion needed to ambulate. In these cases, the toe-off phase of gait is often significantly altered, with an abnormal push-off being the typical presentation. In more severe injuries, often the athlete cannot bear weight.

The great toe complex is often swollen, with significant periarticular edema and bruising around the joint. Ecchymosis along the plantar aspect of the first MTP joint can be a sign of a more significant injury. In the lower-grade injuries, the athlete presents with plantar tenderness, but often that tenderness becomes more global, extending to the dorsal side of the joint as the severity of the injury increases(**Box 1**).

Range of motion of the joint is typically limited because the athletes often self-splint their joints. With manipulation of the joint, pain is elicited. Passive dorsiflexion of the joint causes discomfort on physical examination. Resisted plantarflexion should be tested, and weakness or significant apprehension is noted. The weakness with plantarflexion can signal an injury to the plantar structures, signifying a disruption of the plantar plate, flexor hallucis brevis, and/or the flexor hallucis longus. A vertical Lachman test should also be used. Anderson and Shawen[11] described the use of this test

---

Box 1
Turf toe grade and treatment

Grade	Injury	Treatment	Return to Play
I	Sprain to the plantar structures with attenuation but no loss of continuity Localized edema Minimal to no ecchymosis	RICE Symptomatic treatment Stiff orthotic insert	As tolerated
II	Partial tearing of plantar ligaments Moderate edema Apprehension to dorsiflexion Decreased motion secondary to pain	RICE CAM walking boot Assistance with ambulation as needed	Up to 2–3 wk Turf toe taping Often change of shoewear necessary
III	Disruption of the plantar plate Significant swelling and global ecchymosis Instability with toe Lachman Significant weakness	Casting or surgical repair	14–18 wk Turf toe taping Often change in shoewear necessary

Abbreviation: RICE, rest, ice, compression, and elevation.

Adapted from Anderson RB, Shawen SB. Great-toe disorders. In: Porter DA, Schon LC, eds. Baxter's The Foot and Ankle in Sport. 2nd ed. Philadelphia, PA: Elsevier Health Sciences; 2007: 411 to 433.

to assess the stability of the joint. Typically, the examiner gets 1 good opportunity to assess the stability the joint, with subsequent examinations resulting in apprehension and splinting of the joint.

IMAGING

Initial evaluation of the injury should involve standard radiographic imaging. Anteroposterior, lateral, and axial sesamoid images should be obtained. The radiographs should be weight bearing, with contralateral comparison views taken to assess any differences from the opposite, uninjured side. In the most severe injuries, weight-bearing images may not be possible because of pain; however, every attempt to obtain them should be made. The comparison weight-bearing views allow an assessment of the sesamoid position. Proximal migration, as well as sesamoid fractures, can be assessed on these views. In complete plantar plate ruptures, the sesamoids, 1 or more commonly both, migrate proximally (**Fig. 2**). Typically, in turf toe injuries, the bony structures are normal, with the only notable abnormality being the position of the sesamoids.

Stress fluoroscopy can be useful, when available. Dorsiflexion stress testing can help determine the extent of the injury. This test allows the examiner to evaluate the excursion of the sesamoids, which can be predictive of the severity of the injury (**Fig. 3**). Waldrop and colleagues[12] found that a 3-mm difference in the excursion of the sesamoids relative to the contralateral side is predictive of a higher-grade injury. This difference is determined by the distance from the distal pole of the sesamoids to the proximal plantar aspect of the proximal phalanx. The more severe injuries, involving at least 3 of the 4 ligaments (medial collateral ligament, tibial phalangeal sesamoid ligament, fibular phalangeal sesamoid ligament, and the lateral collateral ligament), can be quantified with dorsiflexion stress testing using this threshold as the standard.

MRI is another imaging modality typically used in this setting. MRI is used to evaluate the extent of the soft tissue damage in this injury. It is used to determine the severity of the injury to the plantar plate, flexor hallucis longus, as well as any intra-articular disorder[13] (**Fig. 4**). An MRI scan is a static test, with the injury being a dynamic injury. With the toe at rest, the extent of the injury is difficult to fully appreciate, whereas other aspects of the injury, including articular and bony injury, can be overstated.[14] Ultimately, all aspects of the imaging contribute to the decision making in how to treat this injury.

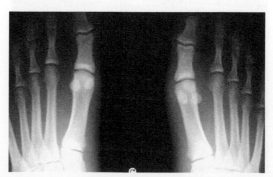

Fig. 2. Weight-bearing contralateral comparison views that show proximal retraction of the sesamoids on the right foot.

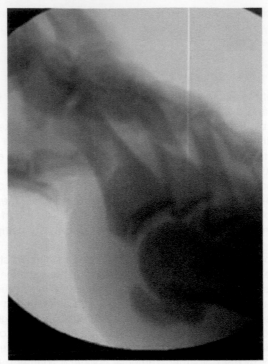

Fig. 3. Stress fluoroscopy image showing widening gap between the base of the proximal phalanx and the sesamoids.

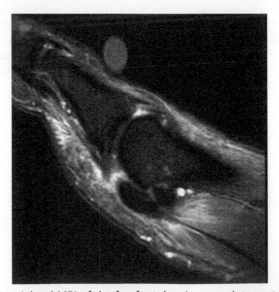

Fig. 4. Sagittal T2-weighted MRI of the forefoot showing complete rupture of the plantar plate, indicating loss of continuity of the phalangeosesamoid ligaments.

NONOPERATIVE TREATMENT

Nonoperative treatment of turf toe injuries is the mainstay of treatment of these injuries. George and colleagues[15] found that only 2% of the 147 turf toe injuries reported to the National Collegiate Athletic Association (NCAA) database for collegiate football players required operative intervention. Rest, ice, compression, and elevation is the standard treatment applied to these injuries to help the initial swelling sustained with the injury. Despite the grade of injury, these modalities and immobilization with a controlled ankle motion (CAM) walker boot can significantly calm the initial symptoms experienced by the athlete. In grade I and grade II injuries, this is typically all that is needed for treatment. There have been many studies with small cohorts that have recommended nonsurgical treatment of these less severe injuries.[1,3,16,17] Once the athlete is transitioned out of the boot, a stiff insole, typically a carbon fiber insert or a Morton extension, is used to limit motion of the first MTP joint. Taping of the first MTP joint can also be useful to take stress off the joint, protecting it from the extreme ranges of motion (**Fig. 5**).

Return to play in athletes with turf toe injury is predicated on a progression of weight-bearing activities, normalizing the gait, and reducing the swelling to allow more normal ranges of motion. Range of motion that exceeds 45° without pain is recommended before returning the athlete to the more sport-specific phases of rehabilitation.[18] Once the athlete can walk without symptoms and the range of motion has returned, a running progression program is initiated. In a grade I injury, or mild grade II injuries, progression through rehabilitation and return to play is typically in the 2-week to 6-week range.[19]

OPERATIVE TREATMENT

Surgical treatment of turf toe injuries is uncommon. Most injuries to the first MTP joint can be treated conservatively. However, there are some injuries that do require stabilization of the joint. Operative treatment of the joint has several indications. These indications include an unstable joint from tearing of the plantar restraints, retraction or

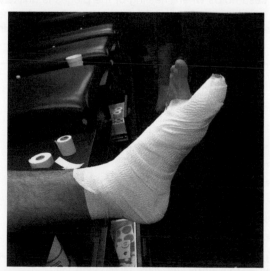

Fig. 5. Turf toe taping to restrict dorsal range of motion, taking stress off the plantar plate.

proximal migration of the sesamoids, diastasis of bipartite sesamoids, dislocation of the joint, intra-articular loose bodies, traumatic hallux valgus, and failed conservative treatment[20] (**Box 2**).

Open repair of turf toe injuries is the standard when surgical repair is required. It is used when there is complete disruption of the plantar restraints. This injury is typically seen distal to the sesamoids, with the injury involving the sesamoid-phalangeal ligaments. Differing approaches can be used, with a plantar J incision or 2 parallel incisions to allow direct repair of the ligaments. If there is enough tissue at the site of the rupture, a direct repair using nonabsorbable suture is advised.[21] If there is not enough tissue to allow a direct repair, suture anchors can be used to reattach the plantar plate back to its insertion on the phalanx.

Injury to the sesamoids can complicate the picture. Various recommendations have been made when the sesamoids are involved in the injury. Although some investigators have recommended nonoperative treatment in these patients, others had concern that fracture or diastasis could impede healing and lead to osteonecrosis, nonunion, or persistent pain.[17] Coughlin[22] recommended that surgical excision of the sesamoids is merited in these patients.[22,23] Surgical excision of the sesamoids can lead to problems because of the important role they play in both stability and strength. A soft tissue reconstruction, with abductor hallucis transfer, should be strongly considered in the case of complete excision of the sesamoid. This plantar transfer of the tendon can fill the void from the defect while both acting as a restraint for stability and contributing to plantarflexion strength of the great toe.[18] This tendon, which is confluent with medial head of the flexor hallucis brevis tendon, is released from its insertion on the proximal phalanx. Careful elevation of the tendon is performed, mobilizing the tendon and the muscle belly by a release of the underlying fascia. Once mobilized, the tendon is transferred plantarly into the defect created by the sesamoid excision. It can be sutured to the surrounding soft tissues or secured back to the proximal phalanx using suture anchors. Sesamoid fractures that lead to instability of the toe can be difficult to treat. Acute fixation of the sesamoids using small cannulated screws has been described but is seldom indicated.[22] Partial sesamoidectomy is another option that can be considered. In cases where the distal piece is much smaller, or cases of diastasis of bipartite sesamoids where healing of the pieces is unlikely, excision of the distal portion is a good option for maintaining the mechanical benefits of the sesamoids while still allowing for restoration of the stability of the joint. Repair of the

---

Box 2
Surgical indications for turf toe

Rupture of the plantar ligaments with unstable MTP joint

Diastasis of bipartite sesamoid

Sesamoid fracture with retraction of proximal poles

Retraction of sesamoids

Traumatic hallux valgus

Loose body in MTP joint

Traumatic osteochondral defect

Failed conservative treatment

From McCormick JJ, Anderson RB. The great toe: failed turf toe, chronic turf toe, and complicated sesamoid injuries. *Foot Ankle Clin.* 2009; 14(2): 135 to 150.

ligaments in these cases can be performed through bone tunnels in the remaining proximal portion of the sesamoid.

Osteochondral lesions are frequently seen in these injuries. Kadakia and Malloy[17] gave a grade B recommendation of surgical management of the osteochondral lesions. Open management of these injuries has shown excellent results in small series. These case reports series have shown excellent results, with microfracture being the most common method of treatment.[24–26] In the setting of turf toe injuries with concomitant acute lesions, debridement of the lesion alone, with or without the addition of the microfracture of the lesion, can be considered.

Traumatic hallux valgus is another of the more common turf toe variants. These injuries occur with a valgus force on the great toe, leading to injury to the medial collateral ligaments in addition to the plantar restraints (**Fig. 6**). This condition can lead to a progressive valgus deformity in these athletes. Surgical repair of this deformity is often necessary. Repair of the medial collateral ligaments with repair of the plantar medial capsule is performed. A direct repair using nonabsorbable suture is the most typical repair, but often a suture anchor in the medial metatarsal head to reattach the collateral ligament to its insertion is also necessary. Although the literature is limited, Anderson[16] recommends acute surgical repair for these athletes with a traumatic bunion. This injury is difficult to treat and has become more prevalent over recent years. As Covell and colleagues[27] reported, although 74% of the athletes were able to return to play, nearly one-quarter of the athletes who sustained this injury were unable to return to play.

As mentioned earlier, 2 different approaches to the plantar plate are commonly used. A medial J incision is the most common of the 2 approaches. The second approach is a dual-incision technique using a combined medial and lateral plantar approach.[17,20] In the plantar medial approach, the plantar medial digital sensory nerve must be identified. Some concern in using this approach is avascular necrosis of the tibial sesamoid because of the proximal to distal vascularization of the sesamoids.[28] If the J incision is used, it is important to avoid a sharp corner at the distal flexor crease with the incision so as to avoid skin necrosis. It is also necessary to develop the flap with full thickness to allow for visualization of the lateral structures. This method is essential to allow access to repair the lateral structures.

Sometimes turf toe injures are missed or inadequately treated, leading to a chronic turf toe condition that makes surgical treatment difficult. In these cases, the athlete

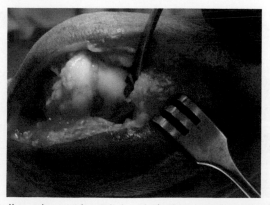

Fig. 6. Traumatic hallux valgus with medial and plantar restraints completely torn and an osteochondral lesion of the first metatarsal head.

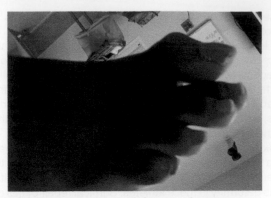

Fig. 7. Chronic turf toe with classic cock-up deformity of great toe.

may have been improperly diagnosed, resulting in continued play. If the injury goes untreated, it can lead to significant deformity. A cock-up toe can result from unrestrained dorsiflexion at the MTP joint as a result of the loss of plantar restraints (**Fig. 7**). The hyperextension is caused by the unopposed pull of the dorsal extensors and the hyperflexion of the interphalangeal joint, which results from the pull of the flexor hallucis longus. Reconstruction is challenging, with various options, including fusion of the interphalangeal joint, mobilization of the flexor hallucis brevis, transfer of the flexor hallucis longus to the proximal phalanx, and dorsal capsulotomy.

CLINICAL OUTCOMES

Most mild to moderate turf toe injuries respond well to nonoperative treatment. George and colleagues,[15] in their query of the NCAA database, found that the average time lost to turf toe injury was 10 days. These injuries are typically more severe than ankle injuries, resulting in a greater time lost from injury.[2] Clanton and colleagues[3] followed 20 athletes after turf toe injuries and found that 50% of the athletes complained of persistent symptoms at least 5 years from the injury. Nihal and colleagues[29] found an incidence of persistent pain similar that of other studies, with nearly 25% of the athletes complaining of pain and stiffness with limited dorsiflexion after 6 months of

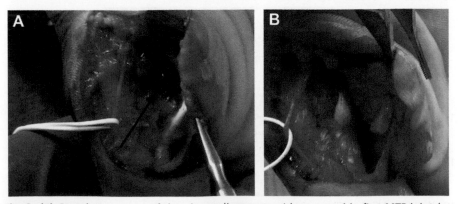

Fig. 8. (*A*) Complete rupture of the plantar ligaments with an unstable first MTP joint (*arrow*). (*B*) Primary repair of the plantar ligaments.

therapy. However, in a more recent study, Smith and Waldrop[30] found more promising outcomes for turf toe injuries.[29] Although many historical studies found turf toe to be a career-threatening injury, Smith and Waldrop[30] reported more promising results with surgical repair of turf toe injuries[16,30] (**Fig. 8**). They found these athletes missed an average of 16.5 weeks, with minimal pain at final follow-up. Players were able to reliably return to play with minimal residual complications.

CLINICS CARE POINTS

- Appropriate evaluation of the athlete and understanding of the athletes is critical in recognizing and diagnosis turf toe injuries in athletes.
- After imaging is completed, treatment is guided by the stability of the joint, which is determined by the extent of the plantar tearing that occurs with the hyperextension.
- Surgical Treatment is critical for good outcomes of unstable plantar plate ruptures.
- With a solid repair and appropriate rehabilitation, good outcomes are expected of athletes that will allow them to return to play at or above their previous level.

DISCLOSURE

The author has nothing to disclose in relation to the content to this article.

REFERENCES

1. Bowers KD Jr, Martin RB. Turf-toe: a shoe-surface related football injury. Med Sci Sports 1976;8(2):81–3.
2. Coker TP, Arnold JA, Weber DL. Traumatic lesions of the metatarsophalangeal joint of the great toe in athletes. Am J Sports Med 1978;6(6):326–34.
3. Clanton TO, Butler JE, Eggert A. Injuries to the metatarsophalangeal joints in athletes. Foot Ankle 1986;7(3):162–76.
4. Rodeo SA, O'Brien S, Warren RF, et al. Turf-toe: an analysis of metatarsophalangeal joint sprains in professional football players. Am J Sports Med 1990;18(3):280–5.
5. Joseph J. Range of movement of the great toe in men. J Bone Joint Surg Br 1954;36:450–7.
6. Stokes IA, Hutton WC, Stott JR, et al. Forces under the hallux valgus foot before and after surgery. Clin Orthop Relat Res 1979;142:64–72.
7. Nigg BM. Biomechanical aspects of running. In: Nigg BM, editor. Biomechanics of running shoes. Champaign (IL): Human Kinetics; 1986. p. 1–25.
8. Mullen JE, O'Malley MJ. Sprains: residual instability of subtalar, Lisfranc joints, and turf toe. Clin Sports Med 2004;23:97–121.
9. Jahss MH. Traumatic dislocations of the first metatarsophalangeal joint. Foot Ankle 1980;1(1):15–21.
10. Munuera PV, Dominguez G, Reina M, et al. Bipartite hallucal sesamoid bones: relationship with hallux valgus and metatarsal index. Skeletal Radiol 2007;36(11):1043–50.
11. Anderson RB, Shawen SB. Great toe disorders. In: Porter DA, Schon LC, editors. Baxter's foot and ankle in sport. 2nd edition. Philadelphia: Elsevier Health Sciences; 2007. p. 423.
12. Waldrop NE 3rd, Zirker CA, Wijdicks CA, et al. Radiographic evaluation of plantar plate injury: an in vitro biomechanical study. Foot Ankle Int 2013;34(3):403–8.

13. Crain JM, Phancao JP, Stidham K. MR imaging of turf toe. Magn Reson Imaging Clin N Am 2008;16(1):93–103, vi.
14. Dietrich TJ, da Silva FL, de Abreu MR, et al. First metatarsophalangeal joint - MRI findings in asymptomatic volunteers. Eur Radiol 2015;25:970–9.
15. George E, Harris AH, Dragoo JL, et al. Incidence and risk factors for turf toe injuries in intercollegiate football: data from the National collegiate athletic association injury surveillance system. Foot Ankle Int 2014;35(2):108–15.
16. Anderson RB. Turf toe injuries of the hallux metatarsophalangeal joint. Tech Foot Ankle Surg 2002;1(2):102–11.
17. Kadakia AR, Molloy A. Current concepts review: traumatic disorders of the first metatarsophalangeal joint and sesamoid complex. Foot Ankle Int 2011;32(8): 834–9.
18. McCormick JJ, Anderson RB. Rehabilitation following turf toe injury and plantar plate repair. Clin Sports Med 2010;29(2):313–323, ix.
19. Mason LW, Malloy A. Turf toe and disorders of the sesamoid complex. Clin Sports Med 2015;34(4):725–39.
20. McCormick JJ, Anderson RB. The great toe: failed turf toe, chronic turf toe, and complicated sesamoid injuries. Foot Ankle Clin 2009;14(2):135–50.
21. McCormick JJ, Anderson RB. Turf toe: anatomy, diagnosis, and treatment. Sports Health 2010;2(6):487–94.
22. Coughlin MJ. Sesamoid pain: causes and surgical treatment. Instr Course Lect 1990;39:23–35.
23. Blundell CM, Nicholson P, Blackney MW. Percutaneous screw fixation for fractures of the sesamoid bones of the hallux. J Bone Joint Surg Br 2002;84(8): 1138–41.
24. Davies MS, Saxby TS. Arthroscopy of the first metatarsophalangeal joint. J Bone Joint Surg Br 1999;81(2):203–6.
25. Debnath UK, Hemmady MV, Hariharan K. Indications for and technique of first metatarsophalangeal joint arthroscopy. Foot Ankle Int 2006;27(12):1049–54.
26. van Dijk CN, Veenstra KM, Nuesch BC. Arthroscopic surgery of the metatarsophalangeal first joint. Arthroscopy 1998;14(8):851–5.
27. Covell DJ, Lareau CR, Anderson RB. Operative treatment of traumatic hallux valgus in elite athletes. Foot Ankle Int 2017;38(6):590–5.
28. Chamberland PD, Smith JW, Fleming LL. The blood supply to the great toe sesamoids. Foot Ankle 1993;14(8):435–42.
29. Nihal A, Trepman E, Nag D. First ray disorders in athletes. Sports Med Arthrosc Rev 2009;17(3):160–6.
30. Smith K, Waldrop N. Operative outcomes of grade 3 turf toe injuries in competitive football players. Foot Ankle Int 2018;39(9):1076–81.

Sports-Related Lisfranc Injuries and Recognition of Lisfranc Variants

Surgical Strategies for Stabilization

Nacime Salomão Barbachan Mansur, MD, PhD[a],*, Eli Schmidt, BS[b]

KEYWORDS

- Lisfranc • Injury • Lesion • Instability • Ligament • Subtle • Flexible • Fixation

KEY POINTS

- Knowledge development has permitted a better diagnosis of Lisfranc injuries and recognition of its variants. Clinical and image assessments are portraying a new scenario for this condition.
- Different lesion patterns have been described meticulously in recent times, helping surgeons with decision making and planning a proper treatment.
- Conservative treatment must be reserved for cases where stability is an absolute certainty. Any doubt must lead patients to operative care, particularly if athletes are the subject.
- Controversy regarding the decision between fusion or fixations remains, because no high-level studies have been published lately.
- Flexible constructions are receiving attention by investigators in search for a more biologic and definitive implant.

INTRODUCTION

Lisfranc injury presents with a wide variety of injury patterns. Unusual mechanisms and presentations may be found, especially when the athletic environment is considered. Advancements in the game technique and player performance portray a new picture for these lesions.[1,2] Although outdated and difficult to replicate nowadays in the professional sports scenario, rate of neglection can vary from 13% to 24% in the general population.[3]

[a] Department of Orthopedics and Traumatology, Escola Paulista de Medicina, Federal University of Sao Paulo, 715 Napoleao de Barros Street-1st Floor, Vila Clementino, São Paulo, São Paulo, SP 04038-002, Brazil; [b] University of Iowa, Carver College of Medicine, 200 Hawkins Drive, John PappaJohn Pavillion (JPP), Room 01066, Lower Level, Iowa City, IA 52242, USA
* Corresponding author.
E-mail address: nacime@nacime.com.br

Foot Ankle Clin N Am 26 (2021) 13–33
https://doi.org/10.1016/j.fcl.2020.11.002

The incidence of Lisfranc injuries is increasing and is reported to be between 9.2/100,000 person-years and 14/100,000 person-years. The unstable lesions are thought to happen in 6/100,000 person years and low-energy traumas now represent the majority of cases.[4,5] Particularly relevant is the increased incidence in sports and the impact on an athlete's career.[6] Football players who sustain a tarsometatarsal (TMT) lesion are prone to shorter careers and often have decreased ability to perform.[7,8] The return to sports also is long and demanding, and evidence suggests the current treatment still is insufficient and not ideal for this group of patients.[9,10]

ANATOMY

Although intrinsically stable due its osseous configuration, the TMT joint is prone to sprains. This may be explained by its rigidity while lying between the very flexible joints of the Chopart and the metatarsophalangeal articulations, along with the natural apex of the Lisfranc when the foot becomes rigid. This topography also is crucial for energy transfer from the rearfoot to the forefoot, adapting the foot to the ground through its 3 columns.[11,12] Traditionally referred to as TMT articulation, it since has been recognized as an anatomically complex injury determined by the naviculocuneiform, cuneiform-navicular, intercuneiform, and intermetatarsal joints.[13]

Bony local anatomy (Roman arch configuration and intricate second metatarsal base), local ligaments, and tendon insertions provide stability for the region. A shallow second TMT mortise is associated with a greater lesion risk.[14] The primary stabilizing structure between the medial (mobile) and intermediate (rigid) columns is the Lisfranc ligament. Originating from the lateral surface of the medial cuneiform, its 3 components (dorsal, intermediate, and plantar) insert at the medial surface of the second metatarsal base.[11,15]

The TMT ligaments are weaker dorsally than on the plantar surface, which explains the common dorsal instability. A lateral Lisfranc ligament (transverse suspensory metatarsal ligament), spanning from the fifth metatarsal base to second metatarsal base, was described recently and, along with the intermetatarsal ligaments (2|3, 3|4 and 4|5), could explain why some of these lateral lesions may behave as a unit. This characteristic also sustains the idea of the middle column reduction allowing lateral column stabilization.[16] Attention also has been given to interosseus ligaments between the cuneiforms and the connections between the navicular and the proximal rows, as these types of damages have become more frequent clinically.[6,17,18]

INJURY MECHANISM AND PATTERNS

Different from the fracture-dislocation scenario, where a high-energy trauma plays a major role in the pathogenesis of these lesions, ligament injuries related to sports are associated with lower forces.[2,10] In sports, indirect trauma is a more common mechanism, but direct dorsal compression over the midfoot may occur, disturbing the plantar ligaments.[19] An axial load applied to a flexed foot fixed to the ground can disrupt the structures at the TMT joint. A twisting movement to the midfoot, secondary to a simple foot torsion, also may cause a Lisfranc injury. Any direction in this type of movement (pronation, supination, flexion, extension, or combination) could cause lesions to the TMT complex. These myriad occurrences demand a mandatory careful clinical assessment to this area in any situation of foot and ankle trauma or sprain.[5,20]

Twisting injury in sports accounts for 21% of these related injuries.[5] A previous large review that included all types of Lisfranc injuries found a breakdown of 43% of motor vehicles accidents; 24% of falls, jumps, and twisting; 13% of crush patterns; and 10%

of sports activities lesions.[21] Video analysis of American football players showed 90% of traumas occurred when a player was engaging another player and frequently included the foot in plantarflexion and the toes dorsiflexed. An axial force was observed while the player tried to push off the ground and this action was combined with some eversion or inversion at the TMT.[22]

Kaar and colleagues[23] divided the lesion configuration into longitudinal and transverse, according to the ligaments involved. Haraguchi and colleagues,[17] using this concept, cataloged 87 lesions and found 38% of the longitudinal type (M1|C1-M2|C2), 30% of the transverse variety (M2-C1|C2), 20% of the transverse with the first TMT lesion form (M1|M2-C1|C2], 6% of longitudinal with transverse-type (M1|C1-M2-C2), 3% of the longitudinal with the first TMT lesion (M1-C1-M2|C2 2% of a longitudinal with transverse with the first TMT pattern (M1-C1-M2-C2), and 13% of a proximal extension form, extending to the naviculocuneiform joints.[17]

Porter and colleagues[6] studied 82 professional athletes' injuries and found 49% of traditional lesions (C1–M1, C2–M1, or C2–M2), 28% of proximal extensions (traditional accompanied by an intercuneiform injury), and 21% of medial column dislocations (C1|M1preserved, instability between the medial and the intermediate columns).

DIAGNOSIS

Lack of reliable information given by a patient and the variety of injury presentations may present a challenge in clinical rationale. Athletes commonly describe a foot sprain, what can be confused with an ankle sprain. A direct hit to the midfoot area and a fall from height also are possible reports.

Objectively, any trauma at the midfoot must have a Lisfranc injury considered in the differential. Physical examination might reveal dorsal edema, plantar ecchymosis, and pain to palpation. A squeezing of the first ray to the fifth ray (force applied to the forefoot), a pronation-supination force, and a piano-key test of the metatarsals (flexion and extension metatarsal movements produced by grasping the metatarsal heads) all may cause pain at the Lisfranc region (**Fig. 1**), supporting a possible diagnosis.[24]

Traditional non–weight-bearing 3-position radiographs can diagnose only severe instabilities; however, bilateral and comparative weight-bearing images may be difficult to obtain soon after the injury. Weight bearing induces stress and reveals mild to moderate instability (**Fig. 2**).[25,26] If pain prevents an adequate radiographic evaluation, then the foot should be immobilized and reevaluated a week later with or without a local anesthetic block.[2,27]

Signs of radiographic instability include incongruity between M1 and C1, between M2 and C2, between M4 and the cuboid, and between M5 and C1 (lateral view). Distances between M1 and M2, C1 and M2, and C1 and C2 commonly are used as well.[24,26,28] A fleck sign, a nutcracker fracture at the cuboid, and other avulsions at the metatarsal bases or the cuneiforms should raise suspicion of an unstable TMT joint.[27] The values and findings are summarized in **Tables 1** and **2**.

The huge variability of the distance between TMT bones in the general population makes it difficult to standardize a specific number for a stable joint.[15,29] These characteristics make bilateral foot radiographs imperative for these patients. Monopodial bilateral radiographs may increase the stress through the joints and help with the diagnosis.

Although having an inherent inability to demonstrate subtle instabilities beacuse of the static and non–weight-bearing characteristics, computerized tomography (CT), ultrasound (US), and magnetic resonance imaging (MRI) may add information to a doubtful scenario.[30,31] Minor incongruities, suggestive of fractures and avulsions,

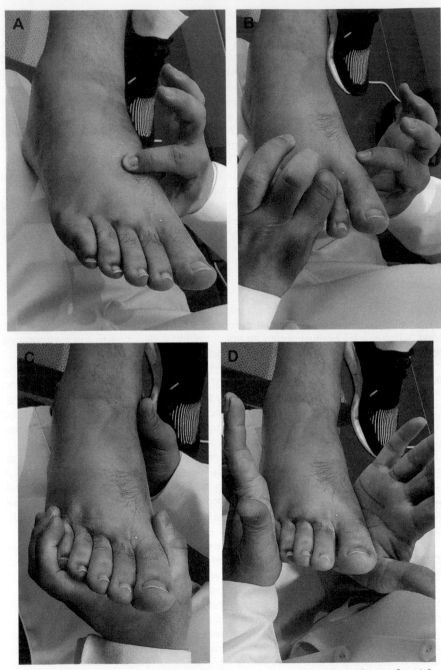

Fig. 1. Examples of maneuvers that may substantiate the clinical hypothesis of a Lisfranc injury. (*A*) Pain at the TMT area (in every ray or column); (*B*) piano-key test, performed by grasping the metatarsal heads and moving them dorsally and plantarly (pain is felt at the Lisfranc joint); (*C*) squeeze forefoot test, executed by grasping the rays by the heads and compressing them against each other (pain at the TMT); and (*D*) forefoot pronation and supination producing pain at the joint.

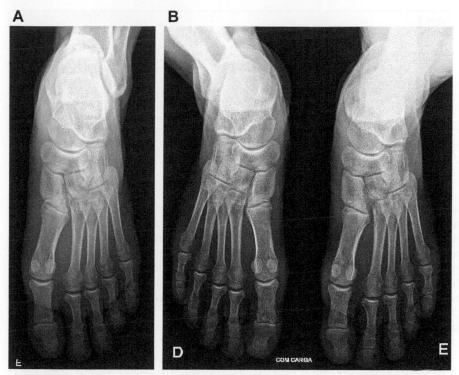

Fig. 2. (*A*) Soccer player with a midfoot sprain and a normal non–weight-bearing radiograph at first evaluation at the emergency room. (*B*) Subsequent weight-bearing comparative radiograph demonstrating a 2-mm opening between medial and middle columns along with a C1 notch sign. D, Right. E, Left.

might be identified in a regular CT scan, but this does not determine the need for surgery. The capability of US to analyze ligaments and bone relations places this examination as an alternative to reduce costs.[30] A Lisfranc ligament rupture seen on an MRI, especially its plantar bundle tear, is suggestive of an unstable injury to the TMT joint.[31] Although very indicative (94% of a positive predictive value), a major or complete Lisfranc ligament injury does not always mean instability, and the ligament's integrity also is not definitive in determining a stable joint (**Fig. 3**).[32]

Table 1 General findings suggesting tarsometatarsal instability	
Anteroposterior and Oblique	**Lateral**
Fleck sign	M5–C1 distance
M5 notch with cuboid	M1–C1 incongruency
Medial M4–cuboid incongruency	Dorsal M1 subluxation
Lateral M1–C1 incongruency	Dorsal M2 subluxation
C1–C2 > 2 mm	
Dorsal M2–C2 opening	
C1 rotation (notch sign)	

Abbreviations: C1, medial cuneiform; C2, intermediate cuneiform; M1, first metatarsal; M2, second metatarsal; M4, fourth metatarsal; M5, fifth metatarsal.

Table 2 Specific findings suggesting tarsometatarsal instability	
Non–Weight Bearing	**Weight Bearing**
Medial or lateral malalignment C2–M2	Medial or lateral malalignment C2–M2
M1–M2 >4 mm	M1–M2 >5 mm
C1–M2 >3 mm	M1–M2 side difference >1 mm
	C1–M2 >5 mm
	C1–M2 side difference >1 mm

Abbreviations: C1, medial cuneiform; C2, intermediate cuneiform; M1, first metatarsal; M2, second metatarsal.

These subsidiary examinations' limitations and particularities still allow room for the use of more aggressive imaging in order to assess stability and allow for better decision making.[23,33] In addition to weight-bearing radiographs, stress images in adduction, abduction, pronation, supination, flexion, and extension have been used to assess TMT instability,[34] but these are limited by pain and feasibility. Additionally, costs and risks impose difficulties on performing these manipulations in a sedated patient. The weight-bearing CT, a current and supported technique that improves diagnoses of foot deformities, may become a tool in assessing Lisfranc injuries and determining joint instability (**Fig. 4**). A cadaveric study has tested the method and could demonstrate relations between staged ligament section and identifiable joint displacements.[35]

Decision over operative and non-operative treatment is based operative treatment or a nonoperative treatment is based on a combination of clinical findings, patient profile, weight-bearing radiographs, MRI, and stress images (if possible).[34,36] Displaced and unstable joints (see **Table 2**) should undergo operative treatment in order to

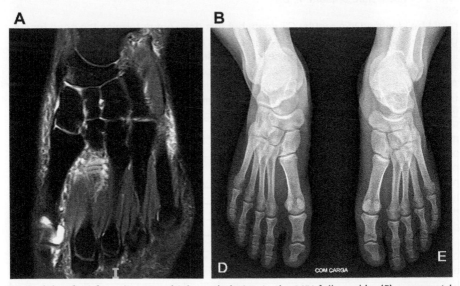

Fig. 3. (*A*) Left Lisfranc ligament high-grade lesion in the MRI followed by (*B*) a symmetric comparative weight-bearing radiograph denoting a stable lesion in a runner. Conservative treatment was proposed, and the patient sustained absence of instability findings during follow-up. D, Right. E, Left.

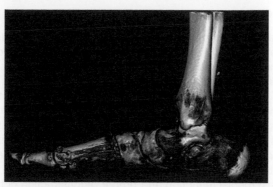

Fig. 4. Weight-bearing CT in a TMT sprain showing a clear instability among medial cuneiform and first metatarsal base in a football player.

restore the local anatomy and biomechanics. Doubt always should lean the judgment toward surgery due to the intrinsic displacement capacity of this lesion.[37,38]

In the authors' experience, athletes experiencing a midfoot trauma should raise a high degree of suspicion for a Lisfranc injury or its equivalents. The patient must be removed from the game or practice immediately. A complete investigation needs to be performed, looking for any sign of displacement or instability, which may direct treatment toward surgical resolution. These injuries by themselves do not need to be characterized as urgent and may wait a day or 2 for proper operative planning. If the clinical findings are solid and instability cannot be confirmed by usual ambulatory images, the player must be taken to the operating room for fluoroscopic stress tests and potential surgery.

CONSERVATIVE MANAGEMENT

If the injury is considered stable and nondisplaced (without any displacement), after a full clinical and radiologic inspection, nonsurgical treatment is ideal.[2,38] Although no reliable study or data support any therapeutics, local immobilization and a non–weight-bearing period are advocated by many investigators.[19,37]

This time frame usually is 6 weeks and during this interval the patient is advised to maintain the TMT area immobilized and to not bear weight. The ankle, toes, and other proximal joints may be mobilized during physical therapy in conjunction with a local and global strengthening program. After this interim, the athlete can start a progressive weight-bearing regimen with a boot (3–4 weeks) followed by wearing a carbon plate insole or a rigid shoe. At this point, the patient is evolving gradually to closed kinetic chain exercises and proprioception training. Return to practice is expected to happen by the twelfth week or, when at a competitive level, by the fourth month after the initial injury.[19,39,40] When considering only stable lesions, conservative treatment demonstrates positive and lasting results.[41,42]

Lack of good support in the literature for these measures and the inherent concept of a stable joint (thus resilient to a controlled stress) may justify placing patients on an early weight-bearing regimen with the assumption that this will continue to be stable in the following weeks.[37,43] However, a study showed that 54% of patients developed instability at a mean of 18 days and required surgery. In this group, the late overall functional results were good and comparable to the nonsurgical subjects with success in other operative series.[37]

SURGICAL MANAGEMENT

Although not always straightforward, from the moment the TMT is decided to be unstable, determination of which specific joints and columns are involved for correct operative planning is necessary. Clinical and imaging evaluations must be taken into consideration. Independent of the type of surgery chosen, some principles must be followed. The injury must be stabilized/fixed from proximal to distal (intercuneiforms before metacuneiforms) and from the intermediate to the medial and lateral columns due the natural capacity of these joints to reduce and stabilize others.[16,44–46] Clamps and pins may be used to maintain joint reductions. The exception for this sequence is when a cuboid fragmentation occurs, shortening the lateral column. In these cases, restoration of the lateral length (plates and external fixator) earlier is mandatory to assist medial reduction and proper reconstruction of the complex.[46]

Intraoperatively, all TMT columns' transverse stabilities, as well as longitudinal and proximal stabilities (see **Table 2**), may be tested directly (open approach) or fluoroscopically by performing local stress maneuvers.[46] Naviculocuneiform involvements usually are easily recognized before surgery, but traction, pivoting, squeezing, and rotation can be applied to the foot in uncertain situations. The lateral column should be checked after medial and proximal stabilization for any residual displacement or gross instability. Temporary (4–6 weeks) Kirschner wire fixation (bridging plates or frames in severe instabilities or comminutions) from the fourth and fifth metatarsals to the cuboid must be carried out in this situation, after articular relations are reestablished.[46,47]

Percutaneous or Open

Percutaneous techniques have gained attention recently in order to minimize wound-related problems.[48–50] Screws, tapes, sutures, grafts, and even plates are described techniques for this type of approach—the first 3 are the most commonly used.[43,51] The joints are reduced by external compression or with a tenaculum, controlled with fluoroscopy, and then fixed. A few retrospective series indicated faster healing and a quicker return to sports with a lower complication rate and functional outcomes that are comparable to the open methods results.[50,52,53] Postoperative radiographs were used to judge reduction in these articles, what may impair proper alignment evaluation. Most studies demonstrated the importance of anatomic reduction for outcomes improvement and arthritis prevention.[9,38,54–58] The advent of endoscopic-assisted reductions may diminish malalignments possibilities when choosing a percutaneous treatment.[38,39,59]

Open approach remains the standard when dealing with Lisfranc injuries due the quality of data available. Current controversies abound with respect to flexible fixation, rigid implants, or fusion constructs concerning surgical costs, complications, stability, and functional results.[60–64] Usually, an incision is centered over the second TMT joint, preventing damage to the neurovascular bundle and allowing visualization of the mortise and the intercuneiform space.[11,65,66] Medial column instability may be accessed by the same incision or by an additional medial one (**Fig. 5**). An unstable lateral column (when not reduced automatically) might need a lateral incision over the fourth and fifth metatarsal base intervals. Proximal lesions (naviculocuneiform) can be handled with a longer longitudinal incision. Transverse incisions have been described for multiple column involvement with similar results and complications.[67,68]

Screws

Crossed screws and Kirschner wires are the most traditional implants for fixation of Lisfranc injuries, including for the pure ligament variants.[69] Debate remains over the

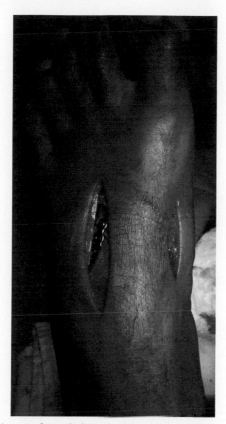

Fig. 5. Intraoperative picture of a wakeboard athlete with a full transverse and longitudinal lesion through the medial and intermediate columns (C1-M1, C2-M2, C3-M3 and C1-M2), demonstrating the traditional longitudinal incision centered at the second ray and an adjuvant medial approach.

inherent stiff characteristics and the need for subsequent removal. The joint lesion concern was a matter of great debate through the past few decades, when investigators, trying to minimize cartilage impairment, advocated the use of smaller-diameter screws and transarticular fixation only from C1 to C3 and from C1 to M2. New published data overturn the concept of articular damage when putting screws through the cuneiforms and from M2 to C1, showing unequivocally that the cartilage areas of this joints are limited and marginal, allowing the implant to be placed without harming cartilaginous tissue.[70,71]

The screw invariably is inserted from the second metatarsal base to the medial cuneiform, stabilizing the TMT mortise.[72] This is the authors' preferred direction, because it brings the smaller (and unstable) fragment to a larger (and constant) fragment. If a longitudinal instability is present, a screw must be placed prior to the step above, inserting a screw from C1 to C2. Residual instability between M2 and C2 or M1 and C1 or M3 and C3 may be treated (**Fig. 6**) with crossing screws (impairing cartilage in this case).[19,27,73] No difference was found between the types (cortical, cannulated, and absorbable) or the diameter of screws.[74,75]

When necessary (and previously to TMT fixation, as stated), a screw construction might be implemented through the naviculocuneiform joints. It is the author's opinion

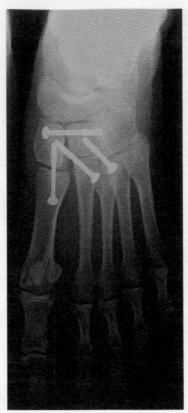

Fig. 6. Example of a screw construct for a Lisfranc ligament injury at the medial and middle columns.

that reduction needs to be carried out directly and, despite the authors' preference for plates in this scenario, screws can be inserted from the medial navicular to C1 and C2 and from C1 to the lateral navicular. Because no exaggerated compression is needed at this area, fully treated (3.5-mm or 2.7-mm) implants are a good option.

Plates

The concept of using bridging plates over the TMT joint to treat ligament injuries was developed in order to increase stability and avoid potential problems with transarticular screws.[76,77] Although commonly used in conjunction with a Lisfranc screw (M2–C1), its use has been supported by articles showing good clinical and radiological outcomes with this approach.[55,78,79] Based on the available clinical and biomechanical evidence at this time, this is the authors' preferred construct when an M2–C1 lesion is not isolated, particularly in athletes and patients with a high body mass index.

Plates usually are constructed from C1 to M1, from C2 to M2, from C3 to M3, and from C1 to other cuneiforms. New anatomic plates (X, H, L, and U formats) were designed to facilitate hardware positioning (**Fig. 7**), even though no data were produced testing these models specifically. Locking plates did not show any superiority over nonlocking implants.[80] Despite its reliable and lasting results, criticism over this method remains as the need for considerable incisions and subsequent implant removal persists.

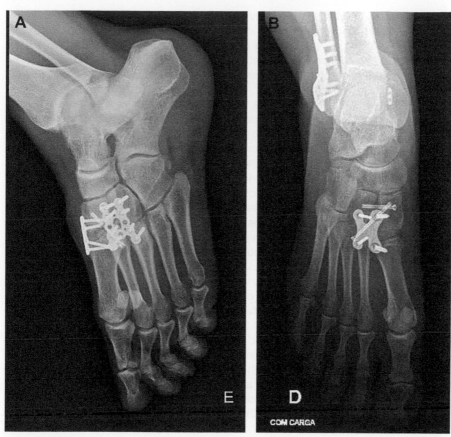

Fig. 7. Different plate configurations for TMT instabilities (*A*) in a soccer player and (*B*) in a handball player.

From the authors' perspective, M2–C1 and C1–C2 pure instabilities may be managed with transarticular screws. If an unstable M1–C1, M3–C3, or M2–C2 relation is still noted after the prior step, bridging plates over these joints are a reasonable option.[45] They provide the necessary strength while avoiding direct cartilage harm.[76] Plate stabilization also is a good indication when mild comminution or small fractures are present, due to its intrinsic capability in securing bone length and to reduce fragments through ligamentotaxis.

A combined medial and intermediate columns instability might receive an anatomic (U, X, H, and so forth) plate from a dorsal incision securing both segments. The addition of an unstable M3–C3 to the situation changes planning, leading the authors to insert a plate (or plates) for M2–C2–M3–C3 from the dorsal approach and to perform a medial incision for an M1–C1 plating. A lateral column bridging plate has its indications when Cub–M4–M5 comminution and shortening is present. A full medial column impairment (Nav–C1–M1) is additionally a fine situation for a long plate because this can reestablish medial length and anatomic relations.

Arthrodesis

Since the article by Ly and Coetzee in 2006,[58] there has been considerable debate over the comparison between internal fixation and fusion for Lisfranc lesions.[58,81]

Notwithstanding the paucity of quality studies, recent literature and systematic reviews examined both techniques in terms of reoperation, costs, and function.[61–63,82–87] When those results are scrutinized and only ligament injuries are considered, no real difference is seen in terms of clinical outcomes. Considering expense and the need of hardware removal, there is an obvious advantage toward the fusion group.[85–87]

The reliability of TMT fusion tempts investigators to proceed with this in athletes. Only Cochran and colleagues[85] compared fusion with internal fixation in the sports population, finding that the arthrodesis group had an earlier return to practice, a faster running pace, and similar functional scores compared with open reduction and internal fixation. MacMahon and colleagues[88] reviewed return to recreational sports in non-athletes submitted to fusion, showing that 75% had no impairment to their activity level, many participating in high-impact activities.

Comminute injuries and late presentations are good indications for primary arthrodesis in players.[27] Although no reliable method was described to state how much comminution is necessary to condemn a joint, many investigators use 20% or 50% of the cartilage surface and the potential association with multiple injuries as factors that subjectively influence this decision. Prior failed surgery, subacute and chronic injuries are also logical candidates for arthrodesis since local scar tissue formation and cartilage damage may hinder fixation outcomes.

When proceeding with fusion, medial (M1–C1) and lateral (Cub–M4–M5) columns usually are spared out of respect for their natural mobility, vital for performance in several sports, especially dancing and gymnastics. The first TMT management was analyzed by Stødle and colleagues[89] in a general, nonathlete population. They found no differences in terms of function when comparing arthrodesis to fixation, despite that the latter group presented better alignment and more radiographic arthritic findings. The investigators' decision for fusion has a low threshold for M2–C2 and M3–C3 (30% of joint destruction) but a high threshold for M1–C1 (50% of joint destruction). Even in a severely comminuted scenario, the Cub–M4–M5 joint is bridged and a late arthrodesis indicated if local arthritic symptoms supports it.

The lack of well-designed articles (more systematic reviews than primary clinical trials are available) places this judgment in obscurity. The mild but natural mobility of the middle and medial columns makes it hard to believe that an arthrodesis might be the final answer in unstable but intact joints (**Fig. 8**). It is in this scenario of uncertainty that newly designed options are gaining space in the literature and in current surgeons' practice.

Flexible Fixation

The necessity of preserving physiologic motion, reproducing the TMT joints' true mechanics, and diminishing the need of hardware removal has led investigators to develop less rigid and more biologic implants. Nery and colleagues[64,90,91] were the first to adopt the concept of flexible fixation when treating Lisfranc instability by using, initially, surgical sutures and, subsequently, tendon autografts. Real progress with this idea was accomplished by the introduction of the suture button technique for these injuries, supported by the consistent results in syndesmotic lesions.[92,93]

Despite the inferior biomechanical results compared with screws, several case series have shown good clinical and radiological results through the past decade.[94–97] Traditionally, the device is passed from C1 to M2 (**Fig. 9**), and is consisted of 2 buttons with a high-resisting suture between both. Other options were created to stabilize the cuneiforms, but the addition of screws is common.[65,66,98] Enduring and trustworthy

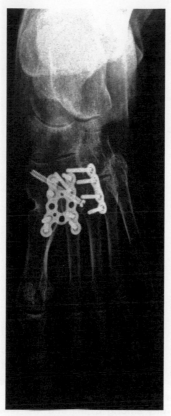

Fig. 8. Arthrodesis over transverse medial and intermediate columns in a Lisfranc neglected injury.

functional outcomes were described in several articles, including when this procedure was applied in athletes.[24,38,99,100]

The development of tunnel ligament reconstruction for graft use was the cornerstone for the advancement of the flexible fixation models.[64,101] New models using passageways and suture tapes were portrayed in pursuit of local mobility preservation along with a high stability construct.[102] The design of these tunnels depends on the lesion pattern, as determined by radiographs and fluoroscopy (**Fig. 10**). They are created crossing cuneiforms and the Lisfranc joints; the tape is passed and secured with interference screws.[102] Cycling and resistance tests comparing this method with conventional ones are starting to present promising findings.[103,104]

Indications for this procedure remain limited, because the technique is still evolving. Absence of structural fractures, lack of comminution, and lesions limited to the medial and intermediate columns (intercuneiforms and TMT) are prerequisites for the tape construction. Higher BMI, chronic lesions, and extreme contact sports (football, rugby, judo, karate, and so forth) also are current relative contraindications to the method. The advantage, besides the lack of necessity to remove the implants, resides in a more biomechanical joint construction, approximating tape placements from the natural ligaments' footprints and configurations.

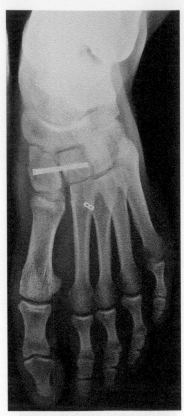

Fig. 9. Lisfranc instability in a basketball player treated with a suture-bottom device stabilizing the longitudinal congruity among C1|M1 and M2. (*Courtesy of* F. C. Raduan, MD, Twin Cities Orthopedics, Minneapolis, MN.)

POSTOPERATIVE CARE

Regardless of the chosen technique, no literature-based postoperative protocol is available for patients undergoing surgery, including athletes.[27,73] A 6-week period of non–weight bearing is advisable by many investigators (splint at first and a boot later). Within this term, patients may begin physical therapy and full mobility at the ankle and toes, keeping the TMT area at rest.[1,38,39] As implants evolved, early protected weight bearing (2–3 weeks) started to be advocated in articles, claiming no loss of correction with this action.[43,53] This is the authors' preferred protocol, starting progressive weight bearing (25 kg/wk) in a boot by the third week and weaning it off at the fifth/sixth week.

Hereafter, patients are prescribed a rigid insole, and progression to mild activities is initiated. During this period, range of motion in any joint other than the TMT is encouraged and performed by a physical therapist. Closed chain exercises are limited until the tenth week. Return to sports in a noncompetitive level usually occurs by 20 weeks. Full resumption to competition is expected to happen approximately 6 months after surgery.[1,8,27] As discussed previously, a high percentage of professional athletes still fail to regain their previous performance levels after a Lisfranc injury.[7,9,60]

IMPLANT REMOVAL

In order to regain the natural mobility at the Lisfranc joint and minimize articular damage, subsequent removal of the hardware has been advocated by many

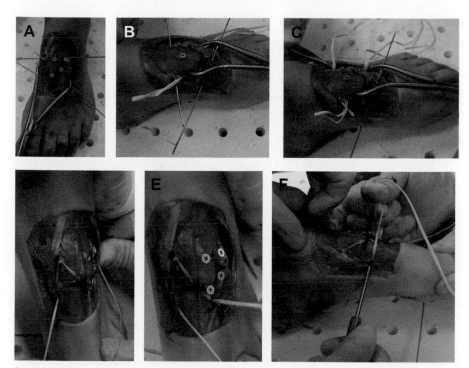

Fig. 10. Image of neoligamentoplasty technique, showing the tunnel configuration where the tapes are introduced. (*A*) Intercuneiform tunnel, M2–C1 tunnel, and M1 base tunnel are created. (*B*) Passage of tape inside tunnel 1 (C1–M2) to reconstruct the Lisfranc ligament and (*C*) passage of tape inside tunnel 2 (C1–C2) to reconstruct the intercuneiform ligaments (inside the loop of the tape); Thereafter, 2 interference screws (3 mm × 8 mm) are inserted (1 in each tunnel 1 and 2) to stabilize the reduction; (*D*) both arms of the tape are passed through the bone tunnel 3 at the base of the first MT—1 from medial to lateral and the other from lateral to medial; (*E*) strong manual tension is applied to each of the tape arms, reducing and stabilizing the first TMT joint; and (*F*) a third interference screw (3 mm × 8 mm) is inserted into tunnel #3 to stabilize the construct. (*Courtesy of* C. A. Nery, MD, PhD, Escola Paulista de Medicina, São Paulo, Brazil.)

investigators.[42,54,69,105] The timing still is uncertain, but 4 months to 6 months after the initial surgery is advisable. Because this procedure demands morbidity and costs, recent publications are vindicating implant maintenance based on good functional scores and possible removal complications.[11,84,106,107]

Nerve injury can reach 15%, and expenses with this second procedure exceed $4000.[84,107] Previous wound complications and local adherences may increase difficulty in removal as well as the potentiality for complications, which may be discussed with patients for proper decision making regarding maintenance or removal of implants. The authors prefer to withdraw plates and screws in 6 months, whenever possible and consented by the patient, so a more natural local biomechanics may be restored. Because this may restore more natural local biomechanics.

Lateral column implants (unless a rare Cub–M4–M5 arthrodesis or an extremely specific situation) always should be removed due joints intrinsic high mobility. Fusion constructions through plates and screws are taken out only if soft tissue rash is present. Flexible implants are required to be withdrawn only in failures or when the material irritates the region.

DISCLOSURE

N.S. Barbachan Mansur and E. Schmidt: Nothing to disclose.

ACKNOWLEDGEMENTS

The authors state their high appreciation to Dr Cesar de Cesar Netto for the inestimable support to this study.

REFERENCES

1. Eleftheriou KI, Rosenfeld PF. Lisfranc injury in the athlete: evidence supporting management from sprain to fracture dislocation. Foot Ankle Clin 2013;18(2): 219–36.
2. Welck MJ, Zinchenko R, Rudge B. Lisfranc injuries. Injury 2015;46(4):536–41.
3. Sherief TI, Mucci B, Greiss M. Lisfranc injury: How frequently does it get missed? And how can we improve? Injury 2007;38(7):856–60.
4. Ponkilainen VT, Laine H-J, Mäenpää HM, et al. Incidence and characteristics of midfoot injuries. Foot Ankle Int 2019 Jan;40(1):105–12.
5. Stødle AH, Hvaal KH, Enger M, et al. Lisfranc injuries: Incidence, mechanisms of injury and predictors of instability. Foot Ankle Surg 2020;26(5):535–40.
6. Porter DA, Barnes AF, Rund A, et al. Injury pattern in ligamentous lisfranc injuries in competitive athletes. Foot Ankle Int 2019;40(2):185–94.
7. Singh SK, George A, Kadakia AR, et al. Performance-based outcomes following lisfranc injury among professional american football and rugby athletes. Orthopedics 2018;41(4):e479–82.
8. Wang D, Weiss LJ, Abrams M, et al. Athletes with musculoskeletal injuries identified at the NFL scouting combine and prediction of outcomes in the NFL: a systematic review. Orthop J Sports Med 2018;6(12). 2325967118813083.
9. McHale KJ, Rozell JC, Milby AH, et al. Outcomes of lisfranc injuries in the national football league. Am J Sports Med 2016;44(7):1810–7.
10. Deol RS, Roche A, Calder JDF. Return to training and playing after acute lisfranc injuries in elite professional soccer and rugby players. Am J Sports Med 2016; 44(1):166–70.
11. Moracia-Ochagavía I, Rodríguez-Merchán EC. Lisfranc fracture-dislocations: current management. EFORT Open Rev 2019;4(7):430–44.
12. Deschamps K, Matricali G, Eerdekens M, et al. The receptive and propulsive behavior of human foot joints during running with different striking strategies. J Appl Biomech 2019;35(5):336–43.
13. Myerson MS. The diagnosis and treatment of injury to the tarsometatarsal joint complex. J Bone Joint Surg 1999;81(5):756–63.
14. Peicha G, Labovitz J, Seibert FJ, et al. The anatomy of the joint as a risk factor for Lisfranc dislocation and fracture-dislocation: An anatomical and radiological case control study. J Bone Joint Surg 2002;84(7):981–5.
15. Thomas JL, Kopiec A, Mark K, et al. Radiographic value of the lisfranc diastasis in a standardized population. Foot Ankle Spec 2019;XX(X). 193864001989073.
16. Mason L, Jayatilaka MLT, Fisher A, et al. Anatomy of the lateral plantar ligaments of the transverse metatarsal arch. Foot Ankle Int 2020;41(1):109–14.
17. Haraguchi N, Ota K, Ozeki T, et al. Anatomical pathology of subtle lisfranc injury. Sci Rep 2019;9(1):14831.
18. Curtis MJ, Myerson M, Szura B. Tarsometatarsal joint injuries in the athlete. Am J Sports Med 1993;21(4):497–502.

19. Shakked RJ. Lisfranc injury in the athlete. JBJS Rev 2017;5(9):e4.
20. Lievers WB, Frimenko RE, McCullough KA, et al. Etiology and biomechanics of midfoot (lisfranc) injuries in athletes. Crit Rev Biomed Eng 2015;43(2–3):213–38.
21. Lievers WB, Frimenko RE, Crandall JR, et al. Age, sex, causal and injury patterns in tarsometatarsal dislocations: A literature review of over 2000 cases. Foot 2012;22(3):117–24.
22. Kent RW, Lievers WB, Riley PO, et al. Etiology and Biomechanics of Tarsometatarsal Injuries in Professional Football Players. Orthop J Sports Med 2014;2(3). 232596711452534.
23. Kaar S, Femino J, Morag Y. Lisfranc Joint Displacement Following Sequential Ligament Sectioning. J Bone Joint Surg 2007;89(10):2225–32.
24. Crates JM, Barber FA, Sanders EJ. Subtle Lisfranc Subluxation: Results of Operative and Nonoperative Treatment. J Foot Ankle Surg 2015;54(3):350–5.
25. Kennelly H, Klaassen K, Heitman D, et al. Utility of weight-bearing radiographs compared to computed tomography scan for the diagnosis of subtle Lisfranc injuries in the emergency setting. Emerg Med Australas 2019;31(5):741–4.
26. Sripanich Y, Weinberg MW, Krähenbühl N, et al. Imaging in Lisfranc injury: a systematic literature review. Skeletal Radiol 2019. https://doi.org/10.1007/s00256-019-03282-1.
27. Lewis JS Jr, Anderson RB. Lisfranc Injuries in the Athlete. Foot Ankle Int 2016;37(12):1374–80.
28. Seo D-K, Lee H-S, Lee KW, et al. Nonweightbearing radiographs in patients with a subtle lisfranc injury. Foot Ankle Int 2017t;38(10):1120–5.
29. Podolnick JD, Donovan DS, DeBellis N, et al. Is pes cavus alignment associated with lisfranc injuries of the foot? Clin Orthop Relat Res 2017;475(5):1463–9.
30. DeLuca MK, Walrod B, Boucher LC. Ultrasound as a diagnostic tool in the assessment of lisfranc joint injuries. J Ultrasound Med 2019. https://doi.org/10.1002/jum.15138.
31. Raikin SM, Elias I, Dheer S, et al. Prediction of midfoot instability in the subtle Lisfranc injury: Comparison of magnetic resonance imaging with intraoperative findings. J Bone Joint Surg Am 2009;91(4):892–9.
32. Penev P, Qawasmi F, Mosheiff R, et al. Ligamentous Lisfranc injuries: analysis of CT findings under weightbearing. Eur J Trauma Emerg Surg 2020. https://doi.org/10.1007/s00068-020-01302-7.
33. Panchbhavi VK, Andersen CR, Vallurupalli S, et al. A minimally disruptive model and three-dimensional evaluation of lisfranc joint diastasis. J Bone Joint Surg Am 2008;90(12):2707–13.
34. Preidler KW, Peicha G, Lajtai G, et al. Conventional radiography, CT, and MR imaging in patients with hyperflexion injuries of the foot: diagnostic accuracy in the detection of bony and ligamentous changes. Am J Roentgenol 1999;173(6):1673–7.
35. Sripanich Y, Weinberg M, Krähenbühl N, et al. Change in the first cuneiform–second metatarsal distance after simulated ligamentous lisfranc injury evaluated by Weightbearing CT Scans. Foot Ankle Int 2020;41(11):1432–41.
36. Mulcahy H. Lisfranc injury: current concepts. Radiol Clin North Am 2018;56(6):859–76.
37. Chen P, Ng N, Snowden G, et al. Rates of displacement and patient-reported outcomes following conservative treatment of minimally displaced lisfranc injury. Foot Ankle Int 2020;41(4):387–91.
38. Escudero MI, Symes M, Veljkovic A, et al. Low-energy lisfranc injuries in an athletic population: a comprehensive review of the literature and the role of

minimally invasive techniques in their management. Foot Ankle Clin 2018;23(4): 679–92.

39. DeOrio M, Erickson M, Usuelli FG, et al. Lisfranc Injuries in Sport. Foot Ankle Clin 2009;14:169–86.

40. Lattermann C, Goldstein JL, Wukich DK, et al. Practical Management of Lisfranc Injuries in Athletes. Clin J Sport Med 2007;17(4):311–5.

41. Shapiro MS, Wascher DC, Finerman GAM. Rupture of lisfranc's ligament in athletes*. Am J Sports Med 1994;22(5):687–91.

42. Nunley JA, Vertullo CJ. Classification, investigation, and management of midfoot sprains. Am J Sports Med 2002;30(6):871–8.

43. Seybold JD, Coetzee JC. Lisfranc injuries: when to observe, fix, or fuse. Clin Sports Med 2015;34(4):705–23.

44. Lau SC, Guest C, Hall M, et al. Do columns or sagittal displacement matter in the assessment and management of Lisfranc fracture dislocation? An alternate approach to classification of the Lisfranc injury. Injury 2017;48(7):1689–95.

45. Mayne AIW, Lawton R, Dalgleish S, et al. Stability of Lisfranc injury fixation in Thiel Cadavers: Is routine fixation of the 1st and 3rd tarsometatarsal joint necessary? Injury 2017;48(8):1764–7.

46. Myerson MS, Cerrato RA. Current management of tarsometatarsal injuries in the athlete. J Bone Joint Surg Am 2008;90(11):2522–33.

47. Uppal HS. Open Reduction Internal Fixation of the Lisfranc Complex. J Orthop Trauma 2018;32(Suppl 1):S42–3.

48. Stavrakakis IM, Magarakis GE, Christoforakis Z. Percutaneous fixation of lisfranc joint injuries: A systematic review of the literature. Acta Orthop Traumatol Turc 2019;53(6):457–62.

49. Raja A, Pena F. Surgical Trends in the Treatment of Lisfranc Injuries Using the American Board of Orthopaedic Surgery (ABOS) Certification Examination Database. Foot Ankle Spec 2019;13(5):392–6.

50. Vosbikian M, O'Neil JT, Piper C, et al. Outcomes after percutaneous reduction and fixation of low-energy lisfranc injuries. Foot Ankle Int 2017;38(7):710–5.

51. Puna RA, Tomlinson MPW. The role of percutaneous reduction and fixation of lisfranc injuries. Foot Ankle Clin 2017;22(1):15–34.

52. Perugia D, Basile A, Battaglia A, et al. Fracture dislocations of Lisfranc's joint treated with closed reduction and percutaneous fixation. Int Orthop 2003; 27(1):30–5.

53. Wagner E, Ortiz C, Villalón IE, et al. Early weight-bearing after percutaneous reduction and screw fixation for low-energy lisfranc injury. Foot Ankle Int 2013; 34(7):978–83.

54. Schepers T, Oprel PP, Van Lieshout EMM. Influence of approach and implant on reduction accuracy and stability in lisfranc fracture-dislocation at the tarsometatarsal joint. Foot Ankle Int 2013;34(5):705–10.

55. Kirzner N, Zotov P, Goldbloom D, et al. Dorsal bridge plating or transarticular screws for Lisfranc fracture dislocations: a retrospective study comparing functional and radiological outcomes. Bone Joint J 2018;100-B(4):468–74.

56. Lau S, Guest C, Hall M, et al. Functional outcomes post lisfranc injury-transarticular screws, dorsal bridge plating or combination treatment? J Orthop Trauma 2017;31(8):447–52.

57. Lau S, Howells N, Millar M, et al. Plates, screws, or combination? radiologic outcomes after lisfranc fracture dislocation. J Foot Ankle Surg 2016;55(4):799–802.

58. Ly TV, Coetzee JC. Treatment of primarily ligamentous Lisfranc joint injuries: primary arthrodesis compared with open reduction and internal fixation. A prospective, randomized study. J Bone Joint Surg Am 2006;88(3):514–20.

59. Lien S-B, Shen H-C, Lin L-C. Combined innovative portal arthroscopy and fluoroscopy-assisted reduction and fixation in subtle injury of the lisfranc joint complex: analysis of 10 cases. J Foot Ankle Surg 2017;56(1):142–7.

60. Robertson GAJ, Ang KK, Maffulli N, et al. Return to sport following Lisfranc injuries: A systematic review and meta-analysis. Foot Ankle Surg 2019;25(5): 654–64.

61. Alcelik I, Fenton C, Hannant G, et al. A systematic review and meta-analysis of the treatment of acute lisfranc injuries: Open reduction and internal fixation versus primary arthrodesis. Foot Ankle Surg 2020;26(3):299–307.

62. Magill HHP, Hajibandeh S, Bennett J, et al. Open reduction and internal fixation versus primary arthrodesis for the treatment of acute lisfranc injuries: a systematic review and meta-analysis. J Foot Ankle Surg 2019;58(2):328–32.

63. Smith N, Stone C, Furey A. Does open reduction and internal fixation versus primary arthrodesis improve patient outcomes for lisfranc trauma? a systematic review and meta-analysis. Clin Orthop Relat Res 2016;474(6):1445–52.

64. Nery C, Réssio C, Marion Alloza JF. Subtle lisfranc joint ligament lesions: Surgical neoligamentplasty technique. Foot Ankle Clin 2012;17:407–16.

65. Briceno J, Stupay KL, Moura B, et al. Flexible fixation for ligamentous lisfranc injuries. Injury 2019;50(11):2123–7.

66. Crates JM, Barber FA. Dual tightrope fixation for subtle lisfranc injuries. Tech Foot Ankle Surg 2012;11(4):163–7.

67. Philpott A, Lawford C, Lau SC, et al. Modified Dorsal Approach in the Management of Lisfranc Injuries. Foot Ankle Int 2018;39(5):573–84.

68. Vertullo CJ, Nunley JA. The transverse dorsal approach to the lisfranc joint. Foot Ankle Int 2002;23(5):420–6.

69. Stavlas P, Roberts CS, Xypnitos FN, et al. The role of reduction and internal fixation of Lisfranc fracture–dislocations: a systematic review of the literature. Int Orthop 2010;34(8):1083–91.

70. Fernandez I, Weiss WM, Panchbhavi VK. Evaluation of the area of the lisfranc ligament damaged by screw fixation. Foot Ankle Spec 2019;12(1):49–53.

71. Jastifer JR, Christianson ER, VanZweden DJ, et al. Feasibility of transosseous nonarticular fixation of lisfranc injuries. Foot Ankle Int 2019;40(6):672–8.

72. Cook KD, Jeffries LC, O'Connor JP, et al. Determining the strongest orientation for "lisfranc's screw" in transverse plane tarsometatarsal injuries: a cadaveric study. J Foot Ankle Surg 2009;48(4):427–31.

73. Weatherford BM, Anderson JG, Bohay DR. Management of Tarsometatarsal Joint Injuries. J Am Acad Orthop Surg 2017;25(7):469–79.

74. Rozell JC, Chin M, Donegan DJ, et al. Biomechanical comparison of fully threaded solid cortical versus partially threaded cannulated cancellous screw fixation for lisfranc injuries. Orthopedics 2018;41(2):e222–7.

75. Ahmad J, Jones K. Randomized, prospective comparison of bioabsorbable and steel screw fixation of lisfranc injuries. J Orthop Trauma 2016;30(12):676–81.

76. Ho NC, Sangiorgio SN, Cassinelli S, et al. Biomechanical comparison of fixation stability using a Lisfranc plate versus transarticular screws. Foot Ankle Surg 2019;25(1):71–8.

77. Krause F, Schmid T, Weber M. Current swiss techniques in management of lisfranc injuries of the foot. Foot Ankle Clin 2016;21(2):335–50.

78. Bansal A, Carlson DA, Owen JR, et al. Ligamentous lisfranc injury: a biomechanical comparison of dorsal plate fixation and transarticular screws. J Orthop Trauma 2019;33(7):e270–5.
79. van Koperen PJ, de Jong VM, Luitse JSK, et al. Functional outcomes after temporary bridging with locking plates in lisfranc injuries. J Foot Ankle Surg 2016; 55(5):922–6.
80. Park YH, Song JH, Choi GW, et al. Comparative analysis of clinical outcomes of fixed-angle versus variable-angle locking compression plate for the treatment of Lisfranc injuries. Foot Ankle Surg 2020;26(3):338–42.
81. Coetzee JC, Ly TV. Treatment of primarily ligamentous Lisfranc joint injuries: primary arthrodesis compared with open reduction and internal fixation. Surgical technique. J Bone Joint Surg Am 2007;89(Suppl 2):122–7.
82. Yammine K, Boulos K, Assi C. Internal fixation or primary arthrodesis for Lisfranc complex joint injuries? A meta-analysis of comparative studies. Eur J Trauma Emerg Surg 2019. https://doi.org/10.1007/s00068-019-01236-9.
83. Buda M, Kink S, Stavenuiter R, et al. Reoperation rate differences between open reduction internal fixation and primary arthrodesis of lisfranc injuries. Foot Ankle Int 2018;39(9):1089–96.
84. Barnds B, Tucker W, Morris B, et al. Cost comparison and complication rate of Lisfranc injuries treated with open reduction internal fixation versus primary arthrodesis. Injury 2018;49(12):2318–21.
85. Cochran G, Renninger C, Tompane T, et al. Primary arthrodesis versus open reduction and internal fixation for low-energy lisfranc injuries in a young athletic population. Foot Ankle Int 2017;38(9):957–63.
86. Weatherford BM, Bohay DR, Anderson JG. Open reduction and internal fixation versus primary arthrodesis for lisfranc injuries. Foot Ankle Clin 2017;22(1):1–14.
87. Henning JA, Jones CB, Sietsema DL, et al. Open reduction internal fixation versus primary arthrodesis for lisfranc injuries : a prospective randomized study. Foot Ankle Int 2009;30(10):913–22.
88. MacMahon A, Kim P, Levine DS, et al. Return to sports and physical activities after primary partial arthrodesis for lisfranc injuries in young patients. Foot Ankle Int 2016;37(4):355–62.
89. Stødle AH, Hvaal KH, Brøgger HM, et al. Temporary bridge plating vs primary arthrodesis of the first tarsometatarsal joint in lisfranc injuries: randomized controlled trial. Foot Ankle Int 2020;41(8):901–10.
90. Nery C, Réssio C, Marion Alloza JF. Neoligamentplasty for the Treatment of Subtle Ligament Lesions of the Intercuneiform and Tarsometatarsal Joints. Tech Foot Ankle Surg 2010;9(3):92–9.
91. Nery CAS, Bruschini S. Diástase traumática dos ossos cuneiformes do tarso. Rev Bras Ortop 1996;31(7):531–7.
92. Cottom JM, Hyer CF, Berlet GC. Treatment of lisfranc fracture dislocations with an interosseous suture button technique: a review of 3 cases. J Foot Ankle Surg 2008;47(3):250–8.
93. Cottom JM, Hyer CF, Philbin TM, et al. Treatment of syndesmotic disruptions with the arthrex tightrope: a report of 25 cases. Foot Ankle Int 2008;29:773–80.
94. Ahmed S, Bolt B, Mcbryde A. Comparison of standard screw fixation versus suture button fixation in lisfranc ligament injuries. Foot Ankle Int 2010;31:892–6.
95. Hopkins J, Nguyen K, Heyrani N, et al. InternalBrace has biomechanical properties comparable to suture button but less rigid than screw in ligamentous lisfranc model. J Orthop 2020;17:7–12.

96. Panchbhavi VK, Vallurupalli S, Yang J, et al. Screw fixation compared with suture-button fixation of isolated lisfranc ligament injuries. J Bone Joint Surg Am 2009;91(5):1143–8.
97. Marsland D, Belkoff SM, Solan MC. Biomechanical analysis of endobutton versus screw fixation after Lisfranc ligament complex sectioning. Foot Ankle Surg 2013;19(4):267–72.
98. Delman C, Patel M, Campbell M, et al. Flexible fixation technique for lisfranc injuries. Foot Ankle Int 2019;40(11):1338–45.
99. Jain K, Drampalos E, Clough TM. Results of suture button fixation with targeting device aid for displaced ligamentous Lisfranc injuries in the elite athlete. Foot 2017;30:43–6.
100. Charlton T, Boe C, Thordarson DB. Suture button fixation treatment of chronic lisfranc injury in professional dancers and high-level athletes. J Dance Med Sci 2015;19(4):135–9.
101. Hirano T, Niki H, Beppu M. Newly developed anatomical and functional ligament reconstruction for the Lisfranc joint fracture dislocations: A case report. Foot Ankle Surg 2014;20(3):221–3.
102. Nery C, Giza E, Wagner E, et al. Dynamic lisfranc joint repair concept: surgical technique for a synthetic neoligamentplasty. Muscles Ligaments Tendons J 2019;09(04):562.
103. Wagner E, Wagner P, Baumfeld T, et al. Biomechanical evaluation with a novel cadaveric model using supination and pronation testing of a lisfranc ligament injury. Foot Ankle Orthop 2020;5(1). 247301141989826.
104. Baumfeld D, Nery C, Baumfeld T, et al. Syntethic neoligamentplasty with fibertape has the same rigididy than transarticular screws in lisfranc subtle lesions. Foot Ankle Orthop 2019;4(4). 2473011419S0010.
105. Alberta FG, Aronow MS, Barrero M, et al. Ligamentous lisfranc joint injuries: a biomechanical comparison of dorsal plate and transarticular screw fixation. Foot Ankle Int 2005;26(6):462–73.
106. VanPelt MD, Athey A, Yao J, et al. Is routine hardware removal following open reduction internal fixation of tarsometatarsal joint fracture/dislocation necessary? J Foot Ankle Surg 2019;58(2):226–30.
107. Meyerkort DJ, Gurel R, Maor D, et al. Deep peroneal nerve injury following hardware removal for lisfranc joint injury. Foot Ankle Int 2020;41(3):320–3.

Proximal Fifth Metatarsal Fractures in Athletes

Management of Acute and Chronic Conditions

David A. Porter, MD, PhD[a,b,]*, Jeff Klott, MD[c,1]

KEYWORDS

- Proximal fifth metatarsal fractures • Athletes • Non-Jones fracture • Jones fracture

KEY POINTS

- Proximal fifth metatarsal fractures are common in the athlete and can be a source of significant, temporary disability and missed playing time. The pattern of fracture can vary, and the type of fracture leads to a significantly different prognosis and treatment.
- Jones fractures of the fifth metatarsal are particularly common and difficult to treat in the athlete, can have recurrence and refracture, and require expertise to heal. Intramedullary screw fixation is currently the preferred method of fixation.
- There is confusion regarding the classification and therefore treatment of other proximal fifth metatarsal fractures, which require careful evaluation and attention to classification and to treat properly. Os vesalianum can be confused with fracture nonunions, which causes mistreatment.
- Most other (non-Jones fractures and os vesalianum) proximal fifth metatarsal fractures can be treated successfully without surgery.

INTRODUCTION

Proximal fifth metatarsal fractures are common in the athlete.[1] These metatarsal base fractures can be a source of significant, temporary disability and missed playing time.[2–6] The pattern of fracture can vary, and the type of fracture leads to a significantly different prognosis and treatment. Certainly, foot *and* ankle injuries are common in sport and athletes, and although the lateral ankle sprain is the most common injury in sport, foot injuries can be particularly debilitating.[7] Metatarsal fractures are common in the athlete, and the highest incidence is the fifth metatarsal.[8,9] In fact, Cakir and colleagues[10] have reported that the fifth metatarsal accounts for more than 50% of the metatarsal fractures in the trauma patient and that is similar in the athletic population.

[a] Methodist Sports Medicine/TOS, Department of Orthopedics, Indiana University, Purdue University, 201 Pennsylvania Parkway, Suite 100, Carmel, IN 46280, USA; [b] Wabash College; [c] Department of Orthopedics, Indiana University, 46280, USA
[1] present address: 10785 Bay Lane, Fishers, IN 46037, USA
* Corresponding author. Methodist Sports Medicine/TOS, Department of Orthopedics, Indiana University, Purdue University, 201 Pennsylvania Parkway, Suite 100, Carmel, IN 46280, USA
E-mail address: dporter@methodistsports.com

Foot Ankle Clin N Am 26 (2021) 35–63
https://doi.org/10.1016/j.fcl.2020.10.007
1083-7515/21/© 2020 Elsevier Inc. All rights reserved.

Fifth metatarsal fractures can occur acutely as well as chronically with repeated stress. Most acute fractures can be treated nonoperatively.[7] However, occult stress fractures and acute on chronic fracturing can be more difficult to treat nonoperatively. Stress fractures at the fifth metatarsal base (**Figs. 1** and **2**) are typically "Jones fractures" and are more common in the athlete than acute diaphyseal or avulsion fracture.[10] It is critical to be able to differentiate between metaphyseal-diaphyseal stress fractures, "Jones fractures," and other fractures and overuse injuries of the fifth metatarsal (see **Fig. 1**). Operative treatment has become the norm for Jones fracture in the athlete and is common in the nonathlete as well.[5,11,12] However, almost all other fractures and "stress fractures" of the fifth metatarsal are treated nonoperatively.

Classification and Differentiation of Base Fractures

Briefly, these base of the fifth metatarsal fracture have been classified by zone I to III injuries (**Fig. 3**). However, this has still led to some confusion regarding treatment. That is, which of these fractures in which zone have a poor outcome? The original Jones fracture was considered only an acute fracture as described by Sir Robert Jones himself.[13] However, Torg and colleagues[14] classified all metaphyseal-diaphyseal base fractures with evidence for a stress-related precursor as Jones fracture (**see Fig. 2**). Porter[15] well described the classification (see **Fig. 2**). The authors think the approach to fifth metatarsal base fracture is better classified by their physiology and prognosis. Thus, they think that all fractures at the metaphyseal-diaphyseal base that are transverse and show evidence of stress should be classified as a Jones fracture, as described by Torg and presented by Porter.[15] The authors also think that slightly

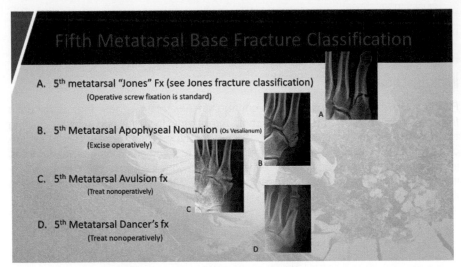

Fig. 1. Proposed fifth metatarsal base classification based on treatment and prognosis. Classification system would use this approach. (*A*) "Jones fracture." All transverse stress fracture from midshaft fifth metatarsal to metaphyseal base. Each of these fractures would be treated with screw fixation. (*B*) "Apophyseal nonunion." Also called "os vesalianum" accessory bone. These accessory bones may be un-united apophysis, and "fracture line" is parallel to the long axis of the shaft and treated with excision. (*C*) "Avulsion fracture." Fractures that are in the metaphysis of the fifth metatarsal base, transverse in alignment, acute in nature, and typically involve some position of the articular surface and treated nonoperatively. (*D*) "Dancer's fracture." Fractures that are long oblique of fifth metatarsal shaft with varying degrees of displacement and are typically treated nonoperatively. Fx, fracture.

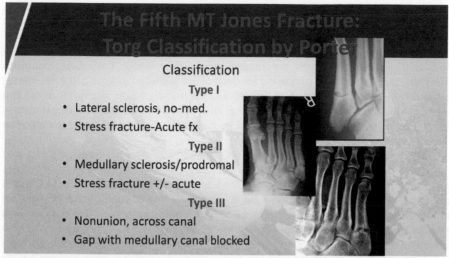

Classification

Type I
- Lateral sclerosis, no-med.
- Stress fracture-Acute fx

Type II
- Medullary sclerosis/prodromal
- Stress fracture +/- acute

Type III
- Nonunion, across canal
- Gap with medullary canal blocked

Fig. 2. Torg classification for fifth metatarsal Jones fractures in the athlete adapted and presented by Porter. Type I is an acute fracture in the presence of a prior partial stress fracture. Type II is a more advanced stress fracture without much of an acute fracture component. Type III is a nonunion with medullary sclerosis. (*From* Porter, DA, Duncan M, Meyer SJF. Fifth metatarsal jones fracture fixation with a 4.5-mm cannulated stainless steel screw in the competitive and recreational athlete: a clinical and radiographic evaluation. Am J Sports Med. 2005;33(5):726-733; with permission.)

more distal fifth metatarsal fractures with transverse fracture lines in the proximal diaphyseal act like and need to be treated like a Jones fracture, even though the authors acknowledge they are a variant. Thus, they propose that fifth metatarsal base fractures be classified as either Jones fracture, fifth metatarsal avulsion fracture, fifth metatarsal apophyseal nonunion, or diaphyseal oblique dancer's fracture (see **Fig. 1**). As discussed further, this leads to a much clearer treatment algorithm.

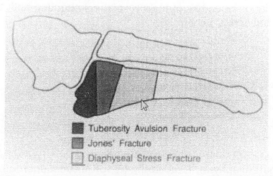

Fig. 3. Schematic fifth metatarsal zones of fracture. Zones I to III of the proximal fifth metatarsal indicating zone I avulsion fracture, zone II Jones fracture, and zone III diaphyseal stress fractures. Note the arrow in zone III, as the area the authors propose has same risk and prognosis as Jones fractures. (*From* Lawrence SJ, Botte MJ. Jones' fracture and related fractures of the proximal fifth metatarsal. Foot Ankle.1993;14(6):358-365; with permission.)

Therefore, the hope in this article is to provide more clarity in definition and classification of the fifth metatarsal fracture. The authors think the correct characterization and classification of fractures of the fifth metatarsal lead directly to a detailed treatment approach. Therefore, having a clear grasp of the fracture classification will lead to more appropriate treatment and expedient healing. They plan to outline more clearly the treatment principles for each of the fracture patterns in the fifth metatarsal base. They propose the reader should not blindly follow a classification, but because each injury can have its own set of considerations, maybe even a certain "feel" to it, each athlete can or should be treated uniquely. Thus, the authors propose the principles within each fracture pattern.

The Jones fracture has the component of repeated stress with sclerotic borders and transverse orientation to the fracture line with different degrees of medullary sclerosis and stress fracture propagation across the base. Historically, it was thought that the more acute fracture overlying a prior partial stress fracture of the fifth could be treated nonoperatively. However, new literature refutes that approach.[16] The authors also discuss the complexities of foot alignment, refractures, and revision surgery as well as new operative techniques and evaluation of screw choice for intramedullary fixation. Likewise, the authors discuss the fifth metatarsal shaft fractures (dancer's fracture) as well as fifth metatarsal base metaphyseal avulsion fractures in both the acute and the chronic setting. Apophyseal nonunion of the base of the fifth metatarsal can be confused with these other fracture patterns and needs to be understood as well. The authors delineate pearls for evaluating these different types of injuries to the fifth metatarsal and the particulars of treatment.

ANATOMY

1. Alignment/contour/articulations (**Fig. 4**A, B)
   a. The base of the fifth metatarsal articulates with both the cuboid proximally and the fourth metatarsal base medially.
   b. The sagittal motion of the fifth metatarsal is significant to allow for accommodation of uneven surfaces with ambulation.
   c. The 1 to 2 tarsometatarsal joints are rigid for better pushoff strength.
   d. The fifth metatarsal is the only metatarsal with an apophysis to allow lateral growth at the base (styloid process).
   e. The metatarsal is curved in both the sagittal and the axial plane of the foot with the most variation occurring in the axial plane, impacting both the starting point and the medial screw penetration.

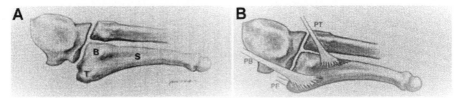

Fig. 4. (*A, B*) Schematic of the fifth metatarsal. (*1*) Bone anatomy lateral foot and fifth metatarsal. B, base; S, shaft (diaphysis); T, tuberosity. (*2*) Soft tissue supporting structures and attachments of the fifth metatarsal base. PB ,peroneus brevis; PF ,lateral band plantar fascia; PT, peroneus tertius. Note that the proximal lateral base of the fifth metatarsal is proximal and inferior to PB attachment. Apophyseal nonunions are often in this location and not involved with PB tendon. (*From* Lawrence SJ, Botte MJ. Jones' fracture and related fractures of the proximal fifth metatarsal. Foot Ankle.1993;14(6):358-365; with permission.)

f. The fifth metatarsal is the only metatarsal with 2 growth plates.

g. Metatarsal growth plate initial closure occurs between 11 and 14 years of age, and complete fusion is usually complete by 17 to 18 years.[17,18]

h. It is a frequent misconception that the peroneus brevis tendon also attaches to the apophysis; the peroneus brevis actually attaches distal and more dorsal on the metatarsal than the apophysis (see **Fig 4**B).

2. Motion/accommodate uneven/sagittal plane

   a. The accommodative fifth metatarsal motion distally with the significant soft tissue attachments proximally leads to inherent increased stress at the metaphyseal-diaphyseal junction, Jones stress fracture.

   b. Fifth metatarsal avulsion fractures and distal oblique metaphyseal fractures (Dancer's fracture) are proximal or distal, respectively, to this added stress location and thus heal well nonoperatively.

   c. The fifth metatarsal diaphyseal shaft and distal shaft and head are vascularized through the nutrient artery[19,20] (**Fig. 5**); transverse fractures in this "watershed area" result in the devascularization of "zone II" injuries.

   d. Intramedullary screw fixation may improve vascularity in "zone II" fractures and stabilize the metatarsal in the longitudinal and sagittal axis.

   e. Hindfoot varus and cavus midfoot alignment transfer weight to both the proximal tuberosity and the fifth metatarsal head, thus increasing plantar lateral stress at the metaphyseal-diaphyseal junction.

   f. Metatarsus adductus creates laterally based tension forces at the midshaft and proximal diaphysis of the fifth metatarsal (**Fig. 6**A–C).

   g. Varus, cavus, and adductus can combine to create a severely overloaded fifth metatarsal and severely impact healing in all fifth metatarsal fractures.[21,22]

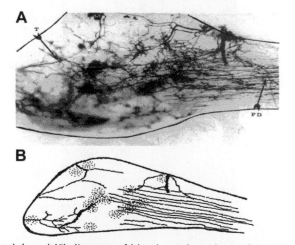

Fig. 5. (*A*) Indium ink and (*B*) diagram of blood supply and vascular anatomy of base fifth metatarsal. Fracture across the metaphyseal-diaphyseal base of the fifth metatarsal interrupts vascular channels at area of fracture leading to increased risk of delayed or nonunion. (*From* Shereff MJ, Yang QM, Kummer FJ, et al. Vascular anatomy of the fifth metatarsal. Foot Ankle. 1991;11(6):350-353 and Smith JW, Arnoczky SP, Hersh A. The intraosseous blood supply of the fifth metatarsal: implications for proximal fracture healing. Foot Ankle. 1992;13(3):143-152; with permission.)

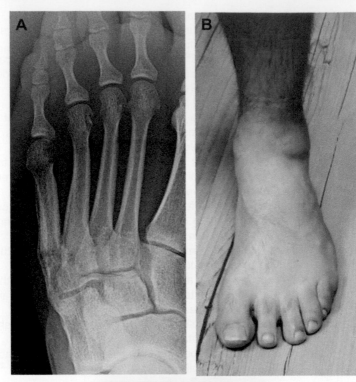

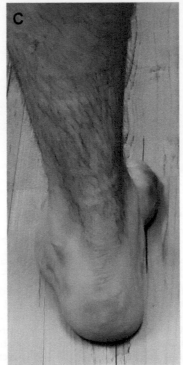

FIFTH METATARSAL META-DIAPHYSEAL "JONES" FRACTURE

Sir Robert Jones, a surgeon himself, is credited with first describing the acute fracture at the base of the fifth metatarsal in the metaphyseal-diaphyseal location.[13] Because of the acute nature of this original injury, historically, only the acute fracture of the fifth metatarsal was classified as a "Jones fracture." However, over time, the detection of other more chronic injuries in this location has rightly been classified as "Jones fractures" because of their similar physiology and response to treatment (see **Fig. 2**). Porter has recently published a thorough review on this topic and a more indepth discussion can be found there.[15]

Athletes typically report acute lateral foot pain at the base of the fifth metatarsal after a twisting injury or landing from a jump. Some patients report prodromal symptoms of mild pain in this area, but often the athlete remembers no prior symptoms. The degree of chronicity of the fracture equates with the amount of acute swelling and bruising. That is, acute complete fractures through a partial stress fracture present with more swelling and ecchymosis. However, more chronic fractures with near complete or complete nonunion present with very little swelling and often no ecchymosis.

A thorough physical examination is imperative to evaluate foot structure and alignment, which can help optimize treatment and prevent nonunion or recurrence, that is, a good, complete evaluation with the athlete standing, evaluating the hindfoot, midfoot, and forefoot alignment to look for mechanical overloading of the lateral foot (see **Fig. 6A–C**). Hindfoot varus[21–23] and first metatarsal plantar flexion both can lead to lateral foot overload and are addressed with foot insert correction. Rarely is surgical correction of the malalignment required except in revision surgery. Hindfoot varus increases the load on the fifth, and therefore, the likelihood of fracture. However, in the initial surgical fixation, the authors' experience has been that the fracture still has a high healing rate with subtle or moderate varus. Thus, they do not do either a first metatarsal osteotomy or a calcaneal osteotomy in the acute setting (see later discussion for revision cases).

Standard 3-view radiographs of the foot are adequate to classify and assess for fracture pattern (see **Fig. 2**). More advanced imaging is typically reserved for the occult fracture, for refractures, for assessment of ongoing healing, or in revision cases. The oblique view is commonly used for classification purposes.

Metabolic assessment of the athlete is also helpful in the athlete with a Jones fracture and probably mandatory to look for correctable causes of fracture susceptibility. That is, a low vitamin D level or menstrual cycle irregularity can lead to fracture predisposition and certainly impair recovery or lead to incomplete healing (see case 2). Up to 50% of division 1 athletes (higher in dark-skinned athletes) have been noted to have abnormal vitamin D levels[24,25] that can be corrected with appropriate nutritional supplementation. Standard bone density testing is not typically required for general assessment. However, in the troublesome recurrent fracture, new technology DEXA scanning allows for more detailed evaluation of the trabecular bone abnormalities.[25]

Fig. 6. (*A–C*) Metatarsus adductus causing lateral foot overload. (*A*) AP radiograph of the athlete with metatarsus showing transverse stress fracture in midshaft fifth metatarsal. (*B*) Clinical view of the athlete with metatarsus adductus through the midfoot and forefoot. Note the mild cavus midfoot and the lateral foot overload because of metatarsus adductus. (*C*) Clinical view of the athlete with neutral hindfoot and mildly plantarflexed first ray causing lateral foot overload.

Classification of Jones Fractures

Torg and colleagues[14] in 1984 classified grades I to III based on the chronicity, degree of medullary sclerosis, presence or absence of prodromal pain symptoms, and extent of the nonunion across the base of the fifth metatarsal (see **Fig. 2**).

Acute type I

The acute type 1 fracture is characterized by no prior prodromal symptoms and typically presents as an acute injury. However, radiographs (see **Figs. 1** and **2**) may show an early transverse stress fracture with an acute fracture line through it. Therefore, it was thought that the stress fracture created a stress riser, and acute injury on the lateral side of the foot, usually from landing or twisting, resulted in a fracture through the existing partial stress fracture. The authors have seen a significant number of athletes present on routine evaluation that have these asymptomatic early partial stress fractures without acute fracture (see case 2). As discussed later, it is likely that many of these will go on to produce an acute fracture if not properly treated and protected.

Chronic type II/III

Both the Torg type II and III fractures are more chronic, are characterized by prior prodromal symptoms (although often minor), and have more extensive radiographic evidence of chronic stress, including medullary sclerosis, and more extensive progression of the nonunion toward the lateral cortex (see **Fig. 2**). With the type III fracture, the radiographic picture is one of a complete nonunion (see **Fig. 2**).

Recurrent

Recurrent fractures are Jones fractures that have received prior treatment, either operative or nonoperative, have progressed to some level of healing, and then have presented with recurrent symptoms and radiographic evidence of refracture or nonunion. Recurrence can occur after appropriate nonoperative treatment, such as non-weight-bearing for 4 to 6 weeks followed by cast or boot treatment for 2 to 3 months with the unfortunate occurrence of recurrent fracturing after return to play. These recurrent fractures can also occur after operative intervention but is typically classified as refractures in that scenario and is discussed next.

Refracture

It is classified as a refracture if an acute fracture episode, similar to the original fracture, occurs after a period of time of complete or near complete healing. Most commonly, this term is used after operative fixation with evidence of a recurrent fracture line in the same or similar location as the original fracture (see case 1). These fractures are particularly troublesome to both the athlete and the treating physician. In the authors' experience, refracture occurs more commonly in the higher-level athlete, such as a division 1 or professional athlete. There has been some evidence that return to play during the same season as the original fracture leads to a higher risk of refracture.[26] In the authors' experience, if there is good radiographic healing, refracture is uncommon after 1 year from the time of definitive operative fixation. Premature return to sport is a known risk for refracture. Previously, the authors had allowed return to sport if there was "progression of healing" and a nontender fracture site. However, in the elite athlete, the authors now require 100% healing on plain radiographs, or if any doubt, a computed tomographic (CT) scan with near full trabeculations to allow return at 3 months to give full clearance. In certain settings, a conversation with the team, training staff, coaches, and agents can allow the athlete to return with radiographic progression and no pain at the fracture site. There must be documented agreement among all parties and the acceptance that refracture can occur and further surgery to bone graft the site required.

Occult Jones fracture

The detection of an early transverse stress fracture in the otherwise asymptomatic foot is considered an "Occult fifth metatarsal Jones fracture" and is often detected as the result of imaging for some other indication. It is occult in that the athlete reports no symptoms and often has no pain on examination. It almost exclusively involves an early transverse lucency in the plantar lateral fifth metatarsal cortex (see case 2 radiographs). This fracture differs from a type I fracture in that there is actually not a complete fracture, but only early osteolysis and minimal transverse "crack."

Treatment

The authors think operative treatment with an intramedullary screw is ideal[5] for Jones fractures of all types. Nonoperative treatment had been advocated, but this is of historic relevance only. Nonoperative treatment should not be considered for the athlete, and if under rare circumstances surgery cannot be performed in the non-athlete, it requires 1 to 2 months of non-weight-bearing until the athlete is nontender at the fracture and followed by 2 to 3 months of boot treatment until follow-up radiographs show healing. Bishop and colleagues[27] and others demonstrated that operative is more effective and preferred by athletes and advocate operative fixation even in the nonathlete.[15,25]

Open reduction, internal fixation

Onlay bone graft Onlay bone grafting was an early technique used to repair fifth metatarsal Jones stress fractures. It is an *uncommon* practice today because the development of intramedullary screw fixation. The onlay graft was a cortical cancellous graft that bridged across the nonunion placed within a trough created in the dorsal lateral aspect of the fifth metatarsal, giving cortical bridging transverse to the axis of stress. This graft required a longer return to sport than is currently observed with intramedullary screws and provided less mechanical resistance to sagittal plane motion.

Intramedullary screw fixation DeLee and colleagues[28] first described intramedullary screw fixation in 1983 with use of a 4.5 malleolar screw.[29] The 4.5 malleolar screw became the "goal standard" for screw fixation.[29] However, that was primarily because there were no other screws that fit in the fifth metatarsal at that time. Operative treatment with intramedullary screw fixation has become the ideal accepted care for the fifth metatarsal Jones fracture in the athlete[5] (**Fig. 7**). Screw fixation is thought to provide more resistance to bending stress and allow natural healing of the fifth metatarsal compared with onlay bone grafting. By counteracting the bending moment centered at the plantar lateral fifth metatarsal base, bone deposition can occur where bone resorption was prominent before. Also, the act of drilling across the fracture with intramedullary screw fixation may improve blood flow also by creating vascular access. The authors think even in the type I fracture this improvement in vascularity can occur despite a "hematoma" in acute fractures. It is possible the impact is less in the acute fracture.

Screw selection, however, is still controversial. Optimal length, diameter, and type have not been determined. However, numerous studies have assessed several screw types and sizes (solid vs cannulated, headless vs traditional head vs low-profile screw head) for pullout strength, cortical purchase, canal size/fill, bending strength, and fatigue resistance.[30–39] Most agree that the largest diameter screw that fits within the

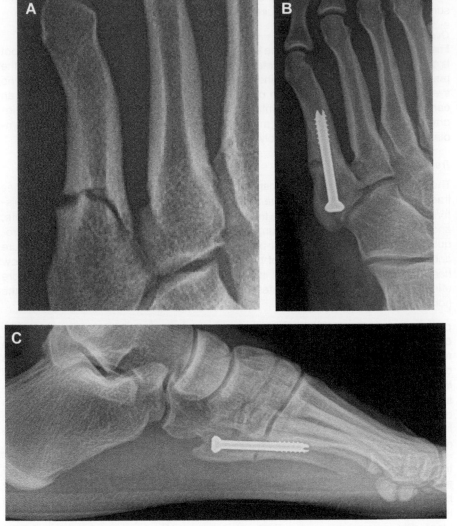

Fig. 7. (A–C) Preoperative and postoperative radiographs of the athlete with fifth metatarsal "Jones" fracture. (A) Preoperative oblique radiograph with acute on chronic transverse fracture. Note that the fracture is just distal to the metaphyseal-diaphyseal junction. (B) Postoperative oblique radiograph showing intramedullary screw fixation with threads past fracture and screw head recessed. (C) Postoperative lateral image of Jones fracture fixation with intramedullary screw.

canal should be used.[6,35,40] Screw length must allow the threads to cross the fracture to engage the diaphysis distal to the fracture. Thread position is particularly important in the Torg type 1 fracture, which is inherently rotationally unstable because of its acute nature. Headless screws have lower pullout resistance. However, it is unclear if a lower pullout resistance relates to failure because screw failure typically is in bending, not pull out. Solid screws have higher resistance to fatigue failure in vitro than cannulated screws.[40] All screws have been shown to fail if fracture healing does not occur. Furthermore, clinical healing rates have not been shown to vary with different screw diameters.[6] Solid screws have been advocated over cannulated screws because of concern for screw breakage and in vitro bending resistance. However, there are no clinical studies to date that have evaluated this theoretic advantage.

Insertion technical tip The starting point for screw placement is critical. The "high and tight" position on the fifth metatarsal base is optimal. The more dorsal the starting point, the more medial and intramedullary the position because of the anatomy of the base. The authors prefer using a threaded guide pin and use an image intensifier controlled by the surgeon to confirm the intramedullary alignment. After initial metaphyseal insertion, the authors place the driver on reverse to decrease the risk of cortical penetration (the pin tends to "bounce off the inner cortex"). If the authors find they mistakenly placed the pin too inferior and lateral, they can place a second pin just dorsal and medial to the first and withdraw the initial pin and then proceed with pin placement. It can be difficult to optimize and maintain intramedullary position in the metatarsus adductus athlete. Occasionally, the authors have to overdrill the initially well-placed pin in the metaphysis with a 3.2-mm drill that then allows them to reposition the pin down the canal without risk of penetration and finish overdrilling after confirmation of full optimal placement of the pin. A cannulated or solid screw can then be placed (solid screw fixation is more popular but not proven clinically to be more effective).

Plantar plate fixation
Plate fixation for Jones fractures has historically been unpopular. However, a new plate designed that is specific for the plantar fifth metatarsal proximal base has generated new interest in plate fixation with reported greater load to failure, higher peak load to failure, and lower gap width in cadaver simulated Jones fracture compared with traditional intramedullary screw fixation.[41,42] Clinical outcomes data are needed to determine if a plantar metatarsal plate location is comfortable for the athlete and if indeed it leads to improved healing.

Bone grafting with open reduction, internal fixation
Traditionally, bone grafting with intramedullary fixation has been reserved for revision cases.[4] It is thought that intramedullary fixation, even with Torg type II/III fractures, do well with screw placement and its mechanical stabilization and improved vascularization. However, on a personal note, there is renewed interest in bone grafting initial cases because of such good results in revision cases and the higher than acceptable delayed/nonunion/refracture in the more elite athlete.[4,26] Cancellous bone graft can be obtained from the iliac crest, proximal tibia, medial malleolus, or calcaneus. The authors use the calcaneus in the high school recreational athlete and reserve the iliac crest for elite athletes (division 1 and professional). Treatment of the elite athlete often combines bone marrow aspirate concentrate (BMAC) with the cancellous graft. The iliac crest is thought to have the highest cell concentration of the sites mentioned.

Revision
There is a paucity of reported data on revision surgery. Hunt and Anderson[4] have written the most complete report. Porter has outlined well the approach the authors take to nonunion after fixation, refracture, and revision surgery.[15] Briefly, they advocate completely taking down the nonunion (unless it is only a screw head impingement), osteotomizing the medial cortex to remove the hinge effect, freshening the nonunion site, bone grafting (typically the iliac crest in elite athletes), and replacing the screw with a larger screw. The authors open the fracture nonunion and use an osteotome to "break through" the medial cortex. The medial cortex can act as a lever to increase

lateral displacement. After taking down this medial cortex, they then drill intramedullary, shingle the outer cortex, and place cancellous graft both intramedullary and dorsal, lateral and plantar lateral to "increase the circumference." The medial take down may slightly shorten the fifth metatarsal, which may decrease plantar pressure (see case 1).

i. Osteotomies: Further preoperative workup to determine cause of nonunion/refracture may alter intraoperative planning (foot osteotomies to correct varus, correcting metabolic deficiencies, shorter or longer screw to optimize fit). Lateral foot overload can occur with either a plantarflexed first ray or a rigid hindfoot varus. An osteotomy is added in the revision case to correct the source for overload, if a Coleman block test shows predominance of first metatarsal plantarflexion, then the authors do a dorsiflexion osteotomy. The authors do a dorsal approach, exposing the first metatarsal base through the extensor hallucis longus and extensor hallucis brevis interval. They place the first cut 1.0 to 1.2 cm distal to the tarsometatarsal (TMT) joint. A second cut is made 2 to 3 mm distal and apex at the plantar cortex. The authors finish the plantar cut with an 8- to 10-mm osteotome and secure the closed down osteotomy with a dorsal 2.7 three-hole, T-plate. If the Coleman block test suggests it is an intrinsic calcaneal varus, a lateral slide or closing wedge is performed. The authors favor a lateral closing Dwyer type. They secure laterally with a 4-hole X-plate. Generally, they have used the first metatarsal osteotomy most commonly, because it is better tolerated in the athlete. A longer period of protected weight-bearing (4–6 weeks) and longer boot immobilization (6–10 weeks) may be required.

ii. Orthobiologics, orthotics: The authors always attempt to get prescription external bone stimulation approval and may use other orthobiologics (platelet-rich plasma or BMAC). However, currently there is no evidence to support the use of platelet-rich plasma or BMAC. Orthotic insert protection in the shoe is always used until the athlete is successfully performing without pain and for the first season. The authors always use a full-length carbon fiber plate (CFP). They use a custom semirigid fabricated orthotic if there is any lateral foot overload to correct hindfoot varus, just as they do in the nonrevision.

iii. Broken or bent screw: A bent screw with a failed fixation always requires exchange. The authors commonly exchange to a 0.5- to 1.0-mm larger-diameter screw. They like the length to be just long enough to have the threads past the fracture site but still within the isthmus of the diaphysis of the fifth metatarsal. A broken screw is more complicated. If the broken screw is cannulated, a broken screw removal set will often allow engagement of the cannula of the screw with a reverse threaded around easy out. The easy out can be introduced proximally through the original entry site after the proximal portion of the screw is removed. If the screw is a solid screw, the authors remove the proximal portion and access the distal portion at the fracture site because they take down the nonunion completely. They hope to be able to engage the distal portion within the fracture site with a needle driver or vice grip–type clamp. Rare instances exist, especially with titanium screws, that the screw (bent or broken) cannot be removed, and then the authors rely on extensive bone grafting only.

FIFTH METATARSAL AVULSION FRACTURE

Avulsion fractures can be misdiagnosed as Jones fractures, but occur more proximally on the fifth metatarsal, at the metaphyseal tuberosity or styloid process (see **Fig. 1**; **Fig. 8A, B**). They are the most common fracture of the proximal fifth metatarsal and

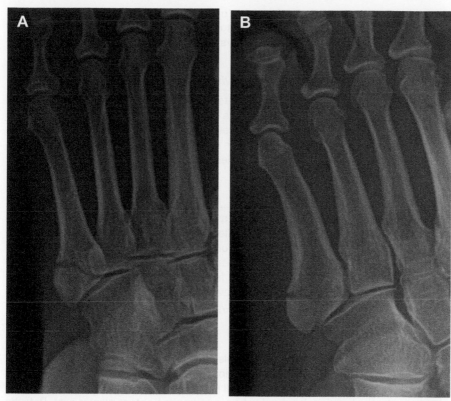

Fig. 8. (*A, B*) Fifth metatarsal acute avulsion fracture. (*A*) AP image showing intraarticular extension but less than 2 mm of displacement. (*B*) Oblique foot radiograph showing nondisplaced fifth metatarsal base avulsion fracture. Images confirm ability to treat nonoperatively.

are usually sustained during an acute supination-inversion injury. They are more common in the recreational and noncompetitive athlete. It is unusual to have avulsion fractures in high-level athletic competition. It is unclear why this is the case. There is lateral swelling and ecchymosis centered along the base of the fifth metatarsal. The fractures are most always closed fractures. (These authors (D.A.P, J.K) have never seen an open avulsion fracture.) Standard 3-view radiographs are typically adequate. The oblique view demonstrates the fracture pattern best (see **Figs. 1** and **8A, B**) but should be visible on all 3 views. However, Pao and colleagues[43] reported that up to 23% of avulsion fractures are not visualized on standard foot views. Because of this, the investigators recommended that if suspicion is high for an avulsion fracture based on mechanism or location of pain, an anterioposterior (AP) view of the ankle, which goes low enough to capture the fifth metatarsal, should be obtained.[41] Advanced imaging (MRI or ultrasound) is reserved for delayed/nonunion or if displacement suggests peroneus brevis involvement with the fracture and a possible tear.

Intraarticular

An avulsion fracture can extend into the metatarsal-cuboid joint. Rosenberg and coworkers[44] recommend surgical fixation for fractures that extend into 30% or more of the joint surface, and incongruence of greater than 2 mm. The authors have not found these fractures to require fixation in most cases unless the peroneus brevis is fully attached to the avulsion and there is 1 cm or more of displacement. Even when there is significant comminution, the authors have had good success with nonoperative treatment (**Fig. 9**A, B).

Lateral Plantar Fascia Versus Peroneus Brevis

As stated in the Anatomy section, the lateral band of the plantar fascia and the abductor digitii quinti minimi (ADQM) are the deforming force for the avulsion fracture. The peroneus brevis attaches more distal (see **Fig. 4**B). Only when the avulsion is more than a centimeter from the joint is the brevis involved with the fractured fragment (see **Fig. 4**B). Operative fixation is required if there is 1 cm or more displacement or if an MRI shows the brevis is attached.

Displaced

Displaced avulsion fractures are classified as those with a gap greater than 2 mm. In addition, comminuted fractures are classified by most as displaced fractures. Most would recommend treating displaced fractures surgically with either open reduction, internal fixation (ORIF), or closed reduction and percutaneous pinning. Surgical intervention should also be considered if the fracture involves more than 30% of the cuboid-metatarsal joint. Some displaced avulsion fractures have a distal extension or a more vertical component. These types are at a higher risk of nonunion (**Fig. 10**A–C).

Treatment

Nonoperative Overall, the prognosis of avulsion fractures with conservative treatment is good, with most patients able to transition into normal activities at 4 to 6 weeks; however, it can take up to 6 months for full recovery.[45] Treatment options consist of a Jones or elastic dressing, hard-sole shoe, pneumatic boot, or plaster cast. Patients can be weight-bearing as tolerated at the time of injury, as Vorlat and associates[46] have demonstrated better outcomes with earlier weight-bearing treatment. Studies by Weiner and colleagues[47] and Zenios and colleagues[48] found significantly better results and quicker return to work when using an elastic wrap compared with a short leg cast. Both groups advised against cast immobilization because of poorer results and inherent cast risks. Of note, some patients may go on to heal with a painless nonunion, which still allows for return to normal activities. The authors have used full weight-bearing in a walking boot for 4 to 6 weeks and then transition to CFP in an athletic shoe with full activity and unrestricted shoe wear at 3 months. The authors have been happy with this approach with a low symptomatic nonunion rate.

Operative For displaced fractures meeting previously described criteria, fixation can be obtained with ORIF, with either interfragment screws (see **Fig. 10**) or tension-band wiring, or closed reduction and percutaneous pinning. Most find these fixation methods for this fracture are not robust enough to allow for early weight-bearing, so further protection with partial weight-bearing (2–4 weeks) and cast or controlled ankle motion (CAM) boot placement (6–8 weeks) has usually been recommended.

Although rare, a painful nonunion persists after nonoperative treatment[49,50] (**Fig. 11**C). The original study by Rettig and associates[49] described ORIF of 3 athletes and excision of the nonunion in 5 athletes. The case series by Ritchie and colleagues[50] described the operative treatment of 6 professional or division I athletes with a painful nonunion subsequently treated with surgical excision and repair of the soft tissues. During planned excision or fixation, one must take care to avoid damage to the lateral dorsal cutaneous branch of the sural nerve. The peroneus brevis can have varied levels of

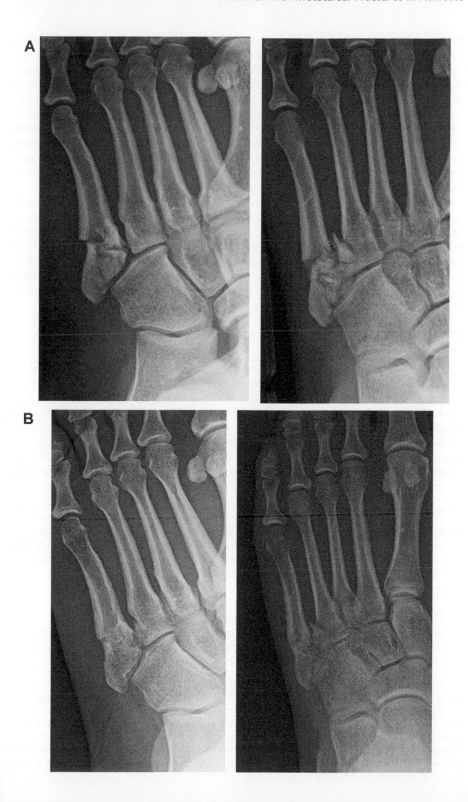

involvement and must be raised dorsally, and the nonunion fragment excised. If a large amount of tendon is attached to the avulsion fragment, the tendon can be elevated off the fragment and repaired back down to the intact tuberosity with drill holes and nonabsorbable suture. Ritchie and associates[50] treated their athletes to non-weight-bearing for a period of 2 weeks postoperatively, but if a brevis repair was done, they were non-weight-bearing for 3 weeks. Following the period of immobilization, the patients were placed in a CAM boot and made weight bearing as tolerated. After the incisions healed, physical therapy commenced consisting of pool therapy, stationary bike, and peroneal tendon strengthening. Patients resumed athletic activities 6 to 8 weeks after the surgery. All patients in this study by Ritchie and coworkers had an uneventful recovery and full functional capacity without symptoms.

In the small series by Rettig,[49] the investigators reported a series of 8 symptomatic nonunions of avulsion fractures of the fifth metatarsal. Five patients had extraarticular fractures where the bone fragment was removed through a lateral incision. They noted care was taken to not disrupt the ligamentous or soft tissue attachments to the remaining bone. They noted that upon evaluation of the fracture fragment, if it articulated with the cuboid, the fragment was fixed with a 4.0 cancellous screw (3 athletes) to restore normal joint anatomy. Of the 8 patients, no complications were experienced, and all were back at sport by 4 months postoperatively.

FIFTH METATARSAL SHAFT (DANCER'S) FRACTURE
Pattern of Fracture

A dancer's fracture is described as a long spiral fracture of the fifth metatarsal diaphysis. It is the most common acute fracture among ballet dancers. It can be caused by a dancer rolling over his or her foot while in a demi-pointe position while the ankle is fully plantarflexed, during the landing phase of a jump (**Fig. 12**). Injury occurs when a torsional force is applied in addition to the axial load on the metatarsal. The athlete presents with acute lateral foot pain with swelling and ecchymosis over the dorsal lateral foot with exquisite tenderness over the area of the fifth metatarsal shaft. Radiographs demonstrate a spiral, oblique fracture starting distal-medial and extending proximal-lateral (**Fig. 13**).

Weight-Bearing Metatarsal Head Position

Despite the often "displaced" fracture on imaging, the critical factor for operative versus nonoperative treatment is the length of the metatarsal and the position of the metatarsal head. A small amount of shortening is tolerated well as long as there is not dorsal translation of the head. Excessive dorsal translation will lead to transfer metatarsalgia of the fourth.

Nonoperative

Initial evaluation for this fracture includes a thorough history and physical examination, and standard 3-view foot radiographs should be obtained with weight-bearing.

Fig. 9. (*A–B*) Proximal fifth metatarsal base comminuted fracture. (*A1*) Oblique and (*A2*) AP radiographs of the foot showing severely comminuted base fifth metatarsal fracture. Note that there is some irregularity of the joint surface but no retraction. The authors decided to treat this nonoperatively because it would be hard to fix with a screw, and even a plate would be difficult to rigidly fix. (*B1*) Oblique and (*B2*) AP images after 3 months of nonoperative treatment with initial boot immobilization and then use of a CFP. The athlete is pain free and active recreationally.

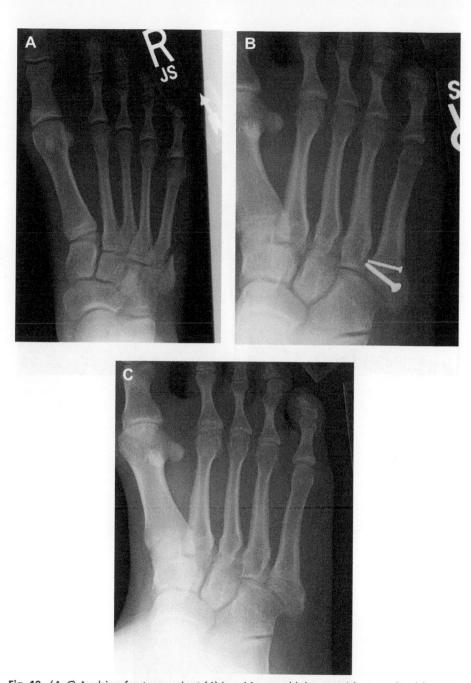

Fig. 10. (*A–C*) Avulsion fracture variant (*A*) in a 14-year-old dancer with more distal fracture component causing rotation of the proximal fragment and necessitating fixation with 2 screws (*B*). (*C*) Follow-up image 1 year after removal of screws showing near normal-appearing fifth metatarsal base.

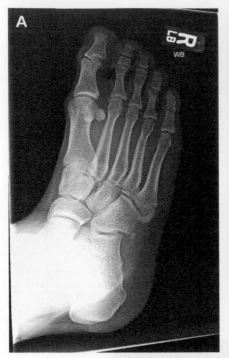

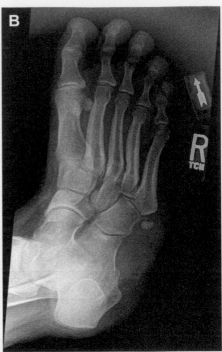

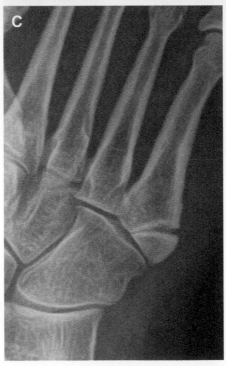

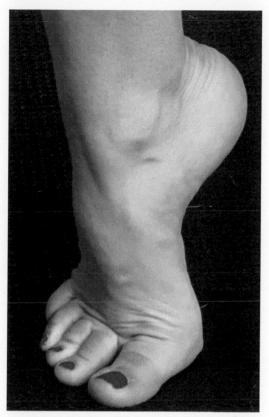

Fig. 12. Dancer's demi-pointe position in classical ballet. Landing in this position can lead to dancer's fracture in ballet. Also, stepping down off a curb or other surface can lead to the same injury in a nondancer athlete.

Dancer's fractures can then be analyzed based on the grading criteria put forward by Shereff,[7] which follows. However, one should recognize that the following cutoffs are not well proven clinically or biomechanically. The criteria state that, if radiographs demonstrate more than 3 to 4 mm of displacement or angulation greater than 10° in the dorsal or planter direction, then a reduction attempt should be attempted. Nondisplaced fractures or fractures that fit inside the listed cutoff criteria can be treated nonoperatively. O'Malley and colleagues[51] performed a study on 35 ballet dancers who sustained a dancer's fracture, 31 of which were treated conservatively and were able to return to professional performance without pain or limitations. Aynardi[52] also

---

Fig. 11. (A–C) (A) Nondisplaced apophyseal nonunion (os vesalianum) of the fifth proximal metatarsal base. Note the more longitudinal nature of the nonunion line. Also, note small os peroneus just lateral to cuboid. (B) Displaced fifth metatarsal base nonunion. Likely old apophyseal nonunion or small styloid fracture nonunion since sclerotic border, but with no recent history of a fracture. (C) Fifth metatarsal metaphyseal avulsion nonunion. Both nonunions in panels (A) and (B) required excision, and the attachment was on the lateral plantar fascia and abductor digiti quinti mini tendon. Nonunion in panel (C) required ORIF with bone graft since involved large portion of articular surface.

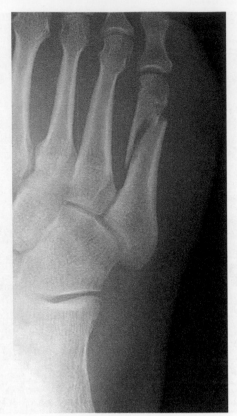

Fig. 13. Displaced fifth metatarsal diaphyseal fracture (dancer's fracture). Note long oblique nature of fracture and mild shortening. Weight-bearing position of the fifth metatarsal head in functional position. This can be treated nonoperatively.

did a retrospective review of 142 patients with a dancer's fracture who were initially treated nonoperatively, 140 of whom went on to heal. Two patients did require open reduction internal fixation for painful nonunion and subsequently healed. These non-displaced fifth metatarsal shaft dancer's fractures can be treated with an elastic dressing, posterior splint, a short leg walking cast, or a hard-sole shoe. These patients can be provided with crutches and made to weight-bear as tolerated. The authors' preference is a walking boot support for 4 to 6 weeks with weight-bearing as tolerated and return to full activity in 6 to 12 weeks.

Operative

Options for surgery include closed reduction and percutaneous K-wire fixation or open reduction internal fixation (authors' preference). If open reduction internal fixation is selected, there are a variety of treatment options, which include lag screw fixation, plate fixation (authors' preference), and hybrid fixation. It is also up to the discretion of the treating surgeon whether the use of bone graft should be used, as there is not good support for or against it at this time. The authors' experience is similar to the literature and rarely is operative fixation necessary. The radiographic appearance can seem concerning, so education of the athlete is imperative.

FIFTH METATARSAL APOPHYSEAL NONUNION (ISELIN DISEASE, OS VESALIANUM, AVULSION NONUNION)

Development

There is confusion, even in the literature, regarding the diagnosis of fifth metatarsal apophysitis (Iselin disease), os vesalianum (accessory bone), and fifth metatarsal metaphyseal avulsion nonunion. It is possible, although not proven, that the metaphyseal apophysitis at the base of the fifth metatarsal can develop into a nonunion and present later as a united apophysis. Os vesalianum is a condition (0.1%–0.4% prevalence) that presents typically in adolescents, but can present later in life, radiographically as an accessory bone at the plantar lateral base of the fifth metatarsal.[53–55] It can be confused for an avulsion fracture nonunion.[56] However, its treatment is more similar to an accessory navicular on the medial side of the foot rather than a fracture nonunion. The os vesalianum has a fibrous union to the plantar lateral fifth metatarsal base and is typically inferior and proximal to the peroneus brevis insertion, which is more dorsal and distal (see **Fig. 1**B; **Fig. 11**A). It is important to recognize the configuration of the nonunion to differentiate between this developmental accessory bone, and a true fifth metatarsal avulsion nonunion (see **Fig. 11**A, C). The articulation of the os vesalianum is more longitudinal and more parallel to the long axis of the fifth metatarsal, similar to the apophyseal growth plate of the fifth. The os vesalianum typically does not involve the TMT articular surface. Avulsion fractures of the fifth metatarsal base typically are transverse to the long axis and extend into the fifth TMT joint (see **Figs.** 1C and **11C**). Treatment of the accessory bone (os vesalianum-apophyseal nonunion) commonly requires surgical excision without fixation (see case 3). The peroneus brevis is often superior to this accessory bone and therefore does not require tendon reattachment unless the accessory bone is very large.

Iselin disease

Osteochondrosis and apophysitis are common conditions in the young athlete. Osteochondroses are bone-cartilage conditions that comprise a heterogenous group of injuries to the epiphyses, physes, and apophyses of children. These injuries have an unknown origin and result from disturbances during endochondral ossification. These conditions are usually self-limited. Proposed mechanisms include rapid growth, hereditary link, anatomic variations, trauma, dietary factors, and vascular supply to the area. These injuries usually follow a common series of events with necrosis of bone and cartilage, revascularization, granulation tissue reorganization, osteoclastic resorption of the necrotic segment, and finally, new bone development.

Apophysitis is a subset of osteochondrosis that occurs where the myotendinous tissue or ligament attaches to bone. An apophysis develops as an accessory ossification center and is evident on plain radiographs. When inflammation and irritation occur at the apophysis, it is called apophysitis. "Traction apophysitis of the 5th metatarsal tuberosity where the peroneus brevis attach is termed Iselin's disease."[57] This condition is thought to be due to a stress reaction and microfractures where the tendon inserts. Is it thought that Iselin disease occurs during a rapid growth period from ages 12 to 13; however, it can appear in girls as young as 8 and boys as young as 10 years of age. Fusion of the apophysis is usually completed by 17 to 18 years. The condition is found more commonly in children playing sports that involve repetitive trauma. Lack of fusion may lead to an os vesalianum.

Athletes with Iselin disease usually present with lateral foot pain during weight-bearing activities and swelling around the fifth metatarsal. Patients will have pain from shoes' pressure directly over the apophysis. Pain may be insidious in nature or acute from an ankle inversion injury.

Radiographs will usually demonstrate a shell-shaped bone fleck running parallel to the long axis of the fifth metatarsal. The affected apophysis may be enlarged on the affected side compared with the contralateral foot radiograph, and there can be evidence of disordered ossification and/or slight separation of the cartilage bone junction. If diagnosis is still in doubt, one could consider obtaining radiographs of the contralateral foot for comparison, or repeating radiographs in 7 to 10 days; at that time, sclerotic changes may be identifiable on radiographs.

Nonoperative if Asymptomatic

If the patient is asymptomatic or this accessory bone or ununited apophysis is an incidental finding, no intervention is necessary. If the athlete presents with acute or subacute complaints of pain and is found to have a traction apophysitis of the fifth metatarsal (apophysitis without a true nonunion), a trial period of nonoperative management can be implemented. One common treatment strategy involves the patient being immobilized in a short leg walking cast or a boot for 2 weeks. After that time, the patient should have repeat radiographs obtained and repeat physical examination. If no radiographic signs of acute fracture are present and/or the patient is symptom free, immobilization can be discontinued. Most patients need 4 weeks of immobilization for symptoms to improve. Once symptom free, patients should progress with a gradual return to activity, which is guided by pain and function. The patient can also participate in a home exercise program that emphasizes strengthening, stretching, and proprioception of the foot and ankle. Sometimes these patients require repeat treatment over the years until final ossification of the apophysis. Operative treatment is reserved for athletes that develop a nonunion after closure of the growth plates. As already mentioned, this may be the evolution of an os vesalianum.

Operative (Excision vs Open Reduction, Internal Fixation)

It is interesting to note that the 2 articles that address nonunions at the base of the fifth metatarsal appear to address both avulsion fracture nonunions and excision of the accessary ossicle, os vesalianum.[49,50] Each article presents radiographs that are consistent with both avulsion fracture nonunions with transverse fracture lines, and images consistent with accessory bone nonunion, os vesalianum. The authors think there is a distinct difference between these 2 "nonunions." Because the avulsion fracture nonunion typically involves a significant portion of the articular surface, operative intervention to retain the fragment is crucial. However, with the accessory bone, because there is no articular surface involvement, and there is rarely significant involvement of the peroneus brevis attachment, excision is the treatment of choice. Also, an avulsion fracture nonunion would require minimal to non-weight-bearing and electrical bone stimulation with prolonged nonoperative treatment if symptomatic. However, in the accessary os vesalianum, bony healing is not possible (see case 3). Therefore, with this accessory bone, an initial short period of immobilization is reasonable, but any persistent pain is best served with operative intervention with excision of the plantar lateral fragment and repair of the lateral plantar fascia and ADQM. The authors think this accessory os vesalianum is actually much more common than a true fifth metatarsal avulsion fracture nonunion. The authors think there is still significant confusion regarding the differentiation of these 2 entities.

CASES STUDIES
Case 1

A division 1 college athlete suffered a fifth metatarsal Jones stress fracture in spring of his junior year. He underwent appropriate ORIF of the fifth metatarsal. He obtained near complete radiographic healing, but as the season progressed, became progressively uncomfortable with cutting and running, and radiographic evidence showed recurrence/refracture with incomplete healing (**Fig. 14**A, B). After the regular season was completed, he underwent revision surgery with exchange screw fixation, calcaneal cancellous bone grafting, and distal tibia BMAC to the fracture (**Fig. 14**C, D). The fracture nonunion was taken down completely and drilled on each side. The authors also took down the medial cortex, which can sometimes cause a hinging effect on the fracture. Taking down the medial cortex can result in a 1- to 2-mm shortening of the fifth metatarsal and improves cortical abutment throughout the fracture. The bone graft was impacted intramedullary at the fracture site as well as around the cortex. A larger 6.5-mm screw was then placed. The large screw compresses the fracture sight. The athlete was able to return to division 1 play and completed his fifth year without difficulty from the fracture.

Case 2

An 18-year-old white female freshman softball player at an NAIA school suffered her second stress fracture. She had had a fourth metatarsal base "Jones" stress fracture

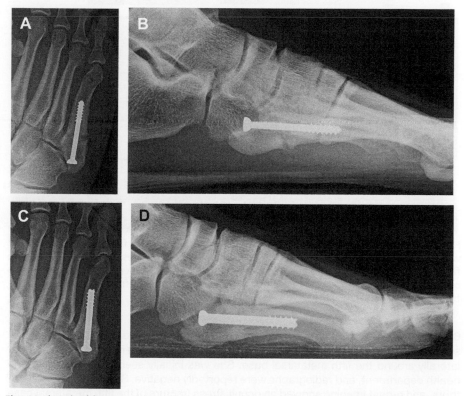

Fig. 14. (*A, B*) Oblique and lateral preoperative view for revision of fifth metatarsal Jones fracture with good placement of intramedullary screw but recurrent fracture with nonunion. (*C, D*) Oblique and lateral postoperative imaging 6 months after revision of fifth metatarsal Jones fracture with excellent complete healing after bone grafting and exchange of screw fixation with larger intramedullary screw. The athlete was able to perform at division 1 level without pain.

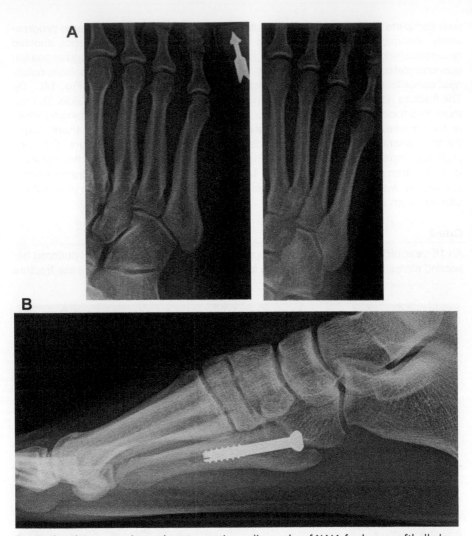

Fig. 15. (*A, B*) Preoperative and postoperative radiographs of NAIA freshman softball player with lateral side foot pain for 1 month. (*A*) Oblique and AP images demonstrating "occult fifth metatarsal base stress fracture consistent with Jones stress fracture." (*B*) Postoperative oblique and lateral images after ORIF fifth metatarsal Jones stress fracture with 5.5-mm intramedullary screw.

6 months earlier, which was treated nonoperatively and healed well. She then presented with a 1-month history of a relatively acute onset of pain in the opposite foot laterally around the fifth metatarsal base. She was initially seen at her college in the health department, and radiographs were reportedly negative. She returned to the authors, and repeat imaging showed an occult stress fracture of the fifth metatarsal base consistent with an early Jones stress fracture (**Fig. 15**A). Because of her history of repeated stress fractures within 1 year, a more detailed history revealed normal menstrual cycles. Laboratory workup identified normal ferritin and iron levels but a vitamin D level of 21 ng/mL, which is severely low (normal is >30 ng/mL, but the authors prefer >40 ng/mL in the athlete). She underwent fifth metatarsal ORIF with a 5.5mm

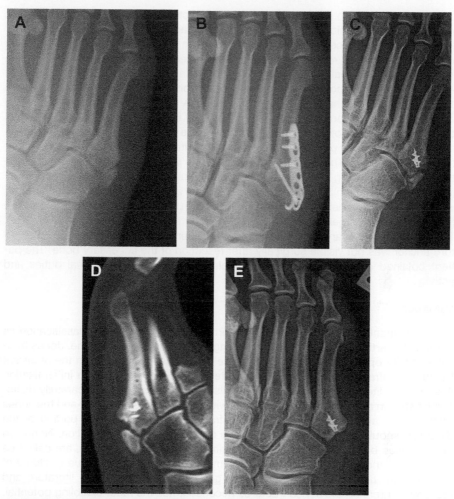

Fig. 16. (*A–E*) Obliques radiographs of the fifth metatarsal base nonunions. (*A*). Preoperative oblique of right foot showing accessory fifth metatarsal base os vesalianum. (*B*) Postoperative oblique image showing hook plate and screw fixation for fifth metatarsal accessory bone mistakenly treated for fracture nonunion. (*C*) Postoperative oblique image after removal of hardware and repair of peroneus longus tendon but continued accessory bone with pain. (*D*) Postoperative CT image after removal of hardware, placement of suture anchor, but clear persistent "nonunion" of accessory os vesalianum with continued pain. (*E*) Postoperative image after excision of os vesalianum with nonvisible suture anchor, healed peroneus brevis tendon, and finally, relief of pain.

screw (**Fig. 15**B). She was also managed with vitamin D supplementation, including 50,000 IU a week for 1 month, and was then maintained on 4000 IU per day until her level of vitamin D was greater than 40 ng/mL. She is in the progress of returning to sports to participate in softball.

Case 3

A patient who injured herself at work who does minimal recreational activity had lateral-sided foot pain after twisting her right foot. The patient presented with pain at the base of the fifth metatarsal with minimal ecchymosis. Images of the right foot were read as a nonunion of the base of fifth metatarsal, although the images appear to be an accessary os vesalianum (**Fig. 16**A). An initial attempt at immobilization was unsuccessful in relieving pain, and the patient then underwent ORIF with a hook plate to try to heal the "nonunion" but had persistent pain (**Fig. 16**B). The patient was referred for a second opinion. The second opinion diagnosed painful hardware and probable tear of the peroneus brevis tendon. A second surgery involved removal of the existing hardware, suture anchor placement in the base of the fifth metatarsal but without removal of the accessory bone at the base of the fifth. Unfortunately, the patient developed persistent lateral foot pain with development of nerve pain after this second surgery. The patient was still unable to participate in any recreational activity or weight-bearing work (**Fig. 16**C). To confirm a painful accessary os vesalianum (apophyseal nonunion), the authors injected local anesthetic at the "nonunion site" with near 100% relief of symptoms. A follow-up CT confirmed the nonunion (**Fig. 16**D). Final surgery involved excision of the apophyseal nonunion (**Fig. 16**E). The nonunion accessory bone was plantar to the peroneus brevis tendon, and the suture anchor was not visible surgically after resection of the accessary bone. The patient obtained excellent relief and was able to return to more normal duties and activity.

SUMMARY

Fifth metatarsal base fractures are common in the athlete. Correct classification as noted in the article will lead to a high healing rate and desired outcome. Jones fractures require operative screw fixation. Bone grafting is always used in the recurrent fracture or refracture. There is renewed interest in bone grafting with initial fixation now, but the literature has not addressed its efficacy. It is crucial to carefully distinguish between avulsion fractures that heal with nonoperative treatment and the Jones fracture. The authors think all transverse fractures that involve any portion of the diaphysis should be treated with operative intramedullary screw fixation. Nonunion of non-Jones base fractures are more commonly an accessory bone, are called os vesalianum, and can be excised if symptomatic. Dancer's long oblique fractures of the shaft are treated nonoperatively with good results. Most of the literature and research centers on the Jones fractures because it has the most disabling potential. Orthobiologics are an emerging area in the treatment of Jones fracture in the athlete.

REFERENCES

1. Kaplan LD, Jost PW, Honkamp N, et al. Incidence and variance of foot and ankle injuries in elite college football players. Am J Orthop 2011;40(1):40–4.
2. Bigsby E, Halliday R, Middleton RG, et al. Functional outcome of fifth metatarsal fractures. Injury, Int J Care Injured 2014;45(12):2009–12.
3. Carreira DS, Sandilands Sm. Radiographic factors and effect of fifth metatarsal Jones and diaphyseal stress fractures on participation in the NFL. Foot Ankle Int 2013;34(4):518–22.
4. Hunt KJ, Anderson RB. Treatment of Jones fracture non-unions in athletes sustaining proximal fifth metatarsal stress fracture. Foot Ankle Int 2010;31(3):203–11.
5. Lareau CR, Anderson RB. Jones fractures: pathophysiology and treatment. JBJS Rev 2015;3(7):e4.
6. Porter DA, Rund AM, Dobslaw R, et al. Comparison of 4.5- and 5.5-mm cannulated stainless steel screws for fifth metatarsal Jones fracture function. Foot Ankle Int 2009;30(1):29–33.

7. Shereff MJ. Complex fractures of the metatarsals. Orthopedics 1990;13:875–82.
8. Kane JM, Sandowski K, Saffel H, et al. The epidemiology of fifth metatarsal fracture. Foot Ankle Spec 2015;8(5):354–9.
9. Petrisor BA, Ekrol I, Court-Brown C. The epidemiology of metatarsal fractures. Foot Ankle Int 2006;27(3):172–4.
10. Cakir H, Van Vliet-Koppert ST, Van Lieshout EM, et al. Demographics and outcome of metatarsal fractures. Arch Orthop Trauma Surg 2011;131(2):241–5. https://doi.org/10.1007/s00402-010-1164-6.
11. Kavanaugh JH, Brower TD, Mann RV. The Jones fracture revisited. J Bone Joint Surg Am 1978;60A:776–82.
12. Weinfeld SB, Haddad SL, Myerson MS. Metatarsal stress fractures. Clin Sports Med 1997;16:319–38.
13. Jones R. Fracture of the base of the fifth metatarsal by indirect violence. Ann Surg 1902;35:695–702.
14. Torg JS, Balduini FC, Zelko RR, et al. Fractures of the base of the fifth metatarsal distal to the tuberosity. Classification and guidelines for non-operative and operative management. J Bone Joint Surg Am 1984;66A:209–14.
15. Porter DA. Fifth metatarsal Jones fractures in the athlete a review. Foot Ankle Int 2018;39(2):250–8.
16. Rouche AJ, Calder JD. Treatment and return to sport following a Jones fracture of the fifth metatarsal. Knee Surg Sports Traumatol Arthrosc 2013;21(6):1307–15.
17. Frush Todd J, Lindenfeld Thomas N. Peri-epiphyseal and overuse injuries in adolescent athletes. Sports Health 2009;1:201–11.
18. Gillespie H. Osteochondroses and apophyseal injuries of the foot in the young athlete. Curr Sports Med Rep 2010;9(5):265–8.
19. Shereff MJ, Yang QM, Kummer FJ, et al. Vascular anatomy of the fifth metatarsal. Foot Ankle 1991;11:350 3.
20. Smith JW, Arnoczky SP, Hersh A. The intraosseous blood supply of the fifth metatarsal: implications for proximal fracture healing. Foot Ankle 1992;13:143–52.
21. Brilakis E, Kaselouris E, Xypnoitos F, et al. Effects of foot posture on fifth metatarsal fracture healing. J Foot Ankle Surg 2012;51(6):720–8.
22. Raikin SM, Slenker N, Ratigan B. The association of a varus hindfoot and fracture of the fifth metatarsal. Am J Sports Med 2008;36(7):1367–72.
23. Yu Shimaski, Nagao M, Miyamori T, et al. Evaluating the risk of a fifth metatarsal stress fracture by measuring the serum 25-hydroxyvitamin D Levels. Foot Ankle Int 2016;37(3):307–11.
24. Villacis D, Yi Anthony, Ryan Jahn BS, et al. Prevalence of abnormal vitamin D levels among division I NCAA Athletes. Sports Health 2014;6(4):340–7.
25. Schwartz EN, Edmundson CP. Medical and metabolic considerations in the Athlete with stress fractures, in Porter and Schon Baxter's the Foot and Ankle in Sports Elsevier Press 2020.
26. Wright RW, Fischer DA, Shively RA, et al. Refracture of proximal fifth metatarsal (Jones) fracture after intramedullary screw fixation in athletes. Am J Sports Med 2000;28:732–6.
27. Bishop JA, Braun HJ, Hunt KJ. Operative versus nonoperative treatment of Jones fractures: a decision analysis model. Am J Orthop 2016;45(3):E69–76.
28. DeLee JC, Evans JP, Julian J. Stress fracture of the fifth metatarsal. Am J Sports Med 1983;11:349–53.
29. Mindrebo N, Shelbourne KD, Van Meter CD, et al. Outpatient percutaneous screw fixation of the acute Jones fracture. Am J Sports Med 1993;21:720–3.

30. DeVries GJ, Cuttica DJ, Hyer CF. Cannulated screw fixation of Jones fifth metatarsal fractures. J Foot Ankle Surg 2011;50:207–12.
31. Glasgow MT, Naranja RJ Jr, Glasgow SG, et al. Analysis of failed operative management of fractures of the base of the fifth metatarsal distal to the tuberosity: the Jones fracture. Foot Ankle Int 1996;17:449–57.
32. Huh J, Glisson RR, Matsumoto T, et al. Biomechanical comparison of intramedullary screw versus low-profile plate fixation of a Jones fracture. Foot Ankle Int 2016;37(4):411–8.
33. Kelly IP, Glisson RR, Fink C, et al. Intramedullary screw fixation of Jones fractures. Foot Ankle Int 2001;22:585–9.
34. Metzl J, Olson K, Davis WH, et al. A clinical and radiographic comparison of two hardware system used to treat Jones fracture of the fifth metatarsal. Foot Ankle Int 2013;34(7):956–61.
35. Ochenjele G, HoB, Switaj PJ, et al. Radiographic study of the fifth metatarsal for optimal intramedullary screw fixation of Jones fracture. Foot Ankle Int 2015;36(3):293–301.
36. Orr JD, Gilsson RR, Nunley JA. Jones fracture fixation. Am J Sports Med 2012;40(3):691–8.
37. Pietropaoli MP, Wnorowski DC, Werner FW, et al. Intramedullary screw fixation of Jones fractures: a biomechanical study. Foot Ankle Int 1999;20:560–3.
38. Scott RT, Hyer CF, DeMill SL. Screw fixation diameter for fifth metatarsal Jones fracture a cadaveric study. J Foot Ankle Surg 2015;54(2):227–9.
39. Shah SN, Knoblich GO, Lindsey DP, et al. Intramedullary screw fixation of proximal fifth metatarsal fractures: a biomechanical study. Foot Ankle Int 2001;22:581–4.
40. Nunley JA, Gilsson RR. A new option for intramedullary fixation of Jones fracture. Foot Ankle Int 2008;29(12):1216–21.
41. Duplantier NL, Mitchell RJ, Zambrano S, et al. A biomechanical comparison of fifth metatarsal Jones fracture fixation methods. Am J Sports Med 2018;46(5):1220–7.
42. Mitchell RJ, Duplantier NL, Delgado DA, et al. Plantar plating for the treatment of proximal fifth metatarsal fractures in elite athletes. Orthopedics 2017;40(3):e563–6.
43. Pao DG, Keats TE, Dussault RG. Avulsion fracture of the base of the fifth metatarsal not seen on conventional radiography of the foot: the need for an additional projection. Am J Roentgenol 2000;175(2):549–52.
44. Rosenberg GA, James J, Sferra. "Treatment strategies for acute fractures and nonunions of the proximal fifth metatarsal. J Am Acad Orthop Surg 2000;8(5):332–8.
45. Egrol K, Walsh M, Rosenblatt BS, et al. Avulsion fractures of the fifth metatarsal base: a prospective outcome study. Foot Ankle Int 2007;28(5):581–3.
46. Vorlat P, Achtergael W, Haentjens P. Predictors of outcome of non-displaced fractures of the base of the fifth metatarsal. Int Orthop 2007;31(1):5–10.
47. Weiner BD, Linder JF, Giattini FG. Treatment of fractures of the fifth metatarsal: a prospective study. Foot Ankle Int 1997;18(5):267–9.
48. Zenios M, Kim WY, Sampath J, et al. Functional treatment of acute metatarsal fractures: a prospective randomised comparison of management in a cast versus elasticated support bandage. Injury 2005;36(7):832–5.
49. Rettig AC, Shelbourne KD, Wilckens J. The surgical treatment of symptomatic nonunions of the proximal (metaphyseal) fifth metatarsal in athletes. Am J Sports Med 1992;20:50–4.

50. Ritchie JD, Shaver C, Anderson RB, et al. Excision of symptomatic nonunions of proximal fifth metatarsal avulsion fractures in elite athletes. Am J Sports Med 2011;39:2466Y9.
51. O'Malley MJ, Hamilton WG, Munyak J. Fractures of the distal shaft of the fifth metatarsal.Dancer's fracture". Am J Sports Med 1996;24:240–3.
52. Aynardi M, Pedowitz DI, Saffel H, et al. Outcome of nonoperative management of displaced oblique spiral fractures of the fifth metatarsal shaft. Foot Ankle Int 2013; 34:1619Y23.
53. Mellado JM, Ramos A, Salvadó E, et al. Accessory ossicles and sesamoid bones of the ankle and foot: imaging findings, clinical significance and differential diagnosis. Eur Radiol 2003;13:L164–77.
54. Coskun N, Yuksel M, Cevener M, et al. Incidence of accessory ossicles and sesamoid bones in the feet: a radiographic study of the Turkish subjects. Surg Radiol Anat 2009;31:19–24.
55. Tsuruta T, Shiokawa Y, Kato A, et al. Radiological study of the accessory skeletal elements in the foot and ankle. Nippon Seikeigeka Gakkai Zasshi 1981;55: 357–70.
56. Kose O. Os vesalianum pedis misdiagnosed as fifth metatarsal avulsion fracture. Emerg Med Australas 2009;21:426.
57. Canale ST, Williams KD. Iselin's disease. J Pediatr Orthop 1992;12:90–3.

Arthroscopic Surgical Technique for Lateral Ankle Ligament Instability

Jorge I. Acevedo, MD[a],*, Peter G. Mangone, MD[b]

KEYWORDS

- Arthroscopy • Brostrom • Lateral ligament repair • Internal brace

KEY POINTS

- Several techniques have been developed to repair the lateral ankle ligaments and effectively treat ankle instability.
- Arthroscopic repair of the lateral ankle ligaments is safe and biomechanically equivalent to open Brostrom-Gould reconstruction.
- An internal brace augmentation can expedite the recovery process as well as strengthen the repair construct and protect it from future injury.

INTRODUCTION

With a frequency of 30,000 per day, ankle sprains are the most commonly occurring injury in physically active patients in the United States.[1] Eighty-five percent of ankle sprains cause injury to the lateral ankle ligaments.[2] The anterior talofibular ligament (ATFL) is involved in 75% of injuries to the ankle, calcaneofibular ligament (CFL) in 41%, and 5% are combined according to an MRI study by Ballal and colleagues.[3] Chronic ankle instability (CAI) can develop in 20% to 40% of patients with these injuries.[1,4] Either open or arthroscopic repair is indicated when nonoperative techniques fail to restore ankle stability. Arthroscopic surgical techniques for lateral ankle instability can generally be categorized into arthroscopic-assisted, all-arthroscopic, and all-inside techniques.[5] Apart from repair of the ankle ligaments, arthroscopic surgical techniques can also address any concurrent lesions, impingement, or synovitis commonly found in unstable and injured ankles.[6] Outcomes from these procedures are promising despite some reports of high complication rates. This article reports an arthroscopic Brostrom procedure with optional internal brace, which is the only

[a] Department of Orthopedics, Southeast Orthopedic Specialists, Foot and Ankle Center, 6500 Bowden Road, Suite 103, Jacksonville, FL 32216, USA; [b] Department of Orthopedics, Blue Ridge Division of EmergeOrtho, Foot and Ankle Center, 2585 Hendersonville Road, Arden, NC 28704, USA
* Corresponding author.
E-mail address: ace4foot@gmail.com

Foot Ankle Clin N Am 26 (2021) 65–85
https://doi.org/10.1016/j.fcl.2020.10.004
1083-7515/21/© 2020 Elsevier Inc. All rights reserved.

technique with published data supporting its biomechanical equivalence to the more traditional open Brostrom-Gould.[7,8]

LATERAL LIGAMENTOUS COMPLEX ANATOMY AND BIOMECHANICS

The 3 main components of the lateral ligamentous complex include the ATFL, CFL, and the posterior talofibular ligament. The weakest of these is the ATFL (ultimate failure, load 138–160 N) and is the most commonly injured in lateral ankle sprains.[9,10] The ATFL is described as a flat, quadrilateral ligament. Sarrafian[11] later described the ligament as having 2 distinct bands. A systematic review by Matsui and colleagues[12] analyzed 10 studies of 263 specimens and found the bundle anatomic variability to be single bundle in 61.6%, double bundle in 35.7%, and triple bundle in 2.7%. The origin of the ATFL has been reported as 10 to 14 mm from the tip of the distal fibula, whereas the insertion is on the lateral portion of the talar neck with a mean length of 11.8 mm to 24.8 mm.[12,13] Based on anatomic studies recently performed, Vega and colleagues[14] proposed that functional instability may be caused by an isolated tear of the superior band of the ATFL, leading to instability symptoms but a normal static ligament examination. In contrast, patients with mechanical instability may have tears in both bands of the ligament.

The CFL originates at a distance of 5 to 8 mm from the tip of the lateral malleolus and courses deep to the peroneal tendons to insert on the lateral wall of the calcaneus. This footprint lays approximately 3 cm posterior and superior to the peroneal tubercle. The CFL's role is to provide subtalar stability extending across the tibiotalar and subtalar joints. However, clinical and biomechanical studies do not suggest direct repair of this ligament to be essential for good outcomes.[3,13,15,16]

The inferior extensor retinaculum (IER) is a Y-shaped structure formed by the stem ligament, an oblique superomedial band, and an oblique inferomedial band and typically is described as a thickening of the crural fascia. An additional superolateral band is formed in up to 64% of cases, giving it an X-shaped morphology.[17] Given the variable nature of the IER, its use in the Brostrom procedure has been questioned. Dalmau-Pastor[17] argued that the Y-shaped morphology does not allow for proper incorporation of the IER but it is the crural fascia that is used, and those with the X-shaped variant are incorporated but the fibers of the oblique superolateral band are weak. In contrast, a prior anatomic study showed inclusion of the IER within the arthro-Brostrom repair and biomechanical studies show how the IER imparts further stability to the modified Brostrom repair because of its calcaneal attachments.[18] This concept is further supported by the studies published by Lee and colleagues[15] in 2011 showing excellent outcomes with ATFL reconstruction using the IER advancement and no CFL reconstruction.

The superficial peroneal nerve (SPN) has been found to run an average distance of 32 mm (24–48 mm) at 90° from the center of the ATFL origin. Because the nerve courses distally, it runs more anterior, therefore placing an accessory incision more distal could serve to reduce the risk of iatrogenic injury.[13] Through the use of palpation and fluoroscopy, Matsui and colleagues[19] have shown that the fibulae obscure tubercle (FOT) is a reliable landmark in 100% of cases and that it may serve as a clinically relevant landmark for location of the ATFL in percutaneous minimally invasive surgery procedures designed to treat chronic lateral ankle instability. The FOT is found on the anterior border of the fibula between the inferior tip and anterior tubercle of the distal fibula. The ATFL origin has a mean measurement of 3.7 mm (range, 0–6.7 mm) proximal to the FOT, whereas the CFL origin has a mean measurement of 4.9 mm (range, 1.1–10.9 mm) distal to the FOT. Clanton and colleagues[20] alternatively suggested that the origin of the ATFL could be placed at 50% of the distance along the anterior fibula border in order to account for the measurement variability in patients who deviate from the mean. This percentage measurement could permit greater accuracy when placing a graft in ankles where the anatomy has been obscured.

INITIAL LIGAMENT RECONSTRUCTION TECHNIQUES IN THE ANKLE

Hawkins[21] was the first to report on arthroscopic ankle stabilization in which he used a staple technique for plication of the lateral ankle ligaments. Despite their promising results, the studies lacked adequate follow-up or outcomes. Kashuk and colleagues[22] modified the technique of Hawkins[21] and produced an arthroscopic technique using suture anchors for repair of the lateral ligamentous complex. Potential benefits of the aforementioned arthroscopic techniques included quicker recovery and decreased morbidity along with a decrease of surgical time and a single approach to address intra-articular pathologic conditions.[4] Although seen as a relatively safe procedure, complication rates are widely varied (0%–29%), including nerve pain, delayed healing of the wound, and deep vein thrombosis (**Table 1**). A systematic review compared the complication rates of open and arthroscopic ligament repair, reporting rates of 8% and 15%, respectively.[23] On further analysis, it was noted that the review included arthroscopic techniques that used accessory incisions[24] and others[25] with heterogeneity in considering complications such as asymptomatic suture knots and transient skin irritation as significantly reportable. Once these variances are taken into consideration and removed, the effective complication rates became similar for both open and arthroscopic ligament repair (8%). In addition, arthroscopic repair has shown comparable functional scores, talar tilt, and return to play compared with open ligamentous repair.[26]

ARTHROSCOPIC REPAIR ANATOMY

Through biomechanical and anatomic evaluation, the IER has been shown to function in stabilization of the subtalar joint similar to the CFL.[16] The Gould modification of the Brostrom procedure involves using the IER, and its use in the repair of the lateral ligament complex has been supported by the data on functional outcomes. However, the Gould augmentation has its detractors; Dalmau-Pastor[17] has called its use into question, as previously mentioned, stating that the crural fascia is inadvertently used rather than the IER. Moreover, the SPN crossed the IER in all their specimens, leading to a possible increased risk of complications. Furthermore, overtightening of the IER can cause stiffness in the posterior subtalar joint.[27] In sharp contrast, Jorge and colleagues[13] suggest that an anteriorly placed accessory portal improves the odds of incorporating the IER instead of the crural fascia, noting that the distance should be less than 22 mm from the lateral malleolus to decrease the risk of injury to the SPN.

In addition to the SPN, the sural nerve and the peroneal tendons may also be at risk during arthroscopic lateral ankle ligament repair. In a cadaveric study by Pitts and colleagues,[28] the accessory lateral portal was located on average greater than 1 cm from all at-risk structures. Because of these structures and their potential for complications, it is important to define a safe zone to avoid entrapment of the at-risk structures. In 2015, Acevedo and colleagues[5] reported that the internervous safe zone between the intermediate branch of the SPN and sural nerve was an average of 51 mm (range, 39–64 mm), whereas the intertendinous safe zone between the peroneus tertius and peroneus brevis was an average of 43 mm (range, 37–49 mm). Santos and colleagues[29] prefer the use of superficial bony landmarks to demarcate the edges of

Table 1
Clinical outcomes of arthroscopic lateral ankle ligament repair

Author, Year	Level of Evidence	Repair Type	Ankles (N)	Follow-up	Time from Injury to Surgery	Preoperative AOFAS/ Karlsson	Postoperative AOFAS/ Karlsson	Satisfaction Rate (%)
Acevedo & Mangone,[38] 2011	IV, retrospective case series	Arthroscopic	24	10.9 mo	NA	NA	NA	95.8
Acevedo et al,[18] 2015	IV, retrospective case series	Arthroscopic	73	28 mo	NA	NA/28.3	NA/90.2	94.5
Cordier et al,[55] 2019	IV, retrospective case series	Arthroscopic	55	29 mo (18–43)	NA	72 (48–84)/ 64 (42–82)	91 (63–100)/ 92 (65–100)	85
Corte-Real & Moreira,[56] 2009	IV, retrospective case series	Arthroscopic	28	27.5 mo (6–48 mo)	7 mo (2–30 mo)	—	85.3 (65–100)	NA
Cottom & Rigby,[40] 2013	IV, case series	Arthroscopic	40	12.13 mo (6–21 mo)	NA	41.2 (23–64)	95.4 (84–100)/ 93.6	NA
Kim,[25] 2011	IV, retrospective case series	Arthroscopic	28	15.9 mo (13–25 mo)	—	60.78	92.48	—
Labib & Slone,[41] 2015	IV, retrospective case series	Arthroscopic	14	3 mo (6–54 wk)	NA	NA	92.8	86
Li et al,[46] 2017	III retrospective cohort	— Arthroscopic Open	60 23 37	— 39.7 mo 35.5 mo	— 16 mo (3–60) 39 mo (3–120)	— 69.3/61.8 69.2/59.7	— 93.3/90.3	—
Nery et al,[57] 2011	IV, retrospective case series	Arthroscopic	38	9.8 y (5–14 y)	9 mo (6–19 mo)	NA	90 (44–100)	94.7
Nery et al,[39] 2017	II, prospective cohort	Arthroscopic	26	27 mo (21–36 mo)	NA	58	90	NA
Song et al,[58] 2017	III, retrospective cohort	— Arthroscopic Reconstruction	28 16 12	— 16.3 mo 19.3	—	— 59.3 61.3	@ 12 mo 93 94.4	—

			N					
Vega et al,[44] 2013	IV, retrospective case series	Arthroscopic	16	22.3 mo (12–35 mo)	NA	67 (59–77)	97 (95–100)	NA
Vega et al,[59] 2020	IV, retrospective case series	Arthroscopic Knotless	24	34.7 mo (18–55)	5 y	65 (52–85)	97 (85–100)	NA
Kim et al,[54] 2019	III, retrospective comparative study	Arthroscopic w/ossicle	125 26	—	—	67.3	@12 mo 85.7	—
		Arthroscopic w/o ossicle	99			65.0	87.0	
Yeo et al,[48] 2016	I, randomized control trial	Arthroscopic	48 25	—	NA	67.5/45.0	@ 12 mo 90.3/76.2	NA
		Open	23		NA	69.9/48.6	89.2/73.5	

Abbreviations: AOFAS, American Orthopedic Foot and Ankle Society; IV, irtravenous; NA, not available.
Data from Refs. [18,25,38–41,44,46,48,54–59]

the safe zone rather than the nerves. Their safe zone landmarks were the tip of the lateral malleolus and the base of the fifth metatarsal, with the peroneus brevis and intermediate dorsal nerve locations derived from the position of the bony landmarks. Of noted importance, a previous study has shown that passing of sutures at least 15 mm anterior to the distal fibula with the ankle held in neutral position improves the likelihood of incorporating a sufficient portion of the IER.[18] Based on this study and others, as well as their own clinical results, the authors maintain the importance of the IER to the lateral ligament complex repair.

BIOMECHANICS OF ARTHROSCOPIC LATERAL LIGAMENT REPAIR VERSUS THE INTERNAL BRACE

In 2013, Drakos and colleagues[7] and Giza and colleagues[8] published data showing biomechanical equivalence of arthroscopic versus open techniques when using matched cadaver pairs. Two anchors were used in the Drakos and colleagues[7] technique, with 1 placed via an accessory portal into the inferior fibula. Giza and colleagues[8] used the arthro-Brostrom all-arthroscopic technique with the standard anteromedial and anterolateral portals. More recently, Lee and colleagues[30] found no significant difference between torque to failure in the open modified Brostrom technique (MBO) (19.9 Nm) and arthroscopic MBO (23.3 Nm). Yoshimura and colleagues[31] investigated optimal suture anchor placement in order to avoid complications with posterior penetration. The investigators recommended the suture anchor should be placed at an angle of less than 45° to the longitudinal axis of the fibula.

Despite the promising results of arthroscopic Brostrom-Gould procedures and the historical results of the traditional open technique, emphasis on early rehabilitation for athletes prompted several investigators to examine the initial strength of open repairs compared with intact ankle ligaments in cadavers. Dong and colleagues[32] found that their arthroscopic reconstruction was not as strong as the intact ankle. In addition, Waldrop and colleagues[33] also investigated the strength of the traditional open Brostrom repair and reported that the repair was at least 50% weaker than the native intact ATFL.

A suture tape internal brace may improve the strength of the repair (**Table 2**). In a study by Viens and colleagues,[34] a repair including a suture tape internal brace was comparable in strength and stiffness with an intact ATFL in cadaveric models. Schuh and colleagues[35] performed 3 repairs on cadavers: traditional Brostrom repair without anchors, suture anchor repair, and suture anchor with internal brace. The highest torque to failure and angle to failure were found in the internal brace group, with both measurements having a statistically significant difference compared with the other 2 groups. Lohrer and colleagues[36] investigated an internal brace alone as repair, finding that it returned the anterior talar drawer to baseline values. Willegger and colleagues[37] randomized 12 cadaveric ankles into a native ATFL group and an internal brace group. In both angle and load to failure, the internal brace group had higher stability. Moreover, the most common mode of failure in the native ATFL was rupture at the midportion of the ATFL, which was absent in the internal brace group. Their results suggest that the internal brace protects against the most common cause of rupture of the ATFL and may help prevent future injuries. Some investigators have voiced concerns about the internal brace construct over-restraining the joint, although the authors have not found that to be an issue when the internal brace construct is placed in the correct anatomic location and strict adherence to the published technique is followed by placing a hemostat under the internal brace before it is secured.

Table 2
Clinical outcomes of internal brace repair

Author, Year	Level of Evidence	Repair Type	Ankles (N)	Follow-up	Preoperative AOFAS/ Karlsson	Postoperative AOFASS/ Karlsson	Outcome
Coetzee et al,[50] 2018	IV, case series	Open with internal brace	81	—	—	94.3	Internal brace provided excellent stability and accelerated rehabilitation
Xu et al,[51] 2019	III, retrospective cohort	— MBA Modified Brostrom (ME)	53 25 28	—	— 68.2 67.3	@ 2 y 97.5 96.3	MBA group had better FAAM scores (functional outcomes). Internal brace reduced ligament elongation
Yoo and Yang,[42] 2016	III, retrospective cohort	— Brostrom with internal brace Brostrom without internal brace	85 22 63	7.4 mo (6–9)	— 65.8 (24–92) 66.7 (44–92)	@ 6 wk 95.9 (87–100) 72.5 (44–97)	Patients with internal brace began rehabilitation earlier. Statistically significant differences in AOFAS were found at 2 wk, 6 wk, and 12 wk

Abbreviations: FAAM, Foot and Ankle Ability Measure; MBA, modified Brostrom with internal brace augmentation.
  Data from Refs.[42,50,51]

ARTHRO-BROSTROM INTRAOPERATIVE TECHNIQUE

- Anesthesia: regional popliteal block (with saphenous block) plus monitored anesthesia care or general anesthesia.
- Examination under anesthesia: a manual examination of the ankle should be performed to assess the hypermobility of the ankle ligamentous complex. This examination serves both to confirm the preoperative diagnosis of instability and to provide the surgeon with important tactile feedback as to the true amount of laxity in the ankle because the patient is relaxed. If too much laxity is encountered, the surgeon should consider whether an arthroscopic ligament procedure is the best procedure versus an augmented-type ligament reconstruction.
- Use of distraction: surgeon preference. If distraction is used, the distraction must be removed before tying the suture construct that tightens the lateral ankle ligament complex.
- Anatomic landmarks: knowledge of the anatomic landmarks is critical for success without complications. The safe zone is drawn on the lateral ankle region. The peroneal tendons, distal fibula, and intermediate branch of the SPN are identified and outlined on the skin. The location of the IER is estimated and drawn using the lateral calcaneal tubercle to help identify the margin of this tissue (**Fig. 1**). The eventual passage of the suture sets will occur in this zone and should be at least 15 mm anterior/distal to the fibula to capture the IER, but should be less than 22 mm from the anterior fibula to minimize nerve entrapment.[10,16]
- Portal placement: use standard anteromedial and anterolateral arthroscopy portals.
- Initial arthroscopic assessment and debridement: the typical diagnostic ankle arthroscopy is performed. This arthroscopy should involve a comprehensive evaluation of the joint combined with the arthroscopic treatment of additional intra-articular pathologic conditions such as osteochondral lesions (OCLs) of the talus or loose body removal. The surgeon must perform a more extensive debridement of the lateral gutter for 2 purposes: to reduce impingement by cleaning out the pathologic fibrotic tissue that usually fills the lateral gutter in patients with CAI, and to allow for adequate visualization of the anterior distal face of the fibula for placement of the anchors.
- Placement of anchors and passage of sutures: the anterolateral gutter is visualized with the 30° arthroscope from the anteromedial portal during this entire sequence. The inferior tip of the fibula is identified with a probe. The first bone anchor is placed 1 cm superior to the tip of the fibula and angled slightly cephalad to avoid drilling through the distal fibular tip. At this point, the sutures are exiting the standard anterolateral portal. The first anchor's set of sutures is passed, 1 at a time, using a sharp-tipped suture passer. This stage can be performed with either an inside-out technique or an outside-in technique. The inside-out technique involves insertion of the sharp-tipped suture passer at the anterolateral portal, and exiting inferiorly, about 1.5 to 2 cm anterior to the distal tip of the lateral malleolus. The outside-in technique involves the insertion of the sharp-tipped suture passer about 1.5 to 2 cm anterior to the distal tip of the lateral malleolus, and exiting at the anterolateral portal. Whether using the inside-out or outside-in technique, the suture passer is merely a means of shuttling sutures from the anterolateral portal through the lateral ligament complex. Care is taken to make sure the suture exit point is at least 15 mm distal to the anterior face of the fibula to ensure capture of the IER. The first of the 2 sutures from this anchor

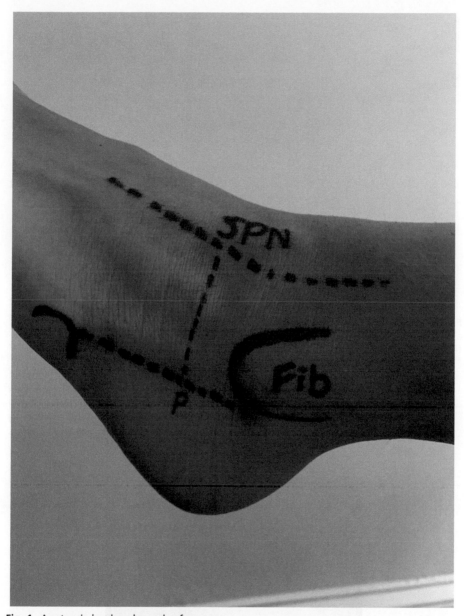

Fig. 1. Anatomic landmarks and safe zone.

is passed just superior to the peroneal tendons, and the second suture is passed 1 cm dorsal/anterior to the first suture along the arc of the IER (**Fig. 2**).

- The second anchor is then placed 1 cm superior to the first anchor in the anterior face of the fibula. This position should be inferior to the level of the talar dome because the ATFL origin is inferior to the talar dome. The second set of sutures is then passed with a sharp-tipped suture passer in the same manner as the first set while visualizing through the arthroscope. The second set of sutures are also

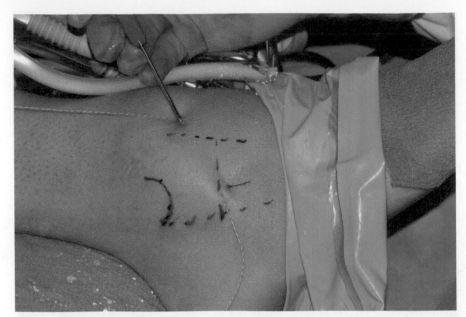

Fig. 2. Passage of the first set of sutures using inside-out technique. The first suture limb is already passed and exiting the skin. The suture passer is noted approximately 1 cm from the first suture limb.

passed individually. The first suture is brought through the tissue 1 cm dorsal/anterior to the last suture from the first anchor along the arc of the IER. The second suture from the second anchor is then passed through the tissue 1 cm dorsal/anterior from the first suture of the second anchor (**Fig. 3**). Care is taken to make sure the sutures are passed entirely within the safe zone to minimize entrapment of the intermediate branch of the SPN (**Fig. 4**).

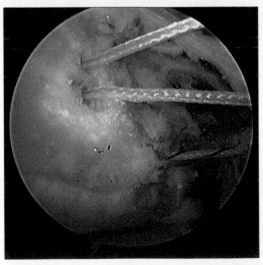

Fig. 3. Arthroscopic visualization of both anchors placed and sutures passed (before tying sutures).

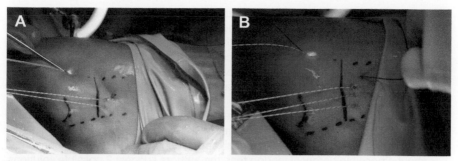

Fig. 4. Passage of a second set of sutures (using outside-in technique) after passage of the first suture set. (*A*) Passage of the first limb of the second anchor. (*B*) Passage of the second limb of the second anchor.

- Tying of suture sets to imbricate lateral ligament complex: a 4-mm incision is made between the 2 sets of sutures. A small arthroscopic probe/hook works best to pass these sutures through the central incision (**Fig. 5**). If an arthroscopic probe does not work, a small hemostat can be used. Should the concern about entrapment of the intermediate branch of the SPN be high, the incision can be made slightly larger and the tissue can be retracted anteriorly to improve visualization of the nerve branches. The ankle is then held in neutral to slight eversion with a slight posterior drawer pressure. The sutures are tied down over the capsule and IER allowing these to imbricate and pull up to the face of the anterior fibula. To confirm satisfactory tissue imbrication to the ATFL origin, the surgeon can either use the arthroscope to watch as the imbrication is being performed or

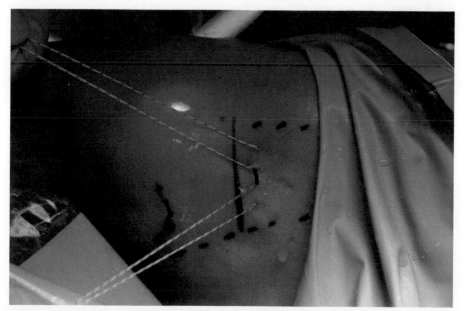

Fig. 5. Half-centimeter incision through which both sets of sutures are passed is marked before the subcutaneous passage and tying of the sutures.

the arthroscope can be removed and then reinserted after the suture sets are tied to assess the intra-articular appearance (**Fig. 6**).

The construct is tested for stability. At this time, supplemental suture techniques, such as a suture bridge or internal brace, can be added as necessary per the surgeon's examination. Should the arthroscopic technique not adequately stabilize the lateral ligament complex, the procedure can easily be converted to an open technique.

- Peroneal tendon disorder: first, we recommend all patients undergoing lateral ankle ligament reconstruction have an MRI scan preoperatively to assess for additional disorder, including peroneal tendon tears. If the surgeon is concerned about a possible peroneal tendon tear, the authors suggest 2 possible solutions. First, a small incision can be made directly over the peroneal tendons to examine and perform a repair as necessary. Usually if a peroneal tendon tear is present, it can be repaired by extending the incision as needed. Second, peroneal tendinoscopy can be used to examine the anatomy and debride through the arthroscope. If a tear is present, then proceed with open incision to perform repair.
- The arthroscopic portals and the small incision for suture tying are then closed with a small nylon mattress suture (**Fig. 7**).
- Postoperative rehabilitation protocol: patients are placed into an initial postoperative splint and held for 7 to 10 days. On return to the office, the sutures can often be removed at the first postoperative visit and the patient can be placed either into a controlled ankle motion (CAM) walker boot or an ankle gauntlet lace-up style brace (depending on the patient's swelling and tenderness). Active dorsiflexion/plantarflexion range of motion is initiated. Inversion is avoided until 6 to 8 weeks after surgery. Fifty-percent weightbearing is started at the first postoperative visit (as long as the patient has no contraindication such as an osteochondritis dissecans lesion of the talus), and the patient is allowed to progress weight bearing over the next several weeks. Gentle inversion/eversion is started at 6 to 8 weeks after surgery and physiotherapy is initiated for leg strengthening and

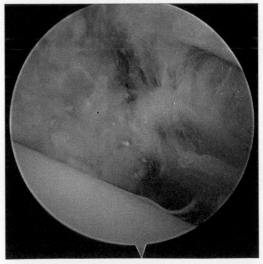

Fig. 6. Repair construct after sutures are tied. The tissue is in direct contact with the anterior fibular face, tightening the lateral ligament complex.

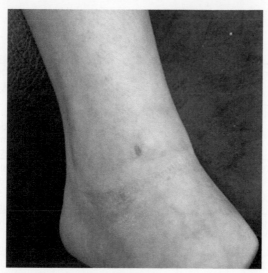

Fig. 7. Postoperative incisions after arthro-Brostrom.

coordination. Most patients are full weight bearing by 3 weeks after surgery. The lace-up style brace is recommended for all weight-bearing activities for the first 3 months. After 3 months, we recommend using the lace-up brace for 6 to 9 months for athletic or rugged activities until such time as the patient has time to fully rehabilitate the leg.

- With the smaller incisions and less soft tissue dissection, immediate postoperative swelling is far less than normal, which usually results in less postoperative pain than with traditional open procedures, and excellent long-term cosmetic appearance.

CURRENT TECHNIQUES AND OUTCOMES FOR ARTHROSCOPIC LATERAL LIGAMENT REPAIR

Arthroscopic lateral ligament repair has progressed in the various methods used over the past decade (**Table 3**). Of the modern approaches, there are 3 distinct techniques: arthroscopic-assisted techniques, all-arthroscopic techniques, and all-inside techniques.

Arthroscopic-Assisted Techniques

Arthroscopic-assisted techniques involve at least 1 accessory portal used to pass bone anchors or sutures through the joint and the ligaments. Numerous clinical studies have reported on the favorable outcomes for patients who are treated with an arthroscopic-assisted repair technique. The first European study, by Corte-Real and Moreira,[24] reported on 28 of 31patients who underwent an arthroscopic-assisted repair. A double-loaded suture anchor and an accessory anterolateral portal were used. Average follow-up was at 24.5 months, with American Orthopaedic Foot and Ankle Society (AOFAS) scores averaging 85.3, and only 2 patients had recurrent instability. Despite a high complication rate (29%), their technique positively contributed to the early development of arthroscopic ligament repair, marking the beginning of the

Table 3
Complications of arthroscopic lateral ligament repair/internal brace repair

Author, Year	Number of Complications (%)	Type of Complications
Acevedo & Mangone,[9] 2015	9 (12.32)	1 residual instability 3 persistent lateral pain 5 neuritis
Coetzee et al,[50] 2018	4 (4.9)	1 slight dehiscence of the incision 1 superficial infection 1 anterior ankle impingement 1 extensor tendinitis
Cordier et al,[55] 2019	5 (9.1)	1 complex regional pain syndrome 2 deep venous thrombosis 1 neuralgia of the SPN 1 dysesthesia of sural nerve and SPN
Corte-Real & Moreira,[24] 2015	9 (29)	3 delayed wound healing 3 neuritis SPN 2 acute ankle sprains
Cottom & Rigby,[40] 2013	3 (7.5)	1 deep vein thrombosis 1 neuritis dorsal cutaneous nerve 1 distal fibular fracture
Kim et al,[54] 2019	4 (3.2)	2 SPN neuropraxia 1 knot pain 1 abscess
Li et al,[46] 2017	1 (4.3)	1 persistent pain
Nery et al,[57] 2011	0	—
Nery et al,[39] 2017	1 (3.8)	1 neuritis SPN
Song et al,[58] 2017		
Reconstruction	1 (8.3)	1 neuritis sural nerve
Repair	2 (12.5)	2 neuritis SPN
Vega et al,[44] 2013	2 (12.5)	1 superficial infection 1 delayed wound healing
Xu et al,[51] 2019		
Internal brace	3 (12)	3 abnormal dorsal foot paresthesia
Without internal brace	2 (7.1)	1 mechanical instability 1 wound infection
Yeo et al,[48] 2016	5 (20)	2 neuritis SPN 1 neuritis sural nerve 2 knot pain
Yoo & Yang,[42] 2016		
Internal brace	0	—
Without internal brace	2 (3.2)	2 neuritis DCN

DCN, Dorsal Cutaneous Nerve.
Data from Refs.[9,24,39,40,42,44,46,48,50,51,54,55,57,58]

modern techniques. Afterward, Kim[25] published the results of a double-loaded suture anchor used on 28 ankles. In contrast with the Corte-Real and Moreira[24] technique, these investigators used a soft tissue penetrator to pass sutures along with an accessory anteroinferior portal. At an average follow-up of 15.9 months, 3 patients were shown to have laxity via stress radiographs but were all able to return to their preinjury levels.

All-Arthroscopic Techniques

All-arthroscopic techniques use only the 2 traditional ankle arthroscopy portals for the passage of bone anchors and/or sutures through the joint and ligaments, but a small incision is used in order to tie the sutures. In 2011, the first fully arthroscopic technique was published,[38] on 24 ankles, that no longer relied on accessory portals or additional incisions for anchor placement or suture passage. Patients reported a 95.8% satisfaction rate at a 10.9-month follow-up. Multiple successive studies with the same technique have reported comparable results.[9,39–42] In the largest study to date, 73 patients were evaluated retrospectively, at an average 28 months with a 94.5% satisfaction rate. The mean Karlsson score increased from a preoperative score of 28.3 to a postoperative score of 90.2.[9] Of the 4 patients who were not satisfied, there was only 1 case of recurrent instability. In 2016, Nery and colleagues[39] published a prospective cohort study that included 26 patients who received an arthroscopic repair with an inside-out technique. The AOFAS score increased from 58 preoperatively to 90 postoperatively at a mean follow-up of 27 months. Regular to poor scores (AOFAS score <80) were found in 4 (15.4%) patients. Pellegrini and colleagues[43] investigated the knotless modification of the Acevedo and Mangone[38] technique, finding it to be safe and reproducible. They reported on 30 patients in 2017 with only 1 complication of complex regional pain syndrome, which resolved 6 months after the procedure. Their study found no cases of recurrent instability.

All-Inside Techniques

All-inside techniques only use the 2 traditional and accessory ankle arthroscopy portals for passage of the bone anchors and/or sutures through the joint and ligaments, but the knot is tied arthroscopically or a knotless technique is used to secure the repair. The development of these techniques is more recent and has shown promising results. Vega and colleagues[44] investigated the use of a knotless suture anchor as a means of preventing complications related to suture prominence (ie, neuritis, suture pain). That study included 16 patients and followed them for an average of 22.3 months (12–35 months). AOFAS scores for the patients improved from an average of 67 (59–77) to 97 (95–100) using an all-inside technique. A superficial infection was present for 1 of the patients and was resolved with conservative management, whereas another patient had a delayed wound healing of the anterolateral portal, which also resolved. There were no major or neurologic complications reported. Furthermore, in 2018, Vega and colleagues[45] found that, in patients with poor ligament tissue quality, the knotless all-inside technique can achieve excellent results. Their technique allows the surgeon to avoid the difficulty of harvesting an autograft as well as avoiding the immunologic response of an allograft. In 2017, Li and colleagues[46] compared 23 patients who underwent arthroscopic repair with 37 patients who underwent open modified Brostrom procedures. Postoperative AOFAS score for the arthroscopic technique was 93.3, Karlsson score 90.3, and Tegner score 5, showing equivalence with open technique scores of 92.4, 89.4, and 5, respectively. Persistent pain was present in 1 (4.3%) patient in the arthroscopic group, with no further complications reported in the group. Rigby and Cottom[47] performed a similar study comparing open Brostrom-Gould with an all-inside arthroscopic repair. Their study also showed the equivalence of outcomes between the open and all-inside arthroscopic repairs. Yeo and colleagues[48] completed the only published randomized controlled trial that compared the open modified Brostrom with an all-inside arthroscopic technique for addressing ankle instability. There were 48 total patients: 25 patients in the arthroscopic group and 23 patients in the open group. The mean Karlsson and AOFAS scores in the arthroscopic group improved from 45 and 76.2 to 67.5 and 90.3, respectively. The open group saw similar score improvements from 48.6 and 73.5 to 69.9 and 89.2. Of the 5 complications present (20%) in the arthroscopic group, 2 were SPN neuritis, 1 was sural neuritis, and 2 were knot pain.

Primary Versus Augmented Repair

Although the Brostrom-Gould procedure remains popular in ankle ligament repair, it has its limitations, including a weaker ATFL compared with a native intact ATFL and a lengthy period of immobilization and rehabilitation. As with other joint ligament reconstructions, the patient often desires to return to play (or work) as soon as possible, which has led to the development of a suture tape internal brace. Mackay and Ribbans[49] performed a Brostrom repair with internal brace with follow-up of outcomes on 20 patients who all had reduced pain, earlier mobilization, and earlier restoration of function compared with the Brostrom repair without an internal brace. Coetzee and colleagues[50] published the outcomes of 81 patients who underwent a Brostrom repair with the internal brace augmentation. Their patients had an average postoperative AOFAS score of 94.3 and were able to participate in an accelerated rehabilitation process allowing athletes to return to sports as early as 8 weeks postsurgery. Yoo and Yang[42] performed a retrospective cohort study that compared the arthroscopic modified Brostrom both with and without the use of an internal brace. The internal brace group consisted of 22 patients, and the group with no internal brace consisted of 63 patients. Patients with the internal brace had AOFAS scores improve from 65.8 to 98, whereas those without the brace improved from 66.7 to 96.5. The internal brace group had no complications and there were 2 (3.2%) cases of dorsal cutaneous neuritis in the group without an internal brace. Despite no statistical difference between the groups in terms of outcomes scores, the internal brace group was able to return to activity and sports sooner. Xu and colleagues[51] compared the Brostrom-Gould with the Brostrom-Gould with internal brace and measured functional outcomes using the Foot and Ankle Ability Measure (FAAM) scale. There was no statistically significant difference in the FAAM scores (93.1 in the internal brace group vs 90.5 without internal brace); however, the FAAM sport scores were statistically different. This difference in return to functionality in sports was attributed to earlier mobilization and rehabilitation as well as the protection against elongation of the ankle ligaments provided by the internal brace. Acevedo and McWilliams[52] presented the results of their investigation on 42 patients who received the internal brace arthroscopically, with a mean follow-up of 33 months. The results showed a significant increase in both AOFAS and FAAM scores with a return to activity of 18 weeks. There were 3 cases of complications, 1 postoperative infection, and 2 episodes of transient neuritis.

Associated Intra-articular Disorders During Arthroscopic Repair

Intra-articular lesions are often associated with CAI, and these may include OCL, loose bodies, or ossicles that can cause pain and osteoarthritis.[53,54] These lesions can be addressed via debridement before the lateral ligament repair. Typically, patients with OCLs have higher rates of dissatisfaction after the procedure. The authors believe that a subset of patients with failed OCL microfracture likely have unrecognized ankle instability that increases rotational shear forces on the articular surface and can affect the healing of the OCL. Consistent with this theory, Jiang and colleagues[53] found that treatment of the OCL along with the Brostrom repair did not present any statistically significant differences in satisfaction compared with patients who did not have any OCL.

Ossicles within the lateral ligament may also present when performing arthroscopy of the ankle. Kim and colleagues[54] found that it was best to perform resection of the surrounding inflamed synovial tissue, followed by dissection and removal of the ossicle. Their study compared the outcomes of patients with and without ossicles and showed no statistically significant difference in outcomes. Both of these studies show that the lateral ligament repair can be safely done alongside any treatment of intra-articular disorders.

SUMMARY

Most of the significant advances in arthroscopic techniques since the 1980s have been focused on ligament reconstruction to stabilize an unstable shoulder and/or knee. During that time, ankle arthroscopy use was primitive, with its primary goal to inspect the joint and provide treatment of intra-articular disorders, such as removal of loose bodies, impingement debridement, and microfracture. A growing understanding of intra-articular pathologic conditions secondary to ankle instability has led to an increase in ankle arthroscopy performed in conjunction with open lateral ligament reconstruction. As was the case with both the knee and shoulder, this combination has motivated several surgeons nationally and internationally to investigate the use of arthroscopic techniques to stabilize the ankle. Significant advances over the last decade have given rise to the development of successful techniques for the treatment of ankle instability via the arthroscope. Notably, the 2-anchor arthro-Brostrom technique described in this article has been the most rigorously studied and currently is the only technique with published data supporting its use as a safe, reproducible, and biomechanically equivalent alternative to the traditional open Brostrom-Gould procedure.[7,8] A suture tape internal brace can add further strength to the repair construct and most closely approximates the strength of an intact ATFL. If the history of arthroscopy in shoulders and knees is any indication for the future of ankle arthroscopy, the next 20 years hold much promise for the further advancement of the techniques and tools involved. With these advancements, it is clear that arthroscopic lateral ankle ligament reconstruction will become the standard of care in foot and ankle orthopedics.

ACKNOWLEDGMENTS

The authors thank Andres Cedeno for assistance with preparation of the article.

DISCLOSURE

Drs J.I. Acevedo and P.G. Mangone are consultants and speakers for Arthrex, Inc, and they receive royalties from the company as well. They are also speakers for Wright Medical.

REFERENCES

1. Freeman MA, Dean MR, Hanham IW. The etiology and prevention of functional instability of the foot. J Bone Joint Surg Br 1965;47:678–85.

2. Shakked RJ, Karnovsky S, Drakos MC. Operative treatment of lateral ligament instability. Curr Rev Musculoskelet Med 2017;10(1):113–21.

3. Ballal MS, Pearce CJ, Calder JD. Management of sports injuries of the foot and ankle: an update. Bone Joint J 2016;98-B(7):874–83.

4. Gribble PA, Bleakley CM, Caulfield BM, et al. 2016 consensus statement of the International Ankle Consortium: prevalence, impact and long-term consequences of lateral ankle sprains. Br J Sports Med 2016;50(24):1493–5.

5. Acevedo JI, Palmer RC, Mangone P. Arthroscopic Treatment of Ankle Instability: Brostrom. Foot Ankle Clin 2018;23(1):555–70.

6. Odak S. Arthroscopic evaluation of impingement and osteochondral lesions in chronic lateral ankle instability. Foot Ankle Int 2015;36(9):1045–9.

7. Drakos M, Behrens S, Hoffman E, et al. A biomechanical comparison of an open vs. arthroscopic approach for the treatment of lateral ankle instability (SS-57). Arthroscopy 2011;27(5):809–15.

8. Giza E, Shin EC, Wong SE, et al. Arthroscopic suture anchor repair of the lateral ligament ankle complex: a cadaveric study. Am J Sports Med 2013;41(11): 2567–72.

9. Acevedo JI, Mangone P. Ankle instability and arthroscopic lateral ligament repair. Foot Ankle Clin 2015;20(1):59–69.

10. Hossain M, Thomas R. Ankle instability: presentation and management. Orthop Trauma 2015;29(2):145–51.

11. Sarrafian SK, Kelikian AS. Syndesmosis. Sarrafian's Anatomy of the Foot and Ankle: Descriptive, Topographic, Functional. 3rd edition. Lippincott Williams and Wilkins; 2011.

12. Matsui K, Takao M, Tochigi Y, et al. Anatomy of anterior talofibular ligament and calcaneofibular ligament for minimally invasive surgery: a systematic review. Knee Surg Sports Traumatol Arthrosc 2017;25(6):1892–902.

13. Jorge JT, Gomes TM, Oliva XM. An anatomical study about the arthroscopic repair of the lateral ligament of the ankle. Foot Ankle Surg 2018;24(2):143–8.

14. Vega J, Pena F, Golano P. Minor or occult ankle instability as a cause of antero-lateral pain after ankle sprain. Knee Surg Sports Traumatol Arthrosc 2016;24(4): 1116–23.

15. Lee KT, Park YU, Kim JS, et al. Long-term results after modified Brostrom procedure without calcaneofibular ligament reconstruction. Foot Ankle Int 2011;32(2): 153–7.

16. Dalmau-Pastor M, Yasui Y, Calder JD, et al. Anatomy of the inferior extensor retinaculum and its role in lateral ankle ligament reconstruction: a pictorial essay. Knee Surg Sports Traumatol Arthrosc 2016;24(4):957–62.

17. Dalmau-Pastor M. X-shaped inferior extensor retinaculum and its doubtful use in the Bröstrom-Gould procedure. Knee Surg Sports Traumatol Arthrosc 2017. https://doi.org/10.1007/s00167-017-4647-y.

18. Acevedo JI, Ortiz C, Golano P, et al. ArthroBrostrom lateral ankle stabilization technique: an anatomic study. Am J Sports Med 2015;43(10):2564–71.

19. Matsui K, Oliva XM, Takao M, et al. Bony landmarks available for minimally invasive lateral ankle stabilization surgery: a cadaveric anatomical study. Knee Surg Sports Traumatol Arthrosc 2017;25(6):1916–24.

20. Clanton TO, Campbell KJ, Wilson KJ, et al. Qualitative and quantitative anatomic investigation of the lateral ankle ligaments for surgical reconstruction procedures. J Bone Joint Surg Am 2014;96(12):e98.

21. Hawkins RB. Arthroscopic stapling repair for chronic lateral instability. Clin Podiatr Med Surg 1987;4(4):875–83.

22. Kashuk KB, Landsman AS, Werd MB, et al. Arthroscopic lateral ankle stabilization. Clin Podiatr Med Surg 1994;11(3):407–23.

23. Guelfi M, Zamperetti M, Pantalone A. Open and Arthroscopic lateral ligament repair for treatment of chronic ankle instability: A systematic review. Foot Ankle Surg 2018;24(1):11–8.
24. Corte-Real NM, Moreira RM. Arthroscopic repair of chronic lateral ankle instability. Foot Ankle Int 2015;5:213–7.
25. Kim ES. Arthroscopic anterior talofibular ligament repair for chronic ankle instability with a suture anchor technique. Orthopedics 2011;34(4). https://doi.org/10.3928/01477447-20110228-03.
26. Matsui K, Takao M, Miyamoto W, et al. Early recovery after arthroscopic repair compared to open repair of the anterior talofibular ligament for lateral instability of the ankle. Arch Orthop Trauma Surg 2016;136(1):93–100.
27. Prisk VR, Imhauser CW, O'Loughlin PF, et al. Lateral ligament repair and reconstruction restore neither contact mechanics of the ankle joint nor motion patterns of the hindfoot. J Bone Joint Surg Am 2010;92(14):2375–86.
28. Pitts CC, McKissack HM, Anderson MC, et al. Anatomical structures at risk in the arthroscopic Brostrom-Gould procedure: A cadaver study. Foot Ankle Surg 2019. https://doi.org/10.1016/j.fas.2019.04.008.
29. Santos FF, Santos NR. Arthroscopic treatment of lateral ankle instability. Is there a safe zone? An anatomic study. Foot Ankle Surg 2020;26(1):61–5.
30. Lee KT, Kim ES, Kim YH, et al. All-inside arthroscopic modified Brostrom operation for chronic ankle instability: a biomechanical study. Knee Surg Sports Traumatol Arthrosc 2016;24(4):1096–100.
31. Yoshimura I, Hagio T, Noda M, et al. Optimal suture anchor direction in arthroscopic lateral ankle ligament repair. Knee Surg Sports Traumatol Arthrosc 2017. https://doi.org/10.1007/s00167-017-4587-6.
32. Dong P, Gu S, Jiang Y, et al. All Arthroscopic remnant-preserving reconstruction of the lateral ligaments of the ankle: A biomechanical study and clinical application. Biochem Biophys Res Commun 2018. https://doi.org/10.1016/j.bbrc.2018.10.041.
33. Waldrop NE, Wijdicks CA, Jansson KS, et al. Anatomic Suture Anchor Versus the Brostrom Technique for Anterior Talofibular Ligament Repair. Am J Sports Med 2012;40(11):2590–6.
34. Viens NA, Wijdicks CA, Campbell KJ, et al. Anterior talofibular ligament ruptures, part 1: biomechanical comparison of augmented Brostrom repair techniques with the intact anterior talofibular ligament. Am J Sports Med 2014;42(2):405–11.
35. Schuh R, Benca E, Willegger M, et al. Comparison of Brostrom technique, suture anchor repair, and tape augmentation for reconstruction of the anterior talofibular ligament. Knee Surg Sports Traumatol Arthrosc 2016;24(4):1101–7.
36. Lohrer H, Bonsignore G, Dorn-Lange N, et al. Stabilizing lateral ankle instability by suture tape - a cadaver study. J Orthop Surg Res 2019;14:175.
37. Willegger M, Benca E, Hirtler L, et al. Biomechanical stability of tape augmentation for anterior talofibular ligament (ATFL) repair compared to the native ATFL. Knee Surg Sports Traumatol Arthrosc 2016;24:1015–21.
38. Acevedo JI, Mangone PG. Arthroscopic lateral ankle ligament reconstruction. Tech Foot Ankle Surg 2011;10(3):111–6.
39. Nery C, Fonseca L, Raduan F, et al. Prospective study of the "inside-out" arthroscopic ankle ligament technique: preliminary result. Foot Ankle Surg 2017. https://doi.org/10.1016/j.fas.2017.03.002.
40. Cottom JM, Rigby RB. The "all inside" arthroscopic Brostrom procedure: a prospective study of 40 consecutive patients. J Foot Ankle Surg 2013;52(5):568–74.

41. Labib SA, Slone HS. Ankle arthroscopy for lateral ankle instability. Tech Foot Ankle Surg 2015;14(1):25–7.
42. Yoo JS, Yang EA. Clinical results of an arthroscopic modified Brostrom operation with and without an internal brace. J Orthop Traumatol 2016;17(4):353–60.
43. Pellegrini MJ, Sevillano J, Ortiz C, et al. Knotless Modified Arthroscopic-Brostrom technique for Ankle Instability. Foot Ankle Int 2019;40(4):475–83.
44. Vega J, Golano P, Pellegrino A, et al. All-inside arthroscopic lateral collateral ligament repair for ankle instability with a knotless suture anchor technique. Foot Ankle Int 2013;34(12):1701–9.
45. Vega J, Montesinos E, Malagelada F, et al. Arthroscopic all-inside anterior talofibular ligament repair with suture augmentation gives excellent results in case of poor ligament tissue remnant quality. Knee Surg Sports Traumatol Arthrosc 2018. https://doi.org/10.1007/s00167-018-5117-x.
46. Li H, Hua Y, Li H, et al. Activity level and function 2 years after anterior talofibular ligament repair: a comparison between arthroscopic repair and open repair procedures. Am J Sports Med 2017;45(9):2044–52.
47. Rigby R, Cottom J. A comparison of the "All-Inside" arthroscopic Brostrom procedure with the traditional open modified Brostrom-Gould technique: A review of 62 patients. Foot Ankle Surg 2017;25(1):31–6.
48. Yeo ED, Lee KT, Sung IH, et al. Comparison of all-inside arthroscopic and open techniques for the modified brostrom procedure for ankle instability. Foot Ankle Int 2016;37(10):1037–45.
49. Mackay G, Ribbans W. The Addition of an "Internal Brace" to augment the Brostrom technique for lateral ankle ligament instability. Tech Foot Ankle Surg 2016; 15(1):47–56.
50. Coetzee J, Ellington J, Ronan J, et al. Functional Results of Open Brostrom Ankle Ligament Repair Augmented with a Suture Tape. Foot Ankle Int 2018;39(3): 304–10.
51. Xu D, Gan K, Li H, et al. Modified Brostrom Repair with and without augmentation using suture tape for chronic lateral ankle instability. Orthop Surg 2019;11(4): 671–8.
52. Acevedo JI, McWilliams JR. Results of Arthroscopic internal brace augmentation Presentation. The Journal of the Japanese Society for Surgery of the Foot; 5th Ankle Instability Group Annual Meeting, Vol. 39 Supplement. Kisarazu, November 3, 2018.
53. Jiang D, Ao Y, Jiao C, et al. Concurrent arthroscopic osteochondral lesion treatment and lateral ankle ligament repair has no substantial effect on the outcome of chronic lateral ankle instability. Knee Surg Sports Traumatol Arthrosc 2018; 26(10):3129–34.
54. Kim W, Lee H, Moon S, et al. Presence of Subfibular Ossicle Does Not affect the Outcome of Arthroscopic Modified Brostrom Procedure for Chronic Lateral Ankle Instability. Arthroscopy 2019;35(3):953–60.
55. Cordier G, Lebecque J, Vega J, et al. Arthroscopic ankle lateral ligament repair with biological augmentation gives excellent results in case of chronic ankle instability. Knee Surg Sports Traumatol Arthrosc 2019;. https://doi: 10.1007/s00167-019-05650-9.
56. Corte-Real NM, Moreira RM. Arthroscopic repair of chronic lateral ankle instability. Foot Ankle Int 2009;30(3):213–7.
57. Nery C, Raduan F, Del Buono A, et al. Arthroscopic-assisted Broström-Gould for chronic ankle instability: a long-term follow-up. Am J Sports Med 2011;39(11): 2381–8.

58. Song B, Changchuan L, Chen N, et al. All-arthroscopic anatomical reconstruction of anterior talofibular ligament using semitendinosus autografts. Int Orthop 2017; 41(5):975–82.
59. Vega J, Malagelada F, Dalmau-Pastor. Arthroscopic all-inside ATFL and CFL repair is feasible and provides excellent results in patients with chronic ankle instability. Knee Surg Sports Traumatol Arthrosc 2020;28(1):116–23.

Modern Open and Minimally Invasive Stabilization of Chronic Lateral Ankle Instability

Tyler Allen, BS[a], Meghan Kelly, MD, PhD[b,c],*

KEYWORDS

- Ankle sprain • Ankle instability • Ligament reconstruction • Ligament repair

KEY POINTS

- The lateral ankle comprises 3 important ligaments: anterior talofibular ligament, calcaneo-fibular ligament, and posterior talofibular ligament. The anterior talofibular ligament is the weakest of the lateral ligament complex.
- Patients should first be evaluated with a thorough history and physical, particularly with an ankle anterior drawer test and talar tilt test. Imaging can aid in the diagnosis.
- Conservative management should be attempted first, but surgery may be required for patients who do not improve. Anatomic repair, particularly direct repair, is the gold standard of management.

INTRODUCTION

It is estimated that 5000 to 27,000 people experience an ankle inversion injury every day in the United States, leading to 7% to 10% of all emergency department visits nationwide and 30% of athletic injuries, making this one of the most common presentations to health care professionals.[1–4] The mainstay treatment of an acute ankle sprain involves conservative management and proprioceptive training; however, the occurrence of an ankle sprain is a significant risk factor in the development of chronic ankle instability (CAI).[5–7]

CAI is defined as the subjective feeling of giving way in combination with recurrent sprains, pain, and swelling, or avoidance of activities that might cause the patient distress about the ankle stability; symptoms that are often revealed during a thorough patient history.[7,8] A key component of CAI is recurrent sprains for at least 1 year following the initial sprain, although many patients reveal a history of multiple sprains

[a] University of Nevada Reno School of Medicine, 1890 Van Ness Avenue, Reno, NV 89503, USA; [b] Department of Orthopedic Surgery University of California at Davis; [c] Department of Orthopedic Surgery, Mount Sinai Icahn School of Medicine, 425 West 59th Street 5th Floor, New York, NY 10019, USA
* Corresponding author. Department of Orthopedic Surgery, Mount Sinai Icahn School of Medicine, 425 West 59th Street 5th Floor, New York, NY 10019, USA
E-mail address: megkellyortho@gmail.com

Foot Ankle Clin N Am 26 (2021) 87–101
https://doi.org/10.1016/j.fcl.2020.11.003

over a period of 10 to 15 years.[9] Patients with CAI often have symptoms of both mechanical and functional instability (abnormal ligamentous laxity on physical examination and the sensation of instability and repeat sprains, respectively).[10] Initial treatment of CAI involves conservative management, particularly functional rehabilitation that uses range-of-motion exercises, peroneal and ankle dorsiflexion strengthening, Achilles tendon stretching, and proprioception training in conjunction with proper ankle immobilization devices.[8] This article discusses the anatomy, pathology, evaluation, treatment, and complications of CAI.

ANATOMY

Ligamentous structures of the subtalar and tibiotalar joints make up the lateral collateral ligament complex of the ankle and hindfoot. The anterior talofibular ligament (ATFL), the calcaneofibular ligament (CFL), and the posterior talofibular ligament (PTFL) make up the lateral collateral ligament complex of the ankle joint, whereas the CFL, the inferior extensor retinaculum, the lateral talocalcaneal ligament, the cervical ligament, and the interosseous talocalcaneal ligament make up the complex within the subtalar joint (**Fig. 1**).

The ATFL is a single-banded or multibanded ligament that originates 13.8 mm from the lateral malleolus' inferior tip on the anterior margin.[11] It courses anteriorly to insert 17.8 mm superior to the apex of the lateral talar process along the anterior border of the talar lateral articular facet. The ATFL is unique because it can be a single band, a bifurcate, or a trifurcate; however, it is unknown whether the anatomic variance has any clinical consequences.[12] The ATFL is the weakest of the 3 lateral ankle ligaments,

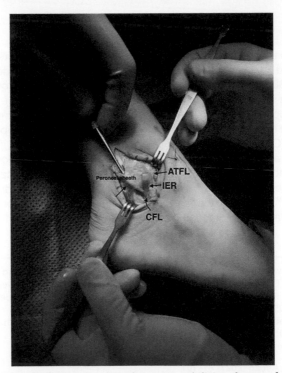

Fig. 1. Intraoperative dissection showing the static stabilizing forces of the lateral ankle. IER, inferior extensor retinaculum.

with a measured mean ultimate load to failure of 154 N (compared with the CFL and PTFL at 345.7 N and 261.2 N, respectively). Characteristics provides an explanation for why the ATFL is the most common ligament to be injured during an acute ankle sprain.[13,14] The CFL originates 5.3 mm anterior to the lateral malleolus' inferior tip and courses posteroinferiorly to cross the subtalar and talocrural joint under the peroneal tendons, inserting 16.3 mm posterosuperiorly from the posterior point of the peroneal tubercle.[11] The PTFL originates 4.8 mm superior to the lateral malleolus' inferior tip on the medial aspect of the lateral malleolus and courses to the posterolateral aspect of the talus.

The position of the foot during an injury is a major determinant of which ligament is primarily damaged. If the foot is in plantar flexion during an inversion injury, the ATFL is most likely injured, whereas the CFL is more likely to be injured in the setting of an inversion injury in dorsiflexion.[8,15] The PTFL does not contribute to lateral ankle stability in a significant capacity.

In addition to the ligaments, the inferior extensor retinaculum (IER) is also noted to provide important stability to the lateral aspect of the ankle and subtalar joint.[6] It is composed of 3 roots that lie within the sinus tarsi, and are labeled the lateral, intermediate, and medial roots. This additional stability is used by the imbrication of the IER over the repaired ATFL during the Broström-Gould procedure.

In addition, the proximal musculotendinous units of the leg are vital to providing stability to the lateral ankle. Other investigators have shown the important role of the peroneal muscles in the maintenance of lateral ankle instability.[16] Therefore, rehabilitation of these muscles is important in order to improve ankle proprioception and to protect the lateral ankle ligamentous complex from further injury.

EVALUATION

The current guidelines for assessing any patient with ankle instability have been suggested by the modified Delphi study, which recommends assessing for 5 components: mechanism of injury, history of previous lateral ankle sprain, weight-bearing status, clinical assessment of bones, and clinical assessment of ligaments.[17]

In patients presenting with signs of CAI, it is imperative to obtain a thorough history. Reports of feelings that the ankle gives way or feelings of instability while traversing unstable terrain or while playing sports strongly indicate CAI. Furthermore, it is important to fully assess the patient for factors that may predispose to CAI. Intrinsic factors, including age, sex, previous ankle injury, aerobic fitness, and foot morphologic characteristics, are important to determine during the history and physical.[5,18] A medical history of conditions pertaining to peripheral neuropathy disorders (Charcot-Marie-Tooth), connective tissue disorders (Marfan, Ehlers-Danlos), or overall ligamentous laxity should be noted because this may have implications in the treatment of the CAI. Furthermore, a chronic history of corticosteroid use or prior use of fluoroquinolone antibiotics may result in poor tendon and ligament quality. In addition, assessing extrinsic factors such as sports participation (indoor courts such as volleyball and basketball convey the highest risk), level of competition, and the use of ankle stabilization (such as taping or braces) during activity aids in the decision making for overall treatment.[18] Additional risk factors, such as supernumerary muscles (most commonly the peroneus quartus) and a posteriorly located fibula may also predispose patients to CAI.[19]

The physical examination is an important step in the assessment of chronic lateral ankle instability. Starting with overall foot alignment, patients with a cavovarus foot or a varus hindfoot alignment often have a history of multiple ankle sprains and clinicians must account for this deformity to achieve a successful outcome.[20] In addition, there is evidence to suggest that injury to the superficial peroneal nerve can occur after repeated inversion injuries because of its anterolateral positioning, thus a careful neurovascular assessment of the ankle and associated ankle eversion strength is important.[8,21] Furthermore, often there is peroneal tendon pain or fullness present, or evidence of a joint effusion.

Two tests that assess for ligamentous integrity are the anterior drawer test and the talar tilt test. The anterior drawer test in 20% of plantar flexion assesses for laxity caused by ATFL disruption, whereas laxity in dorsiflexion suggests disruption in the CFL (**Fig. 2**).[17] The talar tilt test is performed by performing an inversion force with the ankle in a neutral position. A positive test suggests an injury to the ATFL and the CFL (**Fig. 3**). These tests, as well as a careful neurovascular examination, as dictated earlier, should be performed on the contralateral limb as well. Physical examination is important to discern the difference between lateral ligament instability and sinus tarsi syndrome. Sinus tarsi syndrome was first described in 1958 in patients who presented with pain in the sinus tarsi region that alleviated with a local anesthetic. However, the exact cause of sinus tarsi syndrome remains up for debate.[22–24] It has been suggested that it may be a manifestation of subtalar instability, whereas others propose that it is related to fat pad inflammation and synovial herniation into the sinus tarsi causing pain.

Given the overlap in symptoms of lateral ankle instability and sinus tarsi syndrome, appropriate imaging can be helpful for diagnosis. The primary imaging modalities to assess for chronic lateral ankle instability are radiographs and MRI. Initial radiographs should be performed with weight-bearing anteroposterior, lateral, and mortise views. Stress radiographs can be obtained when performing anterior drawer or talar tilt tests; however, laxity can often be assessed with just the physical examination. Studies have suggested that, if there is a 3-mm difference of the anterior translation of the talus relative to the tibia or a 10-mm absolute translation value while performing an anterior drawer test, the test is considered significant on radiographs.[25,26] However, studies indicate that 86% of patients presenting with signs of CAI have more than 5 mm of anterior translation, thus the use of stress radiographs may not be of benefit because this can be detected with physical examination.[27] The CFL can be assessed with anteroposterior imaging while performing the talar tilt test; greater than 3° variation of talar tilt angle from affected to nonaffected side or an absolute of 9° or greater of talar tilt is considered significant.[25] The sensitivity and specificity of stress radiography in determining lateral ankle instability at the tibiotalar joint was 66% and 97% in 1 study,

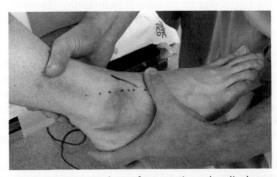

Fig. 2. The anterior drawer test to evaluate for anterior talar displacement relative to the tibia to assess ligamentous laxity.

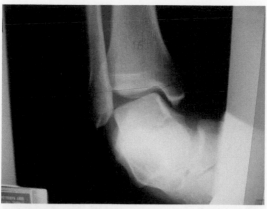

Fig. 3. Anteroposterior radiograph of the ankle showing a positive talar, suggesting injury to the lateral ligamentous complex.

respectively. However, 40% of patients with instability on radiographs also show instability on physical examination, and 40% of those with symptomatic instability appear stable on stress radiographs.[28] Therefore, stress views are a useful adjunct but should not substitute for a carefully performed physical examination.

MRI is a useful imaging modality to assess for lateral ankle instability. The use of MRI allows a three-dimensional assessment of the ATFL and CFL and can show evidence of increased talar tilt (**Fig. 4**). Furthermore, MRI allows the evaluation of associated injuries such as osteochondral lesions, loose bodies, supernumerary muscles, and other potential sources of injury (**Fig. 5**).[19] However, MRI is a higher-cost modality compared with other imaging methods, and its diagnostic ability may depend on magnet strength.[27] Overall, MRI can serve as an adjunct imaging study if a patient is considering surgical intervention given that it allows additional injuries to be identified. Furthermore, if there is concern for sinus tarsi syndrome, MRI may show evidence of synovitis or fibrosis in the sinus tarsi or evidence of interosseus ligament tear. However, as mentioned previously, MRI should not serve as a substitute for a well-performed history and physical because it may not clearly identify chronic injuries to

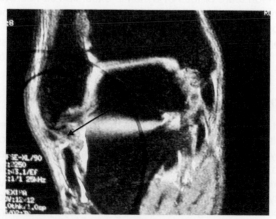

Fig. 4. Coronal T2-weighted MRI showing a CFL tear (*blue arrow*).

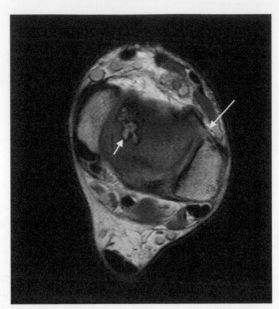

Fig. 5. Axial T2-weighted MRI view showing lateral ligament disruption (*long arrow*) in the setting of an osteochondral lesion (*short arrow*).

the ATFL or CFL that have healed with an increased working length that results in functional instability.

More recently, the use of ultrasonography has increased in popularity. An injured ligament (discontinuity or a hypoechoic ligament) can be observed when performing an anterior drawer test with the transducer placed over the ATFL.[26] A meta-analysis determined that the sensitivity and specificity for diagnosing chronic ATFL injury using ultrasonography were 99% and 91% respectively, whereas the sensitivity and specificity for diagnosing chronic CFL injury were 94% and 91% respectively.[29] The use of ultrasonography can be user dependent and is less accurate in the assessment of concomitant injuries; however, in the hands of an experienced technician, ultrasonography can be a useful adjunct to evaluate for other disorders that result in lateral ankle pain. Peroneal tendon tears or loss of dynamic excursion can be evaluated using ultrasonography and, when paired with an anesthetic injection, can be used to determine the contribution of peroneal tendon injuries in the setting of lateral ankle pain.[30] In addition, diagnostic and therapeutic injections into the sinus tarsi or the ankle joint can also reveal the contributions of sinus tarsi or intra-articular disorder.[22,24]

TREATMENT METHODS

Following an acute ankle sprain, conservative management is the preferred treatment option. One systematic review concluded that RICE (rest, ice, compression, and elevation) therapy with associated immobilization should be the treatment of choice for the first 5 to 7 days during the inflammatory phase of healing and may be augmented with the use of nonsteroidal antiinflammatory drugs (NSAIDs).[31] Following the first 5 to 7 days, the patient should use a semirigid ankle brace to protect against ankle inversion, or use a semirigid orthosis if a grade III injury is present during the proliferation phase of healing. Functional rehabilitation is essential in the treatment of the acute ankle sprain with a focus on progressive muscle strengthening (especially pero-neal muscles and isometric exercises) and proprioception training (with a focus on bal-ance and postural control) for at least 3 months following an injury. Patients should be counseled that they have an increased risk of experiencing additional ankle sprains; however, the likelihood is decreased with neuromuscular training and the use of lace-up ankle braces to provide additional stability.[31] Although there is general agree-ment for conservative management of grade I and II ankle sprains, there has been recent interest in acute surgical management of grade III ankle sprains in professional athletes.[32] In this setting, it has been suggested that acute surgical repair reduces objective instability and may prevent the sequela of chronic instability in the future compared with patients treated using functional rehabilitation.[2,9,33,34] There are no consistent guidelines at this point to advocate surgical versus nonsurgical manage-ment of a grade III sprain in athletes, but conditions such as patient medical history, timing of injury, season, and career stage may all be taken into account to determine the most effective treatment of the individual.

Although most patients improve following nonoperative management with physical therapy, the development of CAI may still occur. Studies report that 35% to 70% of patients may continue to have pain, swelling, or feelings of instability.[35] Resprains can occur in 3% to 34% of patients between 2 weeks and 96 months following the initial insult.[36] As defined earlier, CAI is diagnosed in patients who experience ankle instability following initial trauma for at least 1 year.[9,35] Patients who are diagnosed with CAI usually require surgical intervention if conservative management has failed.[8,35]

Surgical management of CAI can be classified as either anatomic or nonanatomic repairs, and each of these categories can be further divided into augmented or non-augmented techniques. Nonanatomic reconstruction primarily involves the use of the patient's peroneus brevis tendon to stabilize the ankle joint, which include the Evans, Chrisman-Snook, and Watson-Jones procedures.[37]

The Evans procedure involves tenodesis of the peroneus brevis proximally and us-ing the tendon to pass through the distal fibula at an angle that is the average force vector of the ATFL and the CFL. The remaining peroneus brevis is then tenodesed to the peroneus longus.[38] Although early postoperative outcomes showed diminished capacity for an inversion injury, long-term results showed unsatisfactory results, especially compared with anatomic reconstruction.[39,40] The Watson-Jones proced-ure splits the peroneus brevis tendon, passing it through the lateral malleolus and inserting it to the lateral aspect of the talus.[41] The graft then courses backward through a second tunnel and is sutured on itself in the posterolateral aspect of the fibula. Although early results were promising, long-term results showed poor out-comes, including continued radiological instability and incomplete relief of symptoms.[41–43]

In addition, the Chrisman-Snook procedure is a split-tendon transfer of the peroneal brevis through the calcaneus and the fibula, and initial studies suggested excellent outcomes after 10 years.[44,45] Complications such as overtightening, sural nerve in-juries, and wound problems have resulted in this procedure falling out of favor.[45] How-ever, through modifications of the procedure, the use of Chrisman-Snook procedure can be successful, especially in the setting in those patients with poor-quality ligamen-tous material from extrinsic factors such as repeated ankle sprains resulting in subop-timal ligament quality, or intrinsic factors such as connective tissue disorders (eg, Ehlers-Danlos, Marfan).[46,47] As a result, these patients benefit best from either a nonanatomic reconstruction or augmentation in order to restore ankle stability. In addition, other investigators have reported the use of this procedure successfully in the setting of chronic peroneal tendon subluxation, especially in skeletally immature patients.[48,49]

However, given the long-term outcome data, the ideal treatment of CAI remains anatomic repair. Anatomic procedures can be classified into 2 categories: direct repair of the damaged ligament, and anatomic reconstruction using an autograft or allograft. The direct repair technique of the Broström procedure, along with the Gould and Karlsson modifications, is the most popular.[50] The advantages of a direct anatomic repair include its simplicity and the avoidance of donor site morbidity with an autograft; however, the presence of adequate ligamentous tissue is essential for a successful repair. Anatomic reconstruction or a nonanatomic repair, such as the Chrisman-Snook, is preferred in patients who have poor-quality ligaments, have failed a previous lateral ankle repair, have a high body mass index, or have generalized ligamentous laxity.[50]

The Broström procedure is performed by individually dissecting out the ATFL and CFL and reapproximating with the use of heavy suture (**Fig. 6**).[51] The Gould modification reinforces the Broström procedure by the addition of suturing the lateral talocalcaneal ligament to the lateral malleolus and imbrication of the IER to the lateral fibula for additional stability.[52]

Surgical technique for anatomic repair:

- Patient is positioned in the lateral decubitus position with the operative side up. Ensure all bony prominences are padded and a tourniquet is used to enhance visibility.

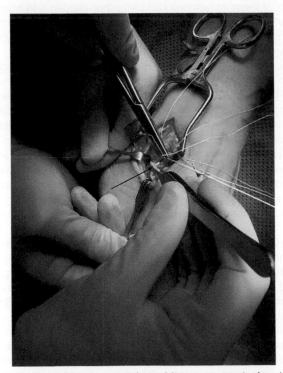

Fig. 6. Intraoperative view of an anatomic lateral ligament repair showing the CFL (*black arrow*).

- A U-shaped incision is created distal to the fibula and taken down through skin and subcutaneous tissue. (If evaluation of peroneal tendons is a concurrent procedure, an incision along the midline of the fibula is used.)
- The extensor retinaculum is dissected off the distal fibula and the peroneal sheath is incised. Once the peroneal tendons are retracted, the CFL is revealed and taken down from its insertion.
- The ATFL is then identified and taken down from its insertion as well.
- The periosteum is lifted off the distal portion of the fibula and a rongeur is used to prepare the bone for placement of the suture anchors.
- Either 1 quad-loaded or 2 dual-loaded anchors are placed in the fibula with 2 sutures being placed in the CFL and the ATFL (**Fig. 7**). The CFL is then repaired while the foot is positioned in eversion and the ATFL is repaired with the foot in dorsiflexion and eversion.
- The extensor retinaculum is then repaired to the periosteum of the fibula for additional stability and the skin closed with Vicryl and nylon sutures.

Following this procedure, it was noted that patients observed a decrease in anterior translation of the talus by 1 mm at 100% body weight and decreased internal rotation of the talus by 3° at 100% body weight.[53] In addition, the Karlsson modification is an anatomic reattachment of the ATFL and CFL through drill holes or anchors into the distal fibula with ligament imbrication, if required, given that the ligaments are often elongated and scarred in patients with CAI.[40,54] Eighty-eight percent of patients receiving the Karlsson modification procedure reported good or excellent results after a mean follow-up period of 3.5 years, and a prospective randomized study investigating outcomes between the Karlsson technique and the Gould technique showed no statistically significant differences after a 2-year period.[54]

Anatomic repair of the lateral ligaments for CAI are important to address the functional impairment for patients; however, they also seem to diminish the development of ankle osteoarthritis that occurs as a result of long-standing altered tibiotalar joint mechanics.[53,55] The increased incidence of ankle osteoarthritis in patients with CAI

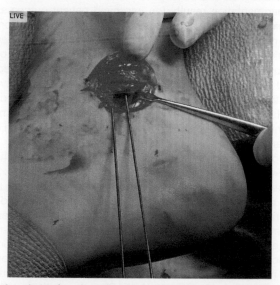

Fig. 7. Intraoperative view of anchor placement for Broström procedure.

is postulated to be caused by unbalanced loading of the medial joint space.[55] In agreement with this phenomenon, studies have demonstrated that patients continued to show improved functional outcomes, as measured by the Foot and Ankle Outcome Score (FAOS), up to a mean of 26 years following the index procedure.[56,57] Furthermore, Tourne and colleagues[58] showed good or very good results in 81% to 96% of patients with a mean follow-up of 11 years.

Anatomic reconstruction is an option for patients who lack adequate capsular tissue and ligamentous tissue.[59] The ATFL or CFL can be anatomically reconstructed using either an autograft plantaris (Anderson technique) or a free autograft of the fascia lata (Elmslie technique) through tunnels in the calcaneus, fibula, and neck of the talus.[60,61] More recently, other investigators have described methods using the gracilis tendons with an interference screw.[62] In addition, a hybrid technique has been described that uses a peroneal longus autograft for anatomic reconstruction of the ATFL along with reapproximation of the native ATFL, which has shown excellent results in a case series of athletes.[63] Allograft tendons can also be used in order to reduce the concern for donor site morbidity and reduce postoperative symptoms. Outcomes from allograft procedures have been excellent with the use of a semitendinosus or gracilis graft.[59,64] Furthermore, Clanton and colleagues[65] showed that the strength of an allograft was similar to that of the native ATFL in a biomechanical study, alleviating concerns that the use of an allograft may not provide the tensile strength that is required for adequate ligament stability.

Although few studies have been performed to directly compare autograft/allograft reconstruction with the anatomic direct repair, the choice of the procedure is still surgeon dependent. Most surgeons favor the use of the anatomic procedure for primary repairs and use the allograft techniques for revision procedures or for patients with connective tissue disorders. Matheny and colleagues,[66] showed similar outcomes when comparing direct repair and anatomic reconstruction after 2 years. Therefore, given the variety in treatments and techniques, further studies are warranted to determine any long-term benefits of one technique compared with another.

Either direct repair or reconstruction of the lateral ligaments can be augmented with favorable results. Coughlin and colleagues[59] showed that a direct repair with a free gracilis tendon augmentation resulted in improved patient outcomes and excellent clinical and radiological stability at 2 years. In addition, the use of nonabsorbable suture tape to augment a direct repair has also been shown to be effective at treating CAI.[13,67] Furthermore, Xu and colleagues[68,69] showed that the use of suture tape to augment the Broström technique results in better outcomes, specifically talar tilt angle, compared with use of the Broström technique alone; however, this has not been a universal finding. In addition, Porter and colleagues[70] revealed in a recent randomized controlled trial that augmentation of a modified Broström-Gould with an extracapsular synthetic ligament showed improved FAOS scores and increased activity scores compared with treatment with repair alone.

However, an open Broström repair does not preclude an arthroscopy before addressing intra-articular disorders. Furthermore, most studies examining arthroscopic versus open Broström procedures show similar results in pain and function between the two procedures.[71–74] Zeng and colleagues[75] showed that using an arthroscopic technique resulted in longer procedure time and increased cost but a smaller scar compared with an open procedure. In addition, some investigators have stated that an arthroscopic procedure has a higher complication rate compared with an open procedure, such as superficial peroneal nerve entrapment with ATFL sutures.[76] A recent meta-analysis determined a statistically significant increase in American Orthopaedic Foot & Ankle Society (AOFAS) scores with an arthroscopic repair versus an open repair (92.2 vs 90.8); however, it remains unknown whether this difference is clinically significant.[77] Surgeon experience is paramount to the choice of the procedure because there is a higher learning curve with the arthroscopic techniques.

SUMMARY

CAI is a common outcome in patients who experience a lateral ankle sprain and can lead to significant debilitation through functional instability. Once conservative measures, including bracing and physical therapy, have failed, surgical methods have provided excellent long-term results. The gold-standard procedure is the anatomic repair, or the Broström, with or without modifications. The purpose of surgical intervention is not only to improve more immediate pain and stability but also to restore proper ankle biomechanics to prevent the onset of osteoarthritis. New methods have emerged incorporating arthroscopic techniques and the addition of various methods of augmentation; however, there do not seem to be significant advantages of these techniques based on comparative studies versus the gold standard.

ACKNOWLEDGMENTS

The authors graciously thank Dr Eric Giza (University of California Davis School of Medicine, Department of Orthopedic Surgery) and Dr Christopher Kreulen (University of California Davis School of Medicine, Department of Orthopedic Surgery) for their guidance and knowledge during the development of this article.

DISCLOSURE

M. Kelly is an AOFAS committee member.

REFERENCES

1. Lynch SA, Renstrom PA. Treatment of acute lateral ankle ligament rupture in the athlete. Conservative versus surgical treatment. Sports Med 1999;27(1):61–71.
2. van den Bekerom MP, Kerkhoffs GM, McCollum GA, et al. Management of acute lateral ankle ligament injury in the athlete. Knee Surg Sports Traumatol Arthrosc 2013;21(6):1390–5.
3. Araoye I, Pinter Z, Lee S, et al. Revisiting the prevalence of associated copathologies in chronic lateral ankle instability: are there any predictors of outcome? Foot Ankle Spec 2019;12(4):311–5.
4. Waterman BR, Owens BD, Davey S, et al. The epidemiology of ankle sprains in the United States. J Bone Joint Surg Am 2010;92(13):2279–84.
5. McKay GD, Goldie PA, Payne WR, et al. Ankle injuries in basketball: injury rate and risk factors. Br J Sports Med 2001;35(2):103–8.
6. Hertel J. Functional anatomy, pathomechanics, and pathophysiology of lateral ankle instability. J Athl Train 2002;37(4):364–75.
7. Guillo S, Bauer T, Lee JW, et al. Consensus in chronic ankle instability: aetiology, assessment, surgical indications and place for arthroscopy. Orthop Traumatol Surg Res 2013;99(8 Suppl):S411–9.
8. Clanton TO, Waldrop NE. Athletic injuries to the soft tissues of the foot and ankle. In: Coughlin MJ, editor. Mann's surgery of the foot and ankle, vol. 1. Philadelphia: Elsevier; 2014. p. 1531–689.
9. Vuurberg G, Hoorntje A, Wink LM, et al. Diagnosis, treatment and prevention of ankle sprains: update of an evidence-based clinical guideline. Br J Sports Med 2018;52(15):956.

10. Ajis A, Maffulli N. Conservative management of chronic ankle instability. Foot Ankle Clin 2006;11(3):531-7.

11. Clanton TO, Campbell KJ, Wilson KJ, et al. Qualitative and quantitative anatomic investigation of the lateral ankle ligaments for surgical reconstruction procedures. J Bone Joint Surg Am 2014;96(12):e98.

12. Milner CE, Soames RW. Anatomical variations of the anterior talofibular ligament of the human ankle joint. J Anat 1997;191(Pt 3):457-8.

13. Viens NA, Wijdicks CA, Campbell KJ, et al. Anterior talofibular ligament ruptures, part 1: biomechanical comparison of augmented Brostrom repair techniques with the intact anterior talofibular ligament. Am J Sports Med 2014;42(2):405-11.

14. Attarian DE, McCrackin HJ, Devito DP, et al. A biomechanical study of human lateral ankle ligaments and autogenous reconstructive grafts. Am J Sports Med 1985;13(6):377-81.

15. Porter DA, Kamman KA. Chronic lateral ankle instability: open surgical management. Foot Ankle Clin 2018;23(4):539-54.

16. Ashton-Miller JA, Ottaviani RA, Hutchinson C, et al. What best protects the inverted weightbearing ankle against further inversion? Evertor muscle strength compares favorably with shoe height, athletic tape, and three orthoses. Am J Sports Med 1996;24(6):800-9.

17. Delahunt E, Bleakley CM, Bossard DS, et al. Clinical assessment of acute lateral ankle sprain injuries (ROAST): 2019 consensus statement and recommendations of the International Ankle Consortium. Br J Sports Med 2018;52(20):1304-10.

18. Hershkovich O, Tenenbaum S, Gordon B, et al. A large-scale study on epidemiology and risk factors for chronic ankle instability in young adults. J Foot Ankle Surg 2015;54(2):183-7.

19. Lotito G, Pruvost J, Collado H, et al. Peroneus quartus and functional ankle instability. Ann Phys Rehabil Med 2011;54(5):282-92.

20. Lintz F, Bernasconi A, Baschet L, et al. Relationship between chronic lateral ankle instability and hindfoot varus using weight-bearing cone beam computed tomography. Foot Ankle Int 2019;40(10):1175-81.

21. O'Neill PJ, Parks BG, Walsh R, et al. Excursion and strain of the superficial peroneal nerve during inversion ankle sprain. J Bone Joint Surg Am 2007;89(5):979-86.

22. Arshad Z, Bhatia M. Current concepts in sinus tarsi syndrome: a scoping review. Foot Ankle Surg 2020.

23. Li SK, Song YJ, Li H, et al. Arthroscopic treatment combined with the ankle stabilization procedure is effective for sinus tarsi syndrome in patients with chronic ankle instability. Knee Surg Sports Traumatol Arthrosc 2018;26(10):3135-9.

24. Frey C, Feder KS, DiGiovanni C. Arthroscopic evaluation of the subtalar joint: does sinus tarsi syndrome exist? Foot Ankle Int 1999;20(3):185-91.

25. Jolman S, Robbins J, Lewis L, et al. Comparison of magnetic resonance imaging and stress radiographs in the evaluation of chronic lateral ankle instability. Foot Ankle Int 2017;38(4):397-404.

26. Oae K, Takao M, Uchio Y, et al. Evaluation of anterior talofibular ligament injury with stress radiography, ultrasonography and MR imaging. Skeletal Radiol 2010;39(1):41-7.

27. Cho JH, Lee DH, Song HK, et al. Value of stress ultrasound for the diagnosis of chronic ankle instability compared to manual anterior drawer test, stress radiography, magnetic resonance imaging, and arthroscopy. Knee Surg Sports Traumatol Arthrosc 2016;24(4):1022-8.

28. Hintermann B. Biomechanics of the unstable ankle joint and clinical implications. Med Sci Sports Exerc 1999;31(7 Suppl):S459–69.
29. Cao S, Wang C, Ma X, et al. Imaging diagnosis for chronic lateral ankle ligament injury: a systemic review with meta-analysis. J Orthop Surg Res 2018;13(1):122.
30. Singh K, Thukral CL, Gupta K, et al. Comparison of high resolution ultrasonography with clinical findings in patients with ankle pain. J Ultrason 2018;18(75): 316–24.
31. Petersen W, Rembitzki IV, Koppenburg AG, et al. Treatment of acute ankle ligament injuries: a systematic review. Arch Orthop Trauma Surg 2013;133(8): 1129–41.
32. Kerkhoffs GM, Tol JL. A twist on the athlete's ankle twist: some ankles are more equal than others. Br J Sports Med 2012;46(12):835–6.
33. Kerkhoffs GM, Handoll HH, de Bie R, et al. Surgical versus conservative treatment for acute injuries of the lateral ligament complex of the ankle in adults. Cochrane Database Syst Rev 2007;(2):CD000380.
34. Kerkhoffs GM, van den Bekerom M, Elders LA, et al. Diagnosis, treatment and prevention of ankle sprains: an evidence-based clinical guideline. Br J Sports Med 2012;46(12):854–60.
35. Song Y, Li H, Sun C, et al. Clinical guidelines for the surgical management of chronic lateral ankle instability: a consensus reached by systematic review of the available data. Orthop J Sports Med 2019;7(9). 2325967119873852.
36. van Rijn RM, van Os AG, Bernsen RM, et al. What is the clinical course of acute ankle sprains? A systematic literature review. Am J Med 2008;121(4):324–31.e6.
37. Guelfi M, Zamperetti M, Pantalone A, et al. Open and arthroscopic lateral ligament repair for treatment of chronic ankle instability: a systematic review. Foot Ankle Surg 2018;24(1):11–8.
38. Evans DL. Recurrent instability of the ankle; a method of surgical treatment. Proc R Soc Med 1953;46(5):343–4.
39. Krips R, Brandsson S, Swensson C, et al. Anatomical reconstruction and Evans tenodesis of the lateral ligaments of the ankle. Clinical and radiological findings after follow-up for 15 to 30 years. J Bone Joint Surg Br 2002;84(2):232–6.
40. Karlsson J, Bergsten T, Lansinger O, et al. Reconstruction of the lateral ligaments of the ankle for chronic lateral instability. J Bone Joint Surg Am 1988;70(4):581–8.
41. Gillespie HS, Boucher P. Watson-Jones repair of lateral instability of the ankle. J Bone Joint Surg Am 1971;53(5):920–4.
42. Hedeboe J, Johannsen A. Recurrent instability of the ankle joint. Surgical repair by the Watson-Jones method. Acta Orthop Scand 1979;50(3):337–40.
43. van der Rijt AJ, Evans GA. The long-term results of Watson-Jones tenodesis. J Bone Joint Surg Br 1984;66(3):371–5.
44. Chrisman OD, Snook GA. Reconstruction of lateral ligament tears of the ankle. An experimental study and clinical evaluation of seven patients treated by a new modification of the Elmslie procedure. J Bone Joint Surg Am 1969;51(5):904–12.
45. Hennrikus WL, Mapes RC, Lyons PM, et al. Outcomes of the Chrisman-Snook and modified-Brostrom procedures for chronic lateral ankle instability. A prospective, randomized comparison. Am J Sports Med 1996;24(4):400–4.
46. Acevedo JI, Myerson MS. Modification of the Chrisman-Snook technique. Foot Ankle Int 2000;21(2):154–5.
47. Kramer D, Solomon R, Curtis C, et al. Clinical results and functional evaluation of the Chrisman-Snook procedure for lateral ankle instability in athletes. Foot Ankle Spec 2011;4(1):18–28.

48. Forman ES, Micheli LJ, Backe LM. Chronic recurrent subluxation of the peroneal tendons in a pediatric patient. Surgical recommendations. Foot Ankle Int 2000; 21(1):51–3.
49. Yang J Jr, Morscher MA, Weiner DS. Modified Chrisman-Snook repair for the treatment of chronic ankle ligamentous instability in children and adolescents. J Child Orthop 2010;4(6):561–70.
50. Yasui Y, Shimozono Y, Kennedy JG. Surgical procedures for chronic lateral ankle instability. J Am Acad Orthop Surg 2018;26(7):223–30.
51. Brostrom L. Sprained ankles. VI. Surgical treatment of "chronic" ligament ruptures. Acta Chir Scand 1966;132(5):551–65.
52. Gould N, Seligson D, Gassman J. Early and late repair of lateral ligament of the ankle. Foot Ankle 1980;1(2):84–9.
53. Wainright WB, Spritzer CE, Lee JY, et al. The effect of modified Brostrom-Gould repair for lateral ankle instability on in vivo tibiotalar kinematics. Am J Sports Med 2012;40(9):2099–104.
54. Karlsson J, Eriksson BI, Bergsten T, et al. Comparison of two anatomic reconstructions for chronic lateral instability of the ankle joint. Am J Sports Med 1997;25(1):48–53.
55. Harrington KD. Degenerative arthritis of the ankle secondary to long-standing lateral ligament instability. J Bone Joint Surg Am 1979;61(3):354–61.
56. Bell SJ, Mologne TS, Sitler DF, et al. Twenty-six-year results after Brostrom procedure for chronic lateral ankle instability. Am J Sports Med 2006;34(6):975–8.
57. Roos EM, Brandsson S, Karlsson J. Validation of the foot and ankle outcome score for ankle ligament reconstruction. Foot Ankle Int 2001;22(10):788–94.
58. Tourne Y, Mabit C, Moroney PJ, et al. Long-term follow-up of lateral reconstruction with extensor retinaculum flap for chronic ankle instability. Foot Ankle Int 2012; 33(12):1079–86.
59. Coughlin MJ, Schenck RC Jr, Grebing BR, et al. Comprehensive reconstruction of the lateral ankle for chronic instability using a free gracilis graft. Foot Ankle Int 2004;25(4):231–41.
60. Elmslie RC. Recurrent subluxation of the ankle-joint. Ann Surg 1934;100(2): 364–7.
61. Anderson ME. Reconstruction of the lateral ligaments of the ankle using the plantaris tendon. J Bone Joint Surg Am 1985;67(6):930–4.
62. Takao M, Oae K, Uchio Y, et al. Anatomical reconstruction of the lateral ligaments of the ankle with a gracilis autograft: a new technique using an interference fit anchoring system. Am J Sports Med 2005;33(6):814–23.
63. Kennedy JG, Smyth NA, Fansa AM, et al. Anatomic lateral ligament reconstruction in the ankle: a hybrid technique in the athletic population. Am J Sports Med 2012;40(10):2309–17.
64. Hua Y, Chen S, Jin Y, et al. Anatomical reconstruction of the lateral ligaments of the ankle with semitendinosus allograft. Int Orthop 2012;36(10):2027–31.
65. Clanton TO, Viens NA, Campbell KJ, et al. Anterior talofibular ligament ruptures, part 2: biomechanical comparison of anterior talofibular ligament reconstruction using semitendinosus allografts with the intact ligament. Am J Sports Med 2014;42(2):412–6.
66. Matheny LM, Johnson NS, Liechti DJ, et al. Activity level and function after lateral ankle ligament repair versus reconstruction. Am J Sports Med 2016;44(5): 1301–8.
67. Cho BK, Park KJ, Kim SW, et al. Minimal invasive suture-tape augmentation for chronic ankle instability. Foot Ankle Int 2015;36(11):1330–8.

68. Xu DL, Gan KF, Li HJ, et al. Modified Brostrom repair with and without augmentation using suture tape for chronic lateral ankle instability. Orthop Surg 2019; 11(4):671–8.
69. Cho BK, Park JK, Choi SM, et al. A randomized comparison between lateral ligaments augmentation using suture-tape and modified Brostrom repair in young female patients with chronic ankle instability. Foot Ankle Surg 2019;25(2):137–42.
70. Porter M, Shadbolt B, Ye X, et al. Ankle lateral ligament augmentation versus the modified Brostrom-gould procedure: a 5-year randomized controlled trial. Am J Sports Med 2019;47(3):659–66.
71. Matsui K, Takao M, Miyamoto W, et al. Early recovery after arthroscopic repair compared to open repair of the anterior talofibular ligament for lateral instability of the ankle. Arch Orthop Trauma Surg 2016;136(1):93–100.
72. Yeo ED, Lee KT, Sung IH, et al. Comparison of all-inside arthroscopic and open techniques for the modified Brostrom procedure for ankle instability. Foot Ankle Int 2016;37(10):1037–45.
73. Li H, Hua Y, Li H, et al. Activity level and function 2 years after anterior talofibular ligament repair: a comparison between arthroscopic repair and open repair procedures. Am J Sports Med 2017;45(9):2044–51.
74. Rigby RB, Cottom JM. A comparison of the "All-Inside" arthroscopic Brostrom procedure with the traditional open modified Brostrom-Gould technique: a review of 62 patients. Foot Ankle Surg 2019;25(1):31–6.
75. Zeng G, Hu X, Liu W, et al. Open Brostrom-Gould repair vs arthroscopic anatomical repair of the anterior talofibular ligament for chronic lateral ankle instability [formula: see text]. Foot Ankle Int 2020;41(1):44–9.
76. Wang J, Hua Y, Chen S, et al. Arthroscopic repair of lateral ankle ligament complex by suture anchor. Arthroscopy 2014;30(6):766–73.
77. Brown AJ, Shimozono Y, Hurley ET, et al. Arthroscopic versus open repair of lateral ankle ligament for chronic lateral ankle instability: a meta-analysis. Knee Surg Sports Traumatol Arthrosc 2020;28(5):1611–8.

Indications and Surgical Treatment of Acute and Chronic Tibiofibular Syndesmotic Injuries with and Without Associated Fractures

Michael P. Swords, DO[a],*, John R. Shank, MD[b]

KEYWORDS

- Syndesmosis • Ankle fracture • Flexible fixation • Incisura • Ankle reconstruction

KEY POINTS

- Syndesmosis injuries may be subtle and require thorough assessment of injuries.
- Failure to reduce and stabilize syndesmotic injuries leads to worse functional outcomes.
- Flexible fixation may allow earlier return to activity but does not improve reduction.
- Fractures of the posterior malleolus, Chaput tubercle of the tibia, and fracture of the Wagstaffe tubercle of the fibula all may represent osseous equivalents to syndesmotic injury and should be recognized and treated with stable internal fixation.
- Anatomic reconstruction of all components of the ankle injury results in improved clinical outcomes in both early and late presentations of syndesmotic injuries.

INTRODUCTION

What Is the Syndesmosis?

The syndesmosis is the complex of osseous and ligamentous structures that maintain the relationship between the fibula and the tibia at the ankle level. The anterolateral (Chaput) tubercle of the tibia, anterior (Wagstaffe) tubercle of the fibula, and the incisura fibularis all contribute to the syndesmotic relationship. The incisura is not consistent in shape and may be either shallow or shallow concave.[1] The anterior inferior tibiofibular ligament (AITFL) originates from the anterolateral tubercle of the tibia (the Chaput tubercle) and attaches to the anterior tubercle of the fibula (Wagstaffe tubercle). The posterior inferior tibiofibular ligament (PITFL) extends from the posterior

---

[a] Michigan Orthopedic Center, 2815 Pennsylvania Avenue, Suite 204, Lansing, MI 48823, USA;
[b] Department of Orthopedic Surgery, Colorado Center of Orthopaedic Excellence, 2446 Research Parkway, Suite 200, Colorado Springs, CO 80920, USA
* Corresponding author.
E-mail address: foot.trauma@gmail.com

Foot Ankle Clin N Am 26 (2021) 103–119
https://doi.org/10.1016/j.fcl.2020.10.006
1083-7515/21/© 2020 Elsevier Inc. All rights reserved.

malleolus to attach along the posterior tubercle of the fibula. The interosseous membrane is located between the tibia and fibula and spans nearly the entire lower leg. The interosseous ligament (IOL) is found in the distal 1 cm of the lower leg and is contiguous with the interosseous membrane. As the number of ligaments that are ruptured increases, the ankle becomes increasingly less stable.[2] A recent study based on arthroscopic evaluation of ligament injury found that AITFL, IOL, and PITFL sectioning were required to create instability in the coronal plane.[3] In a study performed by section of specific ligaments, Ogilvie-Harris and colleagues[4] found that the AITFL provided 35%, the transverse tibiofibular ligament or deep portion of the PITFL 33%, the IOL 22%, and the PITFL 9% of the overall stability. A second sectioning study resulted in significant syndesmotic widening occurring only after the IOL was sectioned.[5]

Why Repair the Syndesmosis?

Patients with isolated malleolar fractures with syndesmotic injury have been reported to have worse functional outcomes (Short Musculoskeletal Function Assessment [SMFA]) at 1 year than patients who had a malleolar fracture without syndesmotic injury.[6] Sagi and colleagues[7] reported worse outcomes at 2 years on both the SMFA and Olerud-Molander ankle score in patients with syndesmotic malreduction, as confirmed by computed tomography (CT) than in patients with an anatomic reduction. Weening and Bhondari[8] have shown that improved SMFA and Olerud-Molander scores were predicted by anatomic reduction of the syndesmosis on radiographic assessment. Small amounts of deformity can lead to significant problems with ankle function.

Biomechanical studies have shown that lateral translation of 1 mm to 2 mm, shortening of 2 mm or more, and external rotation of 5° may result in altered pressure distribution.[9–11] Reconstruction is recommended when syndesmotic rupture is identified in both acute and chronic settings to prevent progression of arthritis and disability. In a successive series of patients undergoing ankle arthrodesis at a tertiary center, 20.3% of patients demonstrated widening of the ankle mortise.[12] Because of the high likelihood of the development of posttraumatic arthritis or malalignment, chronic rupture of the syndesmosis should be identified and addressed to prevent long-term pain, disability, and progression of arthritis.

Acute Syndesmotic Injury

Acute injuries to the syndesmosis may occur as a result of a wide variety of injuries to the lower extremity. Some syndesmotic injuries are obvious, but many are subtle and require due diligence to diagnose the injury accurately. A trial of weight bearing for 7 days to 10 days may reveal instability on follow-up radiographs in cases without associated fracture. In the setting of a fracture to the proximal fibula, tenderness about the distal leg or medial malleolus may indicate a Maisonneuve equivalent injury and warrants further evaluation. Surgical treatment is indicated for all unstable ankle fracture patterns, including trimalleolar, bimalleolar, and unstable lateral malleolar fractures. All operative ankle fractures should be evaluated for associated syndesmosis instability regardless of fracture pattern. Syndesmotic instability is a surgical indication independent of fracture type and may occur in the absence of fracture. High fibula fractures commonly are associated with syndesmotic injury. Although standard treatment principles for ankle fractures require an evaluation of the stability of the syndesmosis in all operatively treated ankle fractures, it is important to recognize other injuries around the ankle may result in syndesmosis disruption. Although rare, syndesmotic injury also may occur in the setting of distal tibia fractures, pilon fractures, talus fractures, and hindfoot injuries with associated dislocation. Careful evaluation of the stability of the syndesmosis should be performed during surgery once fixation of these injuries has been achieved.

Athletic injuries involving the syndesmosis are common. Careful palpation of the syndesmosis and proximal fibula are critical, both on the field and in the clinic, to evaluate for syndesmotic injury. External rotation stress tests can reproduce syndesmotic pain on the field and can be indicative of syndesmotic injury. Bilateral weight-bearing radiographs of the ankle and full-length tibial radiographs are critical in evaluating for syndesmotic injury and are important in ruling out proximal fibula fracture. Stress radiographs can be limited in determining syndesmotic instability secondary to patient guarding. A comparison radiograph of the patient's contralateral ankle is critical in assessing normal radiographic landmarks. For patients without fracture, both magnetic resonance imaging and bilateral CT scans of the ankle are important in gathering data related to ligamentous injury and instability. Syndesmotic sprains, without fracture and with no radiographic instability, generally can be managed nonoperatively with a controlled ankle motion walker and crutches for approximately 6 weeks or until pain symptoms improve. Athletes that have fractures of the proximal fibula and concomitant syndesmotic injuries and syndesmotic injuries with instability by stress test or radiographically should be considered for acute operative syndesmotic stabilization with no return to play for 3 months.

HOW TO ASSESS REDUCTION OF THE SYNDESMOSIS INTRAOPERATIVELY?

Unacceptably high rates of syndesmotic malreduction continue to be reported, regardless of fixation method, with malreduction rates of 0% to 16% reported from review of postoperative radiographs.[8,13–16] Malreduction increases to 22% to 52% with the use of postoperative CT evaluation.[7,17–27] Although most surgeons agree direct reduction of the syndesmosis is necessary, there is poor understanding of how to perform a direct reduction. Reducing the fibula into the incisura may be inaccurate because the incisura is variable in morphology, the distance from the fibula to the incisura of the tibia is greater, and the fit is less predictable moving proximal away from the ankle joint. Two studies suggest individual incisura anatomy may contribute to malreduction.[28,29] Deep and disengaged syndesmoses were more likely to be malreduced by overcompression whereas anteversion and retroversion were associated with anterior and posterior malreductions, respectively.[29]

Generally, all fracture components are reduced and stabilized. The syndesmosis then is evaluated. The tissues often look traumatized and hemorrhagic. Occasionally fracture debris is present in the incisura and needs to be removed prior to any attempt at reduction. Instability may be present by widening in the coronal plane or result in posterior or anterior translation in the sagittal plane. After the syndesmosis is cleared the fibula is reduced by direct reduction. In most Weber B fractures, simply dissecting along the fracture line to the anterior aspect of the fibula leads to the incisura, allowing direct evaluation.

Direct assessment of reduction should be performed just above the level of the ankle joint. In most individuals, there are corresponding small articular facets on the lateral aspect of the tibia and medial aspect of the fibula, which should be congruent after reduction (**Fig. 1**).

A tine of a reduction clamp is placed low and in the midline of the medial malleolus. The reduction is performed manually, with direct visualization of the reduction at the incisura just above the ankle joint. The reduction is maintained by placing the other tine of the reduction clamp on the tip of the lateral malleolus. With the clamp applied

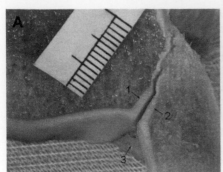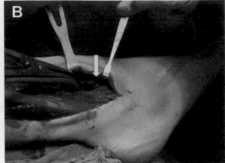

Fig. 1. (A) Direct assessment of reduction should be performed just above the ankle joint. There are corresponding small cartilage facets at the syndesmosis on the tibia (1) and fibula (2). The confluence below the articulation contains posterior aspect of inferior part of anterior tibiofibular ligament (3). (B) Clinical example of the visible articular facet of the tibia used for direct reduction of the syndesmosis. The arrow (*yellow*) points to the articular facet of the tibia. (*Courtesy of* [A] J. Bartoníček, MD, Prague, Czech Republic.)

from the tip of the lateral malleolus to the tip of the medial malleolus, it is in line with the transmalleolar axis, reducing the risk of a sagittal plane mal reduction. The clamp is tightened only to the point it maintains the reduction. The purpose of the clamp is to hold the reduction, not to achieve the reduction. If the clamp is placed higher up on the fibula, over-tightening can result in plastic deformation of the fibula or sagittal malalignment of the fibula in the incisura. A Kirschner (K)-wire then is inserted from the fibula to the tibia above the anticipated level of syndesmotic fixation. This second point prevents the introduction of rotational malalignment with hardware insertion. If a posterior antiglide fibula plate is used for fixation of the fibula fracture, syndesmotic devices may be placed outside of the plate. If the fibula was plated laterally, fixation devices should be placed through the plate.

In athletes, syndesmotic fixation should be placed through a plate. Bicortical fibula screws are placed in the near and far ends of the plate. If, ultimately, the syndesmotic fixation proves bothersome, the plate can be left in when the syndesmotic fixation is removed. The plate provides a stress shield of the holes from where the syndesmotic fixation was removed, allowing return to sport without delay. The plate greatly decreases the risk of fracture occurring at the screw holes in the fibula with early return to sport. In the general population, syndesmotic fixation may be placed either through a plate or independently because there is less demand on a prompt return to sporting activities, reducing the risk of fracture through residual screw holes in the fibula after hardware removal.

MANAGEMENT CONSIDERATIONS IN PROXIMAL FIBULA FRACTURES

Standard treatment of ankle fractures includes reduction and stabilization of all fracture components to restore normal anatomy. This includes establishing correct length, alignment, and rotation of the fibula. The role of reduction of displaced or unstable fracture of the lateral malleolus is well understood and without controversy. Fracture reduction must be performed before assessing the stability of the syndesmosis. Maisonneuve fracture patterns are variable and associated with a posterior malleolus fracture in 80% of cases, medial malleolus fracture in 37% of cases, and a wide variety of displacement patterns at the syndesmosis.[30]

There is significant variation in clinical practice in management of proximal or high fibula fractures and no clear guidelines for treatment.

Ultimately, the goal of treatment of all ankle injuries is restoration of normal anatomy, which, in turn, increases the likelihood of an improved functional outcome. Fibular length is an essential component. Therefore, reduction is necessary of proximal fibula fractures that adversely affect any component of fibular alignment including length, alignment, and rotation.

FIXATION OF LENGTH STABLE PROXIMAL FIBULA FRACTURE PATTERNS
Treatment Considerations

More proximal fractures with length stable patterns may be treated with intramedullary internal fixation. Patterns that are transverse, chevron, or very short oblique fracture patterns are amenable to intramedullary fixation because they are inherently length stable. With relatively simple proximal fibula fractures, reduction clamps are maintained while the syndesmosis is reduced. Provisional fixation consists of both a clamp and a K-wire. A clamp is placed from the tip of the lateral malleolus to the tip of the medial malleolus, paralleling the intermalleolus axis. A K-wire is inserted from the fibula to the tibia to maintain reduction and serve as a second point of fixation, preventing the introduction of rotational or translation deformity when fixation is inserted.

Recommended Fixation Type for Syndesmosis in Length Stable Proximal Fibula Fracture Patterns

Either screws or flexible fixation devices may be used for length stable patterns.

FIXATION OF LENGTH UNSTABLE PROXIMAL FIBULA FRACTURE PATTERNS
Treatment Considerations and Surgical Approach

Comminuted or oblique proximal fibula fractures require the length of the fibula to be restored as part of the surgical reconstruction of the syndesmosis (**Fig. 2**). Accurate length of the fibula may be achieved by direct reduction. Dissection is carried through the skin in line with the fibula. Dissection is carried through the lateral compartment and the peroneal musculature is retracted anteriorly. The superficial peroneal, or, if very proximal, the common peroneal nerve needs to be identified and protected. The fracture is reduced by standard AO reduction techniques.

Flexible syndesmotic fixation is not recommended to treat length unstable patterns without rigid fixation of the fibula fracture. Highly comminuted and length unstable patterns benefit from plate fixation prior to syndesmosis repair. Although locking intramedullary fibular devices are commercially available, many proximal fractures are beyond the working length of these devices making plate fixation necessary. Plate choices include 3.5-mm plates or one-third tubular plates. After length, alignment, and rotation of the fibula have been restored, appropriate syndesmotic relationships are easier to establish. The dissection may be carried distally either by continuing the dissection behind the peroneal musculature to the posterolateral surface of the distal fibula or by dissecting anteriorly to the peroneals in the distal quarter of the fibula to allow access to the lateral surface of the fibula. Dissection anterior to the peroneals allows much easier access to the incisura and allows direct visualization for the reduction of the syndesmotic relationship.

Recommended Fixation Type for Syndesmosis in Length Unstable Patterns

If the fibula is reduced and plated proximally, either screws or flexible fixation may be used.

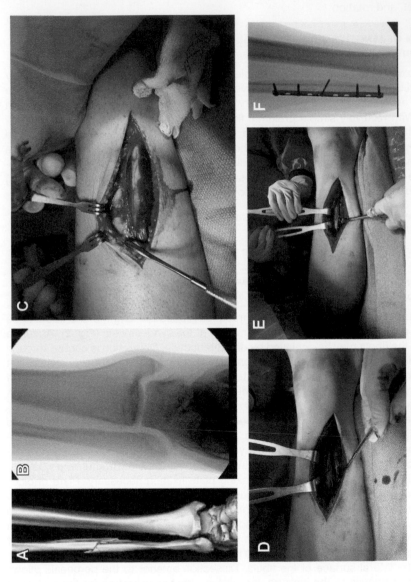

Fig. 2. (*A*) CT and (*B*) mortise radiograph demonstrate a syndesmotic injury with an associated high fibula fracture in a college football player. (*C*) Care must be taken to identify the superficial peroneal nerve during dissection (visible at the tip of the elevator). (*D*) The displaced fibula fracture is seen. (*E*) Clinical and (*F*) radiographic images show anatomic reduction of the fracture with plate fixation.

If the proximal fracture is reduced, but not plated, syndesmosis fixation must consist of rigid screw fixation because use of flexible fixation may result in late displacement or shortening (**Fig. 3**). Hybrid fixation techniques including flexible fixation and a syndesmotic screw have been described for treatment of length unstable Weber C fractures.[31]

Tips for Improving Reduction Accuracy

1. Anatomic reduction is mandatory for all fracture components.
2. Remove debris from syndesmotic region.
3. Align the lateral facet of the tibia to the medial facet of the fibula just above the ankle level.
4. After reduction, 2 provisional points of fixation are necessary until syndesmotic fixation is achieved.

Osseus Causes of Syndesmosis Instability

1. Fracture of the posterior malleolus
2. Fracture of the Chaput tubercle of the tibia
3. Fracture of the Wagstaffe tubercle of the distal fibula

Injury to the syndesmosis may result from fracture of the osseus attachment sites of the various syndesmotic ligaments. These injuries may be posterior or anterior injuries. Preoperative CT scan is helpful in both identifying these injuries and planning surgical management.[32] Fixation of these specific fracture components re-establishes stability to the syndesmosis and as a result traditional syndesmotic fixation is not necessary. This group of fractures includes the following.

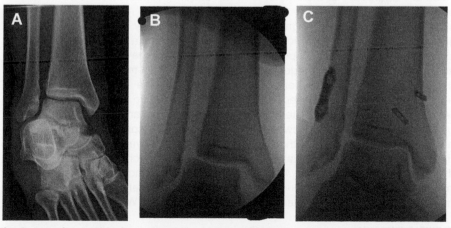

Fig. 3. Length unstable fractures of the proximal fibula must be reduced and stabilized if flexible fixation is going to be used. Use of flexible fixation does not restore or maintain length. This is a clinical example of (*A*) injury radiograph, (*B*), stress radiograph, and (*C*) Post fixation radiograph of a high school athlete with a proximal fibula fracture and syndesmotic injury that has been fixed with flexible fixation while the fibula was not reduced or length stable resulting in malalignment due to the fibula length and rotation not being restored prior to syndesmotic fixation.

FRACTURE OF THE POSTERIOR MALLEOLUS

Fractures of the posterior malleolus have received a significant amount of attention in recent years. Direct reduction of posterior malleolar fractures and internal fixation and are commonly known to play a significant role in re-establishing syndesmotic stability.[33] Lag screw fixation from posterior to anterior is reserved for small fragments. Larger fragments should be treated with plate fixation, often a one-third tubular antiglide plate, after direct reduction. Lag screws are biomechanically inferior to plate fixation for fixation of posterior malleolus fractures.[34]

FRACTURE OF THE CHAPUT TUBERCLE OF THE TIBIA

Fracture of the Chaput tubercle of the tibia results in failure and of the anterior portion of the syndesmosis. This fragment, variable in size, represents an avulsion of the tibial attachment of the syndesmosis (AITFL) and requires fixation. These injuries may be seen in isolation or as a component of a more complex injury. When present, it is necessary to address this injury with direct reduction and fixation. Displacement of this fracture alters the shape of the incisura and may block reduction. This generally is performed using a small anterolateral approach. During the dissection, care is taken to identify and prevent injury to the superficial peroneal nerve. The fragment is reduced and held provisionally with K-wires. A mini–fragment plate then is placed over the wires. The wires then are removed sequentially and replaced by lag screws inserted through the plate to achieve necessary fixation. This fracture may be seen as an isolated injury or part of a more complex ankle injury (**Fig. 4**).

FRACTURE OF THE WAGSTAFFE TUBERCLE OF THE FIBULA

The fracture of the Wagstaffe tubercle of the fibula, when present, often is unrecognized and considered comminution of the fibula fracture. A fracture of the Wagstaffe tubercle represents avulsion of the fibular attachment of the AITFL and must be recognized and addressed at the time of fixation. Anatomic reduction restores the appropriate tension and stability to the syndesmotic ligaments, resulting in syndesmotic stability. Additionally, this fragment may be pulled medially by the AITFL and block standard syndesmotic reduction techniques. After the fibula fracture is reduced and stabilized, typically with a posterior antiglide plate, the Wagstaffe tubercle is addressed. The fracture is reduced and held with K-wires from anterior to posterior through the fibula. If the bone density is poor or the fragment is small and fragile, sutures may be placed in the AITFL and used to aid in reduction. Once reduced, a mini–fragment plate then is slid over the wires and then used for fixation of the fibula. Appropriate screw length results in stable bicortical fixation. Caution is necessary, because screws that are excessively long have the potential to irritate the peroneal tendons. This fixation secures the fibular attachment of the AITFL and, if the fracture is large, the IOL. After fixation is complete, syndesmosis stability should be assessed. Similar to posterior malleolus fractures, typically no additional syndesmotic fixation is necessary after appropriate fixation of the Wagstaffe fracture.

FLEXIBLE FIXATION

There is a growing trend toward flexible fixation of acute syndesmotic disruptions, particularly in the athletic population. This method of treatment potentially lowers the risk of second operation for hardware removal and potentially may lead to earlier return to sport.[35,36] A recent meta-analysis found the functional outcome and complications similar between screws and flexible fixation but flexible fixation might lead to

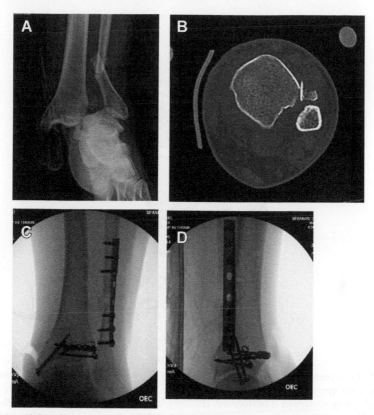

Fig. 4. Injury (*A*) radiograph and (*B*) CT of a trimalleolar equivalent injury with associated fracture of the Chaput tubercle, resulting in anterior osseus instability of the syndesmosis. Post operative (*C*) mortise and (*D*) lateral radiographs. (*C, D*) The patient was treated with direct reduction of all components of the fracture, including direct reduction and plate fixation of the Chaput component. No additionally syndesmotic fixation was necessary.

an earlier return to work.[37] A second meta-analysis found improved functional outcomes and lower rate of syndesmosis malreduction,[38] although a third meta-analysis found a lower rate of implant removal but no discernible difference between the flexible or screw fixation.[39]

Although both screw and flexible fixation both are viable treatment options, flexible fixation may more closely reproduce native ankle mechanics.[40] Flexible fixation alone, however, may not restore rotational stability to the ankle and sagittal plane stability of the fibula.[41,42] A recent prospective randomized trial demonstrated improved functional outcomes and lower reported pain as reported on the visual analog scale.[43] Flexible fixation still requires an accurate reduction as part of successful management. A fixation device is not a reliable method of obtaining an accurate reduction.

The principles and steps of fixation are the same regardless of fixation type and include the following (**Fig. 5**):

1. Restore fibular length and reduce any fibula fracture in anatomic fashion in a length stable fashion.
2. Perform fixation of malleolar fractures, including posterior malleolus.

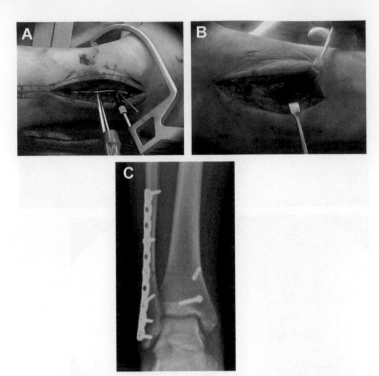

Fig. 5. (A) An intraoperative image demonstrating all fracture components have been sta-bilized and the syndesmosis is reduced and held with both a clamp and wire while flexible fixation of the syndesmosis is performed. (B) The placement of the medial button should be performed in open fashion to prevent injury to medial structures. (C) The final postoperative radiograph demonstrates proper reduction and all ankle landmarks restored with a flexible fixation device used for the syndesmosis.

3. Perform fixation of Chaput or Wagstaffe fractures.
4. Reduce the syndesmosis.
5. Confirm reduction of the syndesmosis.
6. Perform syndesmotic fixation if necessary.

CHRONIC SYNDESMOTIC RUPTURE

Chronic syndesmotic rupture or malreduction must be considered when persistent pain is present after an ankle injury. Weight-bearing ankle radiographs, including ante-roposterior, lateral, and mortise views, are essential. Comparison views of the contra-lateral side may increase the likelihood of noticing subtle malalignment. Ultimately, CT allows the most accurate method of assessment in the chronic setting. In addition to evaluating the syndesmosis, CT is helpful in assessing the presence or absence of osteophytes, malunion of ankle fracture, and posttraumatic arthritic changes. The goal is to provide treatment before significant ankle arthritis is present.

A variety of scenarios may be the cause of chronic syndesmotic rupture, including

1. Malunion of ankle fracture
2. Missed syndesmotic ligament injury
3. Malreduction at the time of fracture fixation

4. Loss of syndesmosis fixation before adequate healing

MALUNION OF THE INITIAL ANKLE FRACTURE

Malunion of the initial ankle fracture injury may result in syndesmotic malalignment. Angular deformities tend to be easiest to correct, whereas rotation deformities are the most difficult. Rotational deformity is difficult to assess using standard fluoroscopy and requires direct visualization of the corresponding articular surfaces of the lateral shoulder of the talus and the distal tibia to best evaluate rotation.[44] Closing wedge osteotomies typically are avoided, because they may result in shortening. Oblique osteotomies may restore length, alignment, and rotation through a single cut if made in the correct plane.[45] Obtaining length may be challenging. Small distractors, specific instrumentation, and/or use of a push screw technique all may aid in gaining length of the fibula. For the push screw technique, a plate is secured to the distal segment of the fibula fracture. A bicortical drill hole is made 3 mm to 4 mm proximal to the plate. The depth is measured with a measuring device; 6 mm is added to the measurement to allow the screw to remain prominent on the near cortex. A lamina spreader then is used to push the screw and plate apart, increasing the length of the fibula. Once appropriate length is achieved, the proximal end of the plate is secured to the fibula.

If using a push screw, it must be bicortical to avoid a fracture from occurring because force is generated when the lamina spreader is opened between the screw and the end of the plate. Regardless of which technique is used to obtain length, it is important to avoid introducing angular deformity as lengthening occurs. The fibula is a straight bone and should appear straight on both anteroposterior and lateral views.

MISSED SYNDESMOTIC LIGAMENT INJURY

Syndesmotic rupture may be subtle and may not be recognized or treated at the time of injury. Sagittal and rotational deformities may not result in widening of the medial clear space and may be difficult to recognize on standard radiographs. Films of the contralateral ankle may identify some small deformities as a result of missed syndesmotic rupture. A CT scan of both ankles is most effective for identifying deformity from missed syndesmotic injury and should be ordered when there is concern that a syndesmotic injury may have been missed. Magnetic resonance imaging is more effective in the acute setting and is less helpful in evaluation of late presentation of missed syndesmotic injury.

MALREDUCTION AT THE TIME OF THE SYNDESMOTIC FIXATION

Even when recognized and treated carefully, malreduction may occur. Postoperative CT scans should be used to ensure appropriate reduction, if uncertain. Intraoperative CT may aid in intraoperative reduction but is not available in most centers.

LOSS OF SYNDESMOTIC FIXATION BEFORE ADEQUATE HEALING

There is no postoperative test to determine if the syndesmosis is adequately healed. Loss of fixation may occur prior to the syndesmosis healing enough to provide necessary stability. This may occur from the hardware breaking or loosening over time. In the author's experience, the most common reason for loss of fixation before adequate healing is due to routine removal of syndesmotic screws. Flexible fixation lessens this risk, because typically it is not removed. Hybrid fixation concepts (screw fixation plus flexible fixation) are gaining popularity because they decrease the likelihood of this occurring, because a flexible device still is present after the screw is removed. This, however, increases the cost of treatment by potential additional surgery to remove the screw coupled with a higher implant cost of the flexible fixation device.

LATE RECONSTRUCTION OF THE SYNDESMOSIS-SURGICAL TECHNIQUE

Numerous techniques have been described for repair of chronic syndesmotic rupture. All techniques involve débridement of the syndesmosis of scar tissue to allow reduction. This débridement generally is done in an open fashion but may be done arthroscopically.[46] The literature consists of case reports and small series. Techniques range from arthrodesis of the syndesmosis,[47–51] to screw fixation after reduction,[48,52–54] and to ligamentous reconstruction.[55,56] Additionally, late reconstruction at the time of ankle arthroplasty has been described.[57] Generally, all series report good results and improvement regardless of the technique used.

A majority of late reconstruction cases are performed with the patient in the supine position. Rarely, a posterior approach to the syndesmosis is required if the preoperative CT scan demonstrates significant posterior fragments that are not be able to be removed from an anterior or lateral approach. The leg is elevated on a positioning pillow to facilitate intraoperative imaging. A bump is placed under the ipsilateral hip. If preexisting syndesmotic or fibular fixation is present, it is removed. Care is taken to look for, and protect, the superficial peroneal nerve, because the position of the nerve is variable.

Any malunion or nonunion present must be addressed, corrected, and stabilized. Dissection is carried over the front of the fibula. The syndesmotic region often is full of scar tissue and may require débridement over approximately the distal 6 cm to 8 cm. Initially, dissection occurs over the fibula anteriorly and scar tissue is removed, allowing the placement of a lamina spreader approximately in the incisura roughly 5 cm to 6 cm above the ankle joint. After the lamina spreader is placed, débridement continues distally toward the distal tibiofibular articulation. The lamina spreader gradually is moved distally to assist with the exposure as scar tissue is removed. Posttraumatic ossification of the syndesmotic region or bone fragments from the initial injury may be present and, if so, must be removed. Occasionally, the incision may need to be lengthened distally to remove any osteophytes present at the anterior ankle level extending off the anterolateral aspect of the tibia or off the fibula.

Osteophyte formation is common in the late reconstruction setting. Osteophytes may be present on the distal tibia, distal fibula, or both. The presence and location of osteophytes are determined from the preoperative CT scan. Osteophytes may be present posteriorly or anteriorly on either the distal fibula or tibia in sagittal plant malreductions and must be removed.

The incisura is débrided carefully all the way down to the ankle joint until the articular cartilage of the talar dome is visible when looking distally between the fibula and tibia. A pituitary rongeur is helpful for this portion of the procedure. A C-arm may be used because the débridement of the syndesmotic region approaches the ankle joint to prevent accidental injury to the talar articular cartilage.

After the syndesmotic region is clear of all impediments for reduction, the ankle joint is addressed. This may be done using a small ankle arthrotomy or by arthroscopy. Soft tissue and chronic scar are removed globally from the ankle and with specific attention to removing any soft tissue in the medial gutter, which blocks reduction. Any osteophytes or loose ossific debris is removed.

The fibula is reduced back into the incisura. This is done with direct visualization and generally can be performed with manual pressure. A pointed reduction clamp then is placed from the tip of the lateral malleolus to the tip of the medial malleolus, recreating the transmalleolar axis, taking care not to over-reduce the syndesmosis. Over-reduction may occur if the clamp is placed above the level of the syndesmosis, resulting in deformation of the fibula as the clamp is tightened. The purpose of the clamp is to hold the reduction, not to achieve the reduction. The pressure applied to the clamp is only what is necessary to maintain the reduction. A

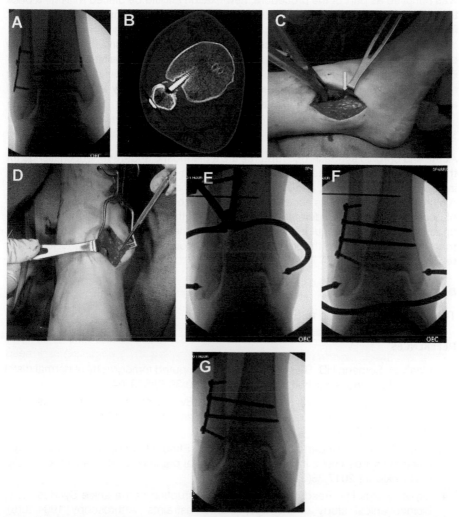

Fig. 6. (*A*) Mortise and (*B*) CT images demonstrating anterior malreduction and fixation failure with screw and flexible fixation construct. (*C*) The incisura is cleaned of debris until the articular cartilage of the talus is visible (*yellow arrow*). (*D*)The medial gutter then is cleaned of all scar and debris. (*F*) The syndesmosis then is reduced and held with a clamp and K-wire while (*E*) fixation is inserted. (*G*) The plate provides stress shielding from the holes from the old fixation and would allow the syndesmotic fixation to be removed without significant time away from sport by retaining the plate.

K-wire then is placed above the level of anticipated syndesmotic fixation to prevent introduction of rotational deformity at the time of implant insertion.

Before implant insertion, reduction is confirmed visually by looking at the relationship between the fibula and tibia. The mortise view is reviewed, and a lateral view may be obtained and compared with the contralateral ankle to help evaluate the fibular position in the sagittal plane by assessing the distance from the posterior cortex of the fibula to the posterior cortex of the fibula. Fixation generally consists of two 4.0-mm cortical screws through all 4 cortices inserted through a one-third tubular plate. Screw trajectory should parallel transmalleolar axis of the reduction clamp. If old hardware was removed as part of the procedure, new fixation should be placed through a plate to avoid loss of fixation or fracture from occurring through the holes in the fibula left from prior fixation devices (**Fig. 6**).

Postoperatively, patients are placed in a splint for 2 weeks and then in a fracture boot for the remainder of treatment. Non–weight bearing generally is maintained for 6 weeks. Flexible fixation devices and screws can be left in indefinitely and are removed only if the hardware proves symptomatic and typically after a minimum of a 6 months. The hardware is maintained in most patients.

SUMMARY

Acute and chronic syndesmotic ruptures are a diagnostic and treatment challenge for the surgeon. These injuries may present in isolation or as components of a multipart injury. Presentations vary, adding to the difficulty of arriving at an accurate diagnosis. A high index of suspicion is necessary. Treatment in both acute and chronic ruptures is of benefit and requires understanding of all contributing factors. Although debate continues on which of the multiple treatment approaches to treat these injuries is best, there is clear consensus that the best clinical outcomes are achieved with anatomic reconstruction.[8,58–60]

DISCLOSURE

The authors have nothing to disclose.

REFERENCES

1. Elgafy H, Semann HB, Blessinger B, et al. Computed tomography of normal distal tibiofibular Syndesmosis. Skeletal Radiol 2010;39(6):559–64.
2. Xenos JS, Hopkinson WJ, Mulligan ME, et al. Evaluation of the ligamentous structures, methods of fixation, and radiographic assessment. J Bone Joint Surg Am 1995;77(6):847–56.
3. Massri-Pugin J, Lubberts B, Vopat BG, et al. Effect of sequential section of ligaments on syndesmotic instability in the coronal plane evaluated arthroscopically. Foot Ankle Int 2017;38(12):1387–93.
4. Ogilvie-Harris DJ, Reed SC, Hedman TP. Disruption of the ankle Syndesmosis: biomechanical study of the ligamentous restraints. Arthroscopy 1994;10(5): 558–60.
5. Bachmann L, Seifert C, Zwipp H. Experimental and clinical diagnosis of ankle injuries with the Syndesmosis spreader. In: Schmidt R, Benesch S, Lipke K, editors. Chronic ankle instability. Ulm (Germany): Libri; 2000. p. 235–8.
6. Egol KA, Pahk B, Walsh M, et al. Outcome after unstable ankle fracture: effect of Syndesmosis stabilization. J Orthop Trauma 2010;24(1):7–11.

7. Sagi HC, Shah AR, Sanders RW. The functional consequence of Syndesmotic joint malreduction at a minimum 2-year follow-up. J Orthop Trauma 2012;26(7): 439–43.

8. Weening B, Bhondari M. Predictors of functional outcome following transsyndes-motic screw fixation of ankle fractures. J Orthop Trauma 2005;(2):102.

9. Ramsey PL, Hamilton W. Changes in the tibiotalar area of contact caused by lateral talar shift. J Bone Joint Surg Am 1976;58:356–7.

10. Zindrick MR, Hopkins DE, Knight GW, et al. The effect of lateral talar shift upon the biomechanics of the ankle joint. Orthop Trans 1985;9:332–3.

11. Thordarson DB, Motamed S, Hedman T, et al. The effect of fibular malreduction on contact pressures in an ankle fracture malunion model. J Bone Joint Surg Am 1997;79(12):1809–15.

12. Grass R, Herzmann K, Biewener A, et al. Injuries of the distal tibiofibular Syndes-mosis. Unfallchirurg 2000;103:520–32 [in German]. 125–9.

13. Yamaguchi K, Martin CH, Boden SD, et al. Operative treatment of syndesmotic disruptions without use of a syndesmotic screw: a prospective clinical study. Foot Ankle Int 1994;15(8):407–14.

14. Hovis WD, Kaiser BW, Watson JT, et al. Treatment of syndesmotic disruptions of the ankle with bioabsorbable screw fixation. J Bone Joint Surg Am 2002;84-A(1): 26–31.

15. Joy G, Patzakis MJ, Harvey JP Jr. Precise evaluation of the reduction of severe ankle fractures. J Bone Joint Surg Am 1974;56(5):979–93.

16. Matuszewski PE, Dombroski D, Lawrence JTR, et al. Prospective intraoperative syndesmotic evaluation during ankle fracture fixation: stress external rotation versus lateral fibular stress. J Orthop Trauma 2015;29(4):e157–60.

17. Berkes MB, Little MTM, Lazaro LE, et al. Articular congruity is associated with short-term clinical outcomes of operatively treated SER IV ankle fractures. J Bone Joint Surg Am 2013;95(19):1769–75.

18. Franke J, von Recum J, Suda AJ, et al. Intraoperative three-dimensional imaging in the treatment of acute unstable syndesmotic injuries. J Bone Joint Surg Am 2012;94(15):1386–90.

19. Gardner MJ, Demetrakopoulos D, Briggs SM, et al. Malreduction of the tibiofibu-lar syndesmosis in ankle fractures. Foot Ankle Int 2006;27(10):788–92.

20. Rammelt S, Zwipp H, Grass R. Injuries to the distal tibiofibular syndesmosis: an evidence- based approach to acute and chronic lesions [vii-viii.]. Foot Ankle Clin 2008;13(4):611–33, vii-viii.

21. Vasarhelyi A, Lubitz J, Gierer P, et al. Detection of fibular torsional deformities af-ter surgery for ankle fractures with a novel CT method. Foot Ankle Int 2006;27(12): 1115–21.

22. Drijfhout van Hooff CC, Verhage SM, Hoogendoorn JM. Influence of fragment size and postoperative joint congruency on long- term outcome of posterior malleolar fractures. Foot Ankle Int 2015;36(6):673–8.

23. Marmor M, Hansen E, Han HK, et al. Limitations of standard fluoroscopy in de-tecting rotational malreduction of the syndesmosis in an ankle fracture model. Foot Ankle Int 2011;32(6):616–22.

24. Miller AN, Carroll EA, Parker RJ, et al. Direct visualization for syndesmotic stabi-lization of ankle fractures. Foot Ankle Int 2009;30(5):419–26.

25. Ruan Z, Luo C, Shi Z, et al. Intraoperative reduction of distal tibiofibular joint aided by three-dimensional fluoroscopy. Technol Health Care 2011;19(3):161–6.

26. Song DJ, Lanzi JT, Groth AT, et al. The effect of syndesmosis screw removal on the reduction of the distal tibiofibular joint: a prospective radiographic study. Foot Ankle Int 2014;35(6):543–8.

27. Garner MR, Fabricant PD, Schottel PC, et al. Standard perioperative imaging modalities are unreliable in assessing articular congruity of ankle fractures. J Orthop Trauma 2015;29(4):e161–5.

28. Cherney SM, Spraggs-Hughes AG, McAndrew CM, et al. Incisura morphology as a risk factor for syndesmotic malreduction. Foot Ankle Int 2016;37(7):748–54.

29. Boszczyk A, Kwapisz S, Krümmel M, et al. Correlation of incisura anatomy with syndesmotic malreduction. Foot Ankle Int 2018;39(3):369–75.

30. Bartonicek J, Rammelt S, Kasper S, et al. Pathoanatomy of Maisonneuve fracture based on radiologic and CT examination. Arch Orthop Trauma Surg 2019;139(4):497–506.

31. Riedel MD, Miller CP, Kwon JY. Augmenting suture-button fixation for Maisonneuve injuries with fibular shortening: technique tip. Foot Ankle Int 2017;38(10):1146–51.

32. Rammelt S, Boszczyk A. Computed Tomography in the diagnosis and treatment of ankle fractures: a critical analysis review. JBJS Rev 2018;6(12):e7.

33. Gardner MJ, Brodsky A, Briggs SM, et al. Fixation of posterior malleolus fractures provides greater syndesmotic stability. Clin Orthop Relat Res 2006;447:165–71.

34. Bennett C, Behn A, Daoud A, et al. Buttress plating versus anterior-to-posterior lag screws for fixation of the posterior malleolus: a biomechanical study. J Orthop Trauma 2016;30(12):664–9.

35. Latham AJ, Goodwin PC, Stirling B, et al. Ankle syndesmosis repair and rehabilitation in professional rugby league players: a case series report. BMJ Open Sport Exerc Med 2017;3:e000175.

36. Colcuc C, Blank M, Stein T, et al. Lower complication rate and faster return to sports in patients with acute syndesmotic rupture treated with a new knotless suture button device. Knee Surg Sports Traumatol Arthrosc 2018;26:3156–64.

37. Chen B, Chen C, Yang Z, et al. To compare the efficacy between fixation with tightrope and screw in the treatment of syndesmotic injuries: a meta-analysis. Foot Ankle Surg 2019;25:63–70.

38. Shimozono Y, Hurley ET, Myerson CL, et al. Suture button versus syndesmotic screw for syndesmosis injuries, a meta-analysis of randomized controlled trials. Am J Sports Med 2019;47(11):2764–71.

39. McKenzie AC, Hesselholt KE, Larsen MS, et al. A systematic review and meta-analysis on treatment of ankle fractures with syndesmotic rupture: suture-button fixation versus cortical screw fixation. Foot Ankle Surg 2019;58:946–53.

40. Pang EQ, Bedigrew K, Palanca A, et al. Ankle joint contact loads and displacement in syndesmosis injuries repaired with Tightropes compared to screw fixation in a static model. Injury 2019;50(11):1901–7.

41. Goetz JE, Davidson NP, Rudert MJ, et al. Biomechanical comparison of syndesmotic repair techniqeus during exernal rotation stress. Foot Ankle Int 2018;39(11):1345–54.

42. Clanton TO, Whitlow SR, Williams BT, et al. Biomechanical comparison of 3 current ankle syndesmosis repair techniques. Foot Ankle Int 2017;38(2):200–7.

43. Andersen MR, Frihagen F, Hellund JC, et al. Randomized trial comparing suture button with single screw for syndesmosis injury. J Bone Joint Surg Am 2018;100:2.

44. Marmor M, Hansen E, Han HK, et al. Limitations of standard fluoroscopy in detecting rotational malreduction of the Syndesmosis in an ankle fracture model. Foot Ankle Int 2011;32(6):616–22.
45. Sangeorzan BJ, Sangeorzan BP, Hansen ST, et al. Mathematically directed single-cut osteotomy for correction of tibial malunion. J Orthop Trauma 1989; 3(4):267–75.
46. Espinosa N, Smerek JP, Myerson MS. Acute and chronic Syndesmosis injuries: pathomechanisms, diagnosis and management. Foot Ankle Clin 2006;11(3): 639–57.
47. Outland T. Sprains and separations of the inferior tibiofibular joint without important fracture. Am J Surg 1943;59:320.
48. Harper M. Delayed reconstruction and stabilization of the tibiofibular Syndesmosis. Foot Ankle Int 2001;22(1):15–8.
49. Katznelson A, Lin E, Militiano J. Ruptures of the ligaments about the tibio-fibular Syndesmosis. Injury 1983;15(3):170–2.
50. Pena FA, Coetzee JC. Ankle syndesmosis injuries. Foot Ankle Clin 2006;11(1): 35–50, viii.
51. Van Dijk CN. Syndesmotic injuries. Tech Foot Ankle Surg 2006;5(1):34–7.
52. Mullins J, Sallis J. Recurrent sprains of the ankle joint with diastasis. J Bone Joint Surg 1958;40-B(2):270–3.
53. Beals T, Manoli A. Late Syndesmosis reconstruction: a case report. Foot Ankle Int 1998;19:485–7.
54. Swords MP, Sands AK, Shank JR. Late treatment of syndesmotic injuries. Foot Ankle Clin 2017;22(1):65–75.
55. Grass R, Rammelt S, Biewener A, et al. Peroneus longus ligamentoplasty for chronic instability of the distal tibiofibular Syndesmosis. Foot Ankle Int 2003; 24(5):392–7.
56. Yasui Y, Takao M, Miyamoto W, et al. Anatomical reconstruction of the anterior inferior tibiofibular ligament for chronic disruption of the distal tibiofibular Syndesmosis. Knee Surg Sports Traumatol Arthrosc 2011;19(4):691–5.
57. Swords M, Brillhaut J, Sands A. Acute and chronic syndesmotic Injury The authors' approach to treatment. Foot Ankle Clin 2018;23:625–37.
58. Scolaro JA, Marecek G, Barei DP. Management of syndesmotic disruption in ankle fractures: a critical analysis review. JBJS Rev 2014;2(12):1–10.
59. Jones CB, Gilde A, Sietsema DL. Treatment of syndesmotic injuries of the ankle: a critical analysis review. JBJS Rev 2015;3(10):1–15.
60. Schepers T, Dingemans SA, Rammelt S. Recent developments in the treatment of acute syndesmotic injuries. Fuß Sprunggelenk 2016;14(2):66–78.

Osteochondral Lesions of the Talus

An Individualized Treatment Paradigm from the Amsterdam Perspective

Quinten G.H. Rikken, BSc[a,b,c],
Gino M.M.J. Kerkhoffs, MD, PhD[a,b,c],*

KEYWORDS

- Osteochondral lesions • OLT • Osteochondral defects • OCD • Ankle • Talus
- Current concepts

KEY POINTS

- Patients with osteochondral lesions of the talus (OLTs) typically present 6 months to 12 months after an initial trauma with deep ankle pain provoked during or after weight-bearing activities.
- Physical examination and imaging (computed tomography or magnetic resonance imaging) are paramount in the diagnosis of an OLT.
- The lesion size and morphology, surgeon and patient preferences, and individual patient aspects guide treatment options for individual patients.
- Conservative treatment is the primary treatment of all OLTs, regardless if surgery is needed.
- Optimal surgical management depends on primary or secondary nature of the lesion, size, morphology, fixability, and presence of a fragment.

INTRODUCTION

Osteochondral lesions of the talus (OLTs) are characterized by damage to the articular cartilage of the talus and its underlying subchondral bone. Up to 75% of OLTs occur after traumatic injuries, such as ankle sprains and ankle fractures.[1–3] Advancements in

a Department of Orthopaedic Surgery, Amsterdam Movement Sciences, Amsterdam UMC, Location AMC, University of Amsterdam, Meibergdreef 9, Amsterdam 1105 AZ, The Netherlands; b Academic Center for Evidence Based Sports Medicine (ACES), Amsterdam, The Netherland; c Amsterdam Collaboration for Health and Safety in Sports (ACHSS), AMC/VUmc IOC Research Center, Amsterdam, The Netherlands
* Corresponding author. Department of Orthopaedic Surgery, Amsterdam Movement Sciences, Amsterdam UMC, Location AMC, University of Amsterdam, Meibergdreef 9, Amsterdam 1105 AZ, The Netherlands.
E-mail address: g.m.kerkhoffs@amsterdamumc.nl

Foot Ankle Clin N Am 26 (2021) 121–136
https://doi.org/10.1016/j.fcl.2020.10.002
1083-7515/21/© 2020 The Author(s). Published by Elsevier Inc. This is an open access article under the CC BY license (http://creativecommons.org/licenses/by/4.0/).

imaging and arthroscopy have provided clinicians with novel insights into optimal treatment indications and has drastically advanced the number of surgical treatments available, as well as improved existing treatment paradigms.[4–7] To date, however, no superior treatment of OLT exists.[4,8] Therefore, an individualized treatment algorithm, guided by patient and lesion characteristics, is the preferred treatment option for OLT management. This current concepts review provides an overview of the available evidence for the diagnosis and treatment of OLTs, current and emerging, and provides evidence-based treatment guidelines from the Amsterdam perspective.

ETIOLOGY

The exact etiology of an osteochondral lesion currently is unknown. The injury mechanism leading to cartilage damage preceding diagnosis is the occurrence of an ankle sprain, where the talus impacts on the distal tibial plafond, thereby creating microfractures (cracks) in the cartilage and subchondral bone plate (**Fig. 1**).[9,10] During weight-bearing, synovial fluid infiltrates these microfractures due to increased pressure, which induces osteonecrosis.[10,11] This causes lesion expansion with, in some cases, the formation of cysts, and leads to pain.[11] These changes alter the ankle joint congruency and biomechanical loading, which can accelerate ankle degeneration further.[12] Juvenile OLT (ie, osteochondritis dissecans) similarly often presents after trauma but seems present from early childhood without being symptomatic.[13] It is hypothesized that, from a morphologic point of view, these specific fragment type lesions are embedded onto the talar dome and held in place by fibrous tissue (**Fig. 2**). Trauma can destabilize this fibrotic connection and initiate a symptomatic process, although it is also possible that these specific morphologic lesions can be considered an accidental finding when a patient presents with complaints nonspecific for an osteochondral lesion in the ankle.

CLINICAL PRESENTATION

Patients typically present 6 months to 12 months after an initial trauma (ankle fracture or sprain), with deep ankle pain provoked during or after load-bearing activities. Additional symptoms may include, but may not be limited to, stiffness, a locking or

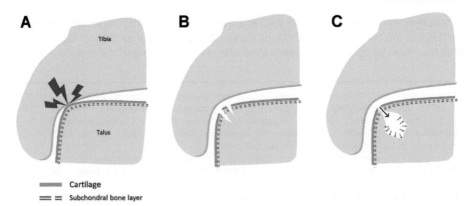

Cartilage
Subchondral bone layer

Fig. 1. The formation of a traumatic OLT. (*A*) The talus has an impact on the tibia in an ankle sprain, for example, (*B*) Microfractures occur in the talus. (*C*) Hydrostatic loading during weight-bearing forms an OLT.

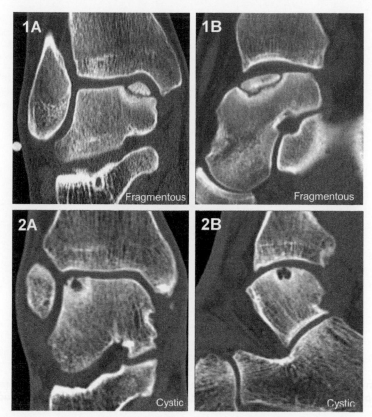

Fig. 2. Illustration of 2 morphologically different OLTs. (*1A*) Coronal and (*1B*) sagittal views of a fragment type lesion amenable for fixation OLT. (*2A*) Coronal and (*2B*) sagittal views of a cystic OLT.

catching sensation (which can indicate a displaced fragment or pseudoimpingement due to the displaced cartilaginous flap), swelling (especially after activities), and reduced range of motion (ROM).[14] The recognizable deep ankle pain can be provoked by forcefully palpating the talar dome with the ankle in full plantar flexion (**Fig. 3**). It must be stated, however, that the sensitivity of this test is unknown and if lesions are located far posteriorly, this test can be false negative due to the inability to palpate the lesion.[15] Thorough physical examination and (hetero)anamnesis are paramount for diagnosis and can aid in deciding further examinations. Further (imaging) examinations of the ankle are justified if clinical suspicion for an OLT is present.

IMAGING

Advancements in imaging have improved the diagnostic accuracy drastically over time. Radiographs are useful only for assessing ankle alignment because its diagnostic accuracy for OLTs is low (**Table 1**).[16] Currently, computed tomography (CT) scans and magnetic resonance imaging (MRI) are the common diagnostic tools, with high sensitivity and specificity (see **Table 1**).[7,16] CT is preferred to assess the bony morphology and size of OLTs and to assess the subchondral bone layer.[7] Additionally, supplementary CT scans with the ankle in maximum plantar flexion can

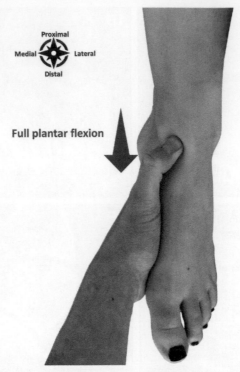

Fig. 3. An example of forced palpation of the medial talus. This can reproduce the recognizable deep ankle pain. Notice that with plantar flexion a larger portion of the talus can be reached.

determine arthroscopic accessibility during preoperative planning.[15] MRI is used to asses ankle cartilage, detect bone marrow edema, or diagnose concomitant soft tissue injuries of the ankle. Preferably, lesion size is determined with CT, because MRI can overestimate the lesion size when bone edema is present.[17]

Radiologists should report the lesion morphology, which includes the presence of loose bodies, cysts (complexes) with or without a bony roof, sclerotic aspects, kissing lesions, fragment type lesion, signs of previous microfracturing, and containment type.

Table 1		
Sensitivity and specificity of imaging modalities for osteochondral lesions of the talus according to Verhagen and colleagues[16]		
Modality	Sensitivity	Specificity
Standard radiograph	0.59	0.91
Mortise view radiograph	0.70	0.94
CT	0.81	0.99
MRI	0.96	0.89

Data from Verhagen RAW, Maas M, Dijkgraaf MGW, et al. Prospective study on diagnostic strategies in osteochondral lesions of the talus. Is MRI superior to helical CT? *J Bone Joint Surg Br.* 2005;87(1):41-46.

Lesion size should be reported in 3 planes (anterior-posterior, medial-lateral, and depth).

TREATMENT

It is paramount that an evidence-based personalized treatment approach is applied to patients with an OLT. A personalized approach incorporates all patient and lesion characteristics to determine the optimal treatment of an individual patient. This approach is depicted in **Fig. 4** and includes patient factors (age, body mass index [BMI], preoperative level of activities, and patient preference), lesion factors (primary or nonprimary [ie, failed previous surgical treatment], lesion size, and morphology) and other pathologies in the ankle (hindfoot alignment, ankle stability, and concomitant injuries). This multilevel algorithm starts with conservative therapy. If patients fail a period of conservative therapy, a further selection for surgical treatment can be made. First, a differentiation between primary and failed primary (secondary) lesions is made and ankle alignment is considered. Second, the lesion size is incorporated, which grossly determines the level of invasiveness of the procedure (in accordance with patient and surgeon preferences). After considering lesions size, the lesion morphology (fixable fragment, [multiple] cysts, focal or diffuse lesions, and location on the talus) is taken into account, combined with the overall treatment goal of a patient, thus allowing for a tailor-made approach.

Conservative Treatment

Conservative management is the primary intervention for all OLTs, regardless of lesion and patient characteristics. It is possible symptoms can improve without the need of a surgical intervention.[18] Conservative treatment is not restricted to a single modality and often consists of a combination of interventions. Restriction of weight-bearing and physical or work activities is the primary intervention of conservative treatment and aims at decreasing symptoms. By unloading the ankle joint, less synovial fluid is forced into the developing OLT. This limits further damage to the cartilage and

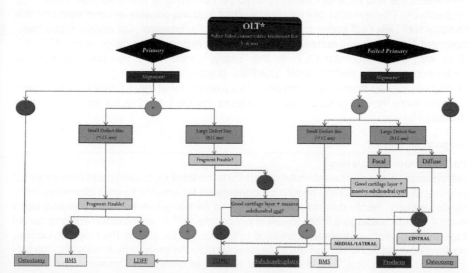

Fig. 4. Flowchart for surgical management of symptomatic OLTs after failed conservative treatment.

subcartilaginous structures, which reduces pain and synovial swelling. Patients who are overweight (BMI >25) are advised to lose weight in order to decrease ankle load. Orthopedic insoles can help with proper load distribution of the ankle joint and improve ROM, thereby aiming at decreasing contact pressure on the OLT. Physiotherapy focusses on strength and balance exercises to reduce symptoms. Hyaluronic acid injections and platelet-rich plasma (PRP) can also be considered. Partial or full (cast) immobilization up to 6 weeks can be used to decrease load bearing. Conservative treatment has the goal of achieving full return to daily activities and sports with slight to moderate pain, noting high-impact sports should be avoided.[18] When patients are restricted to return to high-impact sports or still experience deep ankle pain 3 months to 6 months after the start of conservative therapy, surgical treatment can be considered.

Clinical outcomes for conservative therapy can differ. Seo and colleagues[19] recently published a retrospectively evaluated cohort of 142 symptomatic patients and reported the clinical and radiologic outcomes at mean follow-up of 5.7 years. Patients were not immobilized or restricted in activities in this study. Mean lesion width, length, and depth measured 6.9 mm, 9.4 mm, and 5.4 mm, respectively. The visual analog scale (VAS) decreased significantly, from 3.8 to 0.9, whereas the American Orthopaedic Foot & Ankle Society (AOFAS) score improved slightly (from 86 to 91). Of the 83 patients who underwent CT scan at final follow-up, lesion size did not change in 69 (83.2%), 5 (6%) decreased, and 9 (10.8%) increased but were significantly deeper pretreatment compared with the other groups. No progression of ankle osteoarthritis (OA) was found on radiographs at final follow-up. Similarly, Klammer and colleagues[20] reported the natural history of a retrospective case series with 48 untreated patients (50 ankles) with a minimum follow-up of 2 years. Average mediolateral and anteroposterior diameter and depth at initial MRI were 9.6 mm, 15.8 mm, and 8.3 mm, respectively. No significant size changes were found at mean follow-up of 52 months. At initial visit, 13 (61.9%) of 21 available patients showed no signs of OA. At mean 50 months follow-up of all cases, radiographic evaluation found grade 1 OA and grade 2 OA (according to van Dijk and colleagues[21]) in 27% of cases each. At final follow-up, however, 24% and 62% of cases reported no pain (VAS 0) and mild pain (VAS 1–3), respectively. These results point to the need for a strong consideration of conservative therapy with new OLT patients. Up to 55% of OLTs, however, fail conservative management.[22] Reilingh and colleagues[13] published a retrospective case series of 37 children with a symptomatic OLT. In this study, conservative therapy consisted of restriction of sports and physical activities, physiotherapy, taping, or casting; 92% of children initially treated with conservative therapy for at least 6 months underwent surgery, even though children are considered the best candidates for conservative therapy.[23]

Surgical Treatment

Bone marrow stimulation

Arthroscopic bone marrow stimulation (BMS) is the treatment used most frequently for primary OLTs.[4] BMS ideally should be considered for small (<15-mm diameter), noncystic, primary, nonfixable lesions but can also be considered and the treating team do not wish to undergo a more invasive procedure.[24,25] After débridement and curettage of the defective cartilaginous tissue to the base of the lesion, the sclerotic bone is perforated or drilled to disrupt the intraosseous blood vessels, which mitigates the formation of a fibrin clot.[14,26] Through the release of multipotent mesenchymal stem cells, revascularization is promoted, subsequently initiating the formation of fibrocartilage rather than hyaline-like cartilage.[26]

Clinical outcomes after BMS can be considered successful (AOFAS score ≥80 points) in 82% of primary OLTs, according to a recent systematic review from Dahmen and colleagues.[4] Toale and colleagues[27] found a weighted mean postoperative AOFAS score of 89.9 at midterm follow-up (71.9 months) in their systematic review. This review also found a low complication rate of 3.4% and a reoperation rate of 6.0%.

When specifically considering sports outcomes, Steman and colleagues[28] reported a pooled return to sport (RTS) rate at any level and preinjury level of 88% and 79%, respectively. This review found a time to RTS after BMS that ranged from 15 weeks to 26 weeks. The weighted mean time to RTS at any level was found to be 4.5 months by a systematic review from Hurley and colleagues.[29]

Long-term outcomes of BMS have been reported sparsely in the literature. van Bergen and colleagues[30] published the longest follow-up cohort to date. This study included 50 patients with primary OLTs treated with BMS or débridement at a mean 141 months' follow-up. A median AOFAS score of 88 (range: 64–100) was reported. At final follow-up, 63% and 4% of patients were found to have grade 1 OA and grade 2 OA, according to the van Dijk classification,[21] respectively. Moreover, progression of OA by 1 grade was reported in 33% of patients.

The development of OA due to the deterioration of fibrocartilage over time, altered joint biomechanics, and subchondral bone damage are concerns in the current literature and daily clinical practice. Multiple investigators have reported the occurrence of OA in their cohorts treated with BMS. In a retrospective case series, Ferkel and colleagues[31] reported the clinical and radiologic outcomes of 50 arthroscopically treated patients at a mean follow-up of 72 months. This study found 34% of patients developed OA or progressed by 1 or more stage of the van Dijk classification,[21] most often to grade 1. From a subgroup of 17 previously studied patients 35% had deteriorating modified Weber scores. Solely those patients with a grade 2 OA or grade 3 OA showed an association with inferior clinical outcomes in this study.

The progression of OA after BMS can be explained partly by the inferior wear characteristics of fibrocartilage compared with the native hyaline cartilage.[32,33] Additionally, a depressed subchondral bone plate after BMS has been proposed to be associated with poor outcomes. Reilingh and colleagues[34] found a depressed subchondral bone plate in 79% of patients as assessed per 1-year follow-up CT. In a different study, this group found lesion dimensions unchanged 1-year postoperatively compared with preoperatively (except for lesion depth).[35] Subchondral bone healing was reported to be poor in 37% of patients, indicating a limited healing capacity following BMS. Moreover, this study also reported incomplete sclerotic bone perforation or cysts to not be (fully) débrided in 13 of 58 OLTs, as assessed on 1-year postoperative CT.[35] These findings warrant further research in BMS indication and sustainability of results in long-term follow-up studies.

Secondary lesions (ie, failed primary surgical treatment) treated with BMS are reported less frequently in the literature than their primary counterparts.[4,8] Repeat BMS in 12 patients reported by Savva and colleagues[33] improved the AOFAS score from 42.4 preoperatively to 80.5 at a mean follow-up of 5.9 years. This study excluded cystic lesions as Robinson and colleagues[36] found poor results after repeat BMS in 50% of patients with mostly cystic lesions. A paucity in the literature is present, however, and controversy remains about the effectiveness of repeat BMS compared with the primary procedure.

Treatment after BMS generally consists of partial weight-bearing in the first 2 weeks postoperatively.[29] ROM exercises are encouraged immediately after surgery but may be limited due to postoperative swelling. Full weight-bearing generally is allowed

6 weeks postoperatively. At this point, physical therapy can be started. Initially, strength and balance exercises with the gradual building of load are encouraged. In this phase (3–4 months postoperatively), no peak axial forces are allowed. With the help of a physiotherapist, patients increase ankle load and strength toward their desired rehabilitation goal.

A novel frontier in the ongoing development of (surgical) treatment strategies for OLTs is adjunct therapies (ie, biologicals). These therapies are administered during the end stage of the BMS procedure or as a stand-alone treatment. PRP and bone marrow aspirate concentrate (BMAC) both are autologous blood products aiming at improving the quality of cartilage and subchondral bone repair and thereby associated clinical outcomes.[18] Preclinical evidence exists for the delay of OA after adjunct therapy administration.[37] Although with a low number of patients, clinical studies have shown the effectiveness of these therapies. Prospective comparative studies with sufficient power and in a randomized setting are highly necessary to define the pure effectiveness of these adjunct treatment options.[38,39]

Fixation techniques

When OLT fragments are fixable, acute primary cases and chronic cases can be considered for fixation.[40] According to experts, an osteochondral fragment diameter of at least 10 mm and depth of 3 mm is a minimum threshold for a technically feasible fixation.[40] For acutely displaced lesions and the skeletally immature, fixation should be considered first. Acute symptomatic but stable lesions and chronic lesions first should be treated conservatively. Contraindications for fixation are ankle OA (grade ≥2), advanced osteoporosis, or septic arthritis.[41]

The advantages of fixation over other surgical treatments are the ability to restore the congruency of the talus and the preservation of hyaline cartilage and subchondral bone.[6,34,40] Additionally, if fixation fails, BMS still can be considered as a follow-up intervention. OLT fixation can be performed arthroscopically in case the lesion can be reached through an anterior or posterior approach and in case the fragment can be fixed perpendicular to the articular cartilaginous talar dome. Open OLT fixation can be considered if lesions are not fixable through arthroscopy or in cases of surgeon preference.

Open fixation of an OLT starts with an arthrotomy to visualize the lesion. Depending on the lesion location, a medial malleolar osteotomy is performed to reach the lesion and to obtain working space.[42–44] Hereafter, the osteochondral fragment is removed and the underlying site and/or cyst curetted or drilled. Bone grafts are collected from the distal tibia or other non–weight-bearing areas of the joint. These bone plugs are used to fill the excavated site, after which the fragment is reduced and fixated. Different techniques have been described for filling and fixating OLTs, such as the use of bone pegs or cancellous bone grafts and screw fixation or the use of Kirschner wires.[6,42,43,45,46]

Outcomes for open fixation of OLTs have been reported in multiple studies. At a mean follow-up of 7 years, good Berndt and Harty scores were found for 24 (89%) out of 27 patients by Kumai and colleagues.[42] In a retrospective study of 20 patients treated with open internal fixation, Schuh and colleagues[43] found excellent and good results according to the Ogilvie-Harris score in 80% and 20% of patients, respectively. Haraguchi and colleagues[46] found a mean Japanese Society for Surgery of the Foot (JSSF) ankle/hindfoot score of 93 out of 100 points at 2 years postoperatively for 44 patients. This study found no correlation between the JSSF score and lesion size or chronicity, meaning that chronic lesions, therefore, are amenable for fixation from an evidence-based perspective. An excellent mean postoperative AOFAS score of

98.5 and VAS score of 0 (meaning no pain) was reported in 83% of patients at 1-year follow-up using bioabsorbable pins by Nakasa and colleagues.[44] The aforementioned study found osteolytic changes in approximately 28% of implants, which was correlated to a shallower insertion angle. This could pose a risk for treatment failure at long-term follow-up and is inherent to fixation procedures. Surgeons, therefore, should carefully insert the fixation screw perpendicular to the osteochondral fragment at a 90° angle to minimize this risk. Disadvantages of the open procedure are need of a longer immobilization period and nonunion or delayed union after an osteotomy.[47,48] These disadvantages prompted the recent development of arthroscopic fixation techniques.[6,49]

Arthroscopic fixation is a technically demanding procedure. Determining the fixation angle is difficult under the scope but is considered a crucial step and as such should be reserved for advanced arthroscopists.[44] The lift, drill, fill, and fix (LDFF) procedure is a novel arthroscopic fixation technique (which can also be performed open) developed by Kerkhoffs and colleagues.[6] The procedure combines the advantages of fixation with marrow stimulation for increased healing potential and consolidation of the fragment.[6,41] Visualization and working space can be created through standard anteromedial and anterolateral portals, or posterior portals if the lesion is located far posteriorly.[6,15,49] First, an osteochondral bone flap is created, which should stay attached posteriorly. By means of a chisel, the flap is lifted and functions like a lever through its posterior attachment (lift), a crucial step, as depicted in **Fig. 5**. Second, the lesion site is débrided and perforated through the sclerotic bone to promote revascularization (drill). In the following step, cancellous bone grafts are harvested from non–weight-bearing areas of the distal tibia and used to pack the lesion site (fill). Similarly to the hood of a car, the osteochondral flap is relocated to its original position with an adequate compression fixated through using a biocortical screw (fix).[6] Rehabilitation after the arthroscopic and open LDFF procedures consists first of a short-leg nonweightbearing cast for 4 and 6 weeks, respectively.[6,41] This then is changed for a

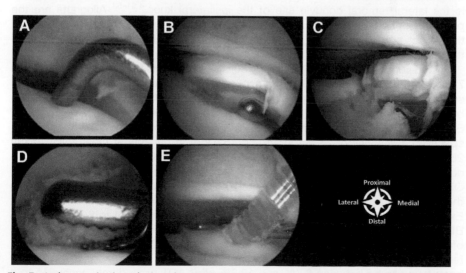

Fig. 5. Arthroscopic view during the LDFF procedure. (*A*) Lesion in situ. (*B*) With the posterior margin of the flap still attached, the lesion is lifted (lift). (*C*) Perforating of sclerotic subchondral bone with a chisel (drill), (*D*) filling of the lesion with cancellous autograft (fill), and (*E*) fixation of the lesion while applying axial pressure for flap stabilization (fix).

walking cast with full weight-bearing allowed. The walking cast can be removed after a period up to 4 weeks for arthroscopically treated cases and 6 weeks for open LDFF cases. Physical therapy can be started at this point, focusing on a return to full weight-bearing in approximately 2 weeks.

The arthroscopic LDFF procedure has shown promising outcomes. Lambers and colleagues[41] published a prospective cohort of 27 ankles and found a postoperative numeric rating scale during running of 2.9 compared with the preoperative numeric rating scale of 7.8 at mean follow-up of 27 months after LDFF fixation, indicating a significant decrease in pain. Fragment fusion was complete on CT scans in 92% of cases at 1-year follow-up, indicating a successful integration of the subchondral bone layer and preservation of hyaline cartilage. Reilingh and colleagues[34] found that the subchondral bone plate was depressed in 28% of LDFF patients on 1-year follow-up CT compared with 79% found in patients treated with BMS. The restoration of the subchondral bone plate and preservation of hyaline cartilage in fixation has been hypothesized to delay the onset or progression of OA compared with marrow stimulation.[41] Midterm to long-term outcomes for fixation techniques, however, are needed to evaluate these premises and to determine the optimal fixation procedure.

Osteo(chondral) transplantation

Autologous or allogenic osteo(chondral) transplantation (AOT) is a restorative technique that replaces the damaged bone–chondral unit. Additionally, it repairs the weight-bearing capacities of the talus.[14] AOT generally is used for larger (>15 mm in diameter), (massive) cystic, primary, and secondary lesions of the talus.

An open approach through an arthrotomy or osteotomy (for medial lesion) is needed for proper visualization. During the conventional AOT procedure, a single cylindrical graft or multiple cylinders (ie, mosaicplasty) are harvested and subsequently implanted into the fully débrided and excised lesion site. Both autografts and fresh allografts are available for transplantation.[4,8,50,51] The primary donor site for autografts is the lateral femoral condyle site of the ipsilateral knee.[4,51–53] Allografts are the preferred option for patients with knee OA, a history of knee infections, or when the defect size exceeds the possibility of a safe sized harvesting procedure from the knee.[50]

Pooled success rates (AOFAS score ≥80) after autografts have been reported to be 77% for primary lesions and 90% for secondary lesions, according to 2 comprehensive systematic reviews.[4,8] The pooled clinical success rate of allografts was found to be 55% in secondary lesions and ranged from 20% to 100% for primary lesions.[4,8] Shimozono and colleagues[53] reported the clinical and radiologic outcomes of a retrospective case-series of 25 autograft and 16 allograft patients at mean follow-up of 26 months and 22 months, respectively. This study found autografts to show significantly superior Foot and Ankle Outcome Scores (FAOS) and Magnetic Resonance Observation of Cartilage Repair Tissue (MOCART) scores over allografts. Additionally, they found an allograft failure rate of 25% compared with no failures for autografts. Extensive research has found the use of greater than or equal to 3 grafts, a high BMI, and uncontained lesion type associated with inferior clinical outcomes either of the ankle or the donor kee.[51,52,54] Even though knee function seems to be unaffected, according to Paul and colleagues,[52] donor-site morbidity of the knee has been found to be between 6.7% and 10.8% after AOT procedures, according to a meta-analysis by Hurley and colleagues.[29]

In recent years, these concerns have caused the emergence of other transplantation sites, such as the iliac crest.[5] Iliac crest transplants are hypothesized to support the regeneration of articular cartilage through the bone-periosteal membrane, which acts as a natural scaffold and possesses local growth factors as well as resemble the natural curvature of the talus.[5,55,56] Hu and colleagues[57] treated 17 cystic OLTs with osteoperiosteal cylindrical grafts from the iliac crest with a mean postoperative AOFAS score of 90 and mean VAS of 0.9 at 33 months follow-up. At second-look arthroscopy, the mean International Cartilage Repair Society (ICRS) score was 9. A preclinical study by Sung and colleagues[58] demonstrated the ability of articular cartilage repair in all subjects after periosteal grafting. Another novel procedure is the talar osteoperiosteal grafting from the iliac crest (TOPIC) technique.[5]

The TOPIC procedure is an individualized treatment that can be considered for primary and secondary lesions greater than 10 mm in diameter. The TOPIC technique is ideal for lesions located at the medial and lateral edges of the talar dome (**Fig. 6**). Preoperatively, a CT scan is made to determine the location, size, and accessibility of the OLT and if an osteotomy is needed. In most cases, an osteotomy is performed to gain access to the joint. Hereafter, the lesion site is inspected, and the OLT excised fully until healthy bone and prepared for graft receipt by microdrilling the subchondral bone base. Drilling facilitates the introduction of marrow cells, which aid the integration of the TOPIC graft. The donor site then is measured for graft harvesting. An

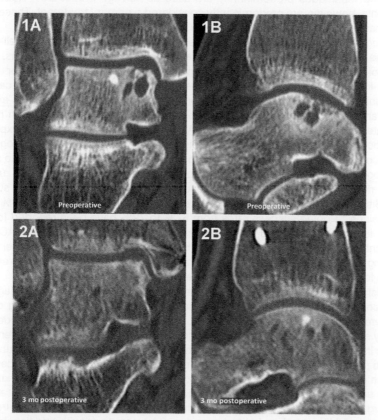

Fig. 6. Preoperative and 3 months postoperative CT scans of a patient treated with the TOPIC procedure. Preoperatively a large posteromedial lesion on (*1A*) coronal and (*1B*) sagittal images. (*2A, 2B*) Three months postoperatively. the graft is well incorporated.

oversized graft (by 1 mm in all directions of the prepared donor site) is harvested from the anterior superior iliac crest. The graft then is prepared to press-fit shape, which allows the surgeon to mimic the size, depth, and curvature of the excised lesion site. This allows for minimal chondral damage during the procedure and accurate fit of the graft. Due to the press-fit preparation of the graft no additional screws are necessary for graft fixation but can be considered if deemed biomechanically appropriate. Postoperatively, patients are placed in a nonwalking cast for 6 weeks, after which they are placed in a walking boot for another 6 weeks. At 12 weeks postoperatively, a CT scan is made to asses graft incorporation and osteotomy healing. This allows aftertreatment to be individualized, if necessary. After this period physical therapy is started to assist recovery.

Results of an initial 10-patient prospective cohort study found an AOFAS score improvement from 50 to 83 points at 1 year postoperatively.[5] Pain during running (VAS) was found to improve from 7.1 to 2.6 at final follow-up. All patients showed consolidation of the graft and osteotomy.

Regenerative and retrograde treatments

Multiple treatment modalities remain and have been used throughout the world. The cell-based techniques predominantly are used as salvage procedures. Retrograde treatments, however, are predominantly considered a primary treatment. These treatments have varying indications and results, as discussed further.

Cartilage transplantation and chondrogenesis-inducing techniques are cell-based therapies used in larger (>15-mm diameter), cystic, and secondary lesions. Either autologous chondrocytes from non–weight-bearing areas of the ankle or blood/marrow-like products are used to resurface the OLT. In the first-generation cartilage transplantation technique, autologous chondrocyte implantation (ACI), cells are harvested and externally expanded for reimplantation. The second-generation matrix-associated chondrocyte implantation (MACI) combines a scaffold with expanded chondrocytes for reimplantation. Autologous matrix–induced chondrogenesis (AMIC) combines microfracturing with a biodegradable collagen membrane to induce chondrogenesis.[59] Bone marrow–derived cell transplantation (BMDCT) uses a platelet-rich fibrin and BMAC-injected scaffold. The treatment success (AOFAS score ≥80 points) rate for these treatments range from 56% to 100% in primary lesions.[4] Pooled success rates from 57% to 72% have been reported for secondary lesions.[18] The need for 2-stage procedures with ACI and MACI is a disadvantage. These techniques and the biomaterials used, however, currently are emerging, with increasing literature published, and could prove a valuable treatment options for secondary and larger primary lesions.[23]

For defects with a good articular cartilage layer (as assessed per MRI or diagnostic arthroscopy) and a (massive) cyst, subchondroplasty or retrograde drilling can be considered.[14,60] During retrograde drilling, a nontransarticular approach under fluoroscopy allows for drilling up to the subcartilaginous cyst and its débridement. This initiates intraosseous blood vessel disruption similarly to BMS and initiates subarticular bone filling of the cyst. Retrograde drilling has been found to have a success rate between 68% and 100% in primary OLTs.[4] Subchondroplasty historically has been used in subchondral bone defects of the knee and recently has been pioneered for OLT surgery.[60] During the procedure, calcium phosphate is injected via a retrograde approach to fill the subchondral lesion and may be combined with additional arthroscopic treatments of the OLT.[61] Only few short-term clinical outcomes are available, and show differing results.[60,61] Avascular necrosis can be a serious complication after subchondroplasty.[62] Future research will determine the efficacy and safety of this technique.

ACKNOWLEDGMENTS

The authors would like to thank Jari Dahmen for his valuable contribution to this work.

DISCLOSURE

No authors reported receiving funding for this study or any other conflict of interest.

REFERENCES

1. Hintermann B, Boss A, Schäfer D. Arthroscopic findings in patients with chronic ankle instability. Am J Sports Med 2002;30(3):402–9.
2. Hintermann B, Regazzoni P, Lampert C, et al. Arthroscopic findings in acute fractures of the ankle. J Bone Joint Surg Br 2000;82(3):345–51.
3. Kerkhoffs GMMJ, Kennedy JG, Calder JDF, et al. There is no simple lateral ankle sprain. Knee Surg Sports Traumatol Arthrosc 2016;24(4):941–3.
4. Dahmen J, Lambers KTA, Reilingh ML, et al. No superior treatment for primary osteochondral defects of the talus. Knee Surg Sports Traumatol Arthrosc 2018; 26:2142–57.
5. Kerkhoffs G, Altink J, Stufkens S, et al. Talar OsteoPeriostic grafting from the Iliac Crest (TOPIC) for large medial talar osteochondral defects: operative technique. Oper Orthop Traumatol 2020. https://doi.org/10.1007/s00064-020-00673-9.
6. Kerkhoffs GMMJ, Reilingh ML, Gerards RM, et al. Lift, drill, fill and fix (LDFF): a new arthroscopic treatment for talar osteochondral defects. Knee Surg Sports Traumatol Arthrosc 2016;24(4):1265–71.
7. van Bergen CJ, Gerards RM, Opdam KT, et al. Diagnosing, planning and evaluating osteochondral ankle defects with imaging modalities. World J Orthop 2015; 6(11):944–53.
8. Lambers KTA, Dahmen J, Reilingh ML, et al. No superior surgical treatment for secondary osteochondral defects of the talus. Knee Surg Sports Traumatol Arthrosc 2018;26:2158–70.
9. Kerkhoffs GMMJ, Karlsson J. Osteochondral lesions of the talus. Knee Surg Sports Traumatol Arthrosc 2019;27(9):2719–20.
10. van Dijk CN, Reilingh ML, Zengerink M, et al. Osteochondral defects in the ankle: Why painful? Knee Surg Sports Traumatol Arthrosc 2010;18(5):570–80.
11. Van der Vis HM, Aspenberg P, Marti RK, et al. Fluid pressure causes bone resorption in a rabbit model of prosthetic loosening. Clin Orthop Relat Res 1998;350: 201–8.
12. Blom RP, Mol D, van Ruijven LJ, et al. A single axial impact load causes articular damage that is not visible with micro-computed tomography: an ex vivo study on caprine tibiotalar joints. Cartilage 2019. https://doi.org/10.1177/1947603519876353.
13. Reilingh ML, Kerkhoffs GMMJ, Telkamp CJA, et al. Treatment of osteochondral defects of the talus in children. Knee Surg Sports Traumatol Arthrosc 2014; 22(9):2243–9.
14. Reilingh M, van Bergen C, van Dijk C. Diagnosis and treatment of osteochondral defects of the ankle. SA Orthop J 2009;8(2):44–50.

15. Van Bergen CJA, Tuijthof GJM, Maas M, et al. Arthroscopic accessibility of the talus quantified by computed tomography simulation. Am J Sports Med 2012; 40(10):2318–24.

16. Verhagen RAW, Maas M, Dijkgraaf MGW, et al. Prospective study on diagnostic strategies in osteochondral lesions of the talus. Is MRI superior to helical CT? J Bone Joint Surg Br 2005;87(1):41–6.

17. Yasui Y, Hannon CP, Fraser EJ, et al. Lesion size measured on MRI does not accurately reflect arthroscopic measurement in talar osteochondral lesions. Orthop J Sports Med 2019;7(2). 2325967118825261.

18. Dombrowski ME, Yasui Y, Murawski CD, et al. Conservative management and biological treatment strategies: proceedings of the international consensus meeting on cartilage repair of the ankle. Foot Ankle Int 2018;39(1_suppl):9S–15S.

19. Seo SG, Kim JS, Seo D-K, et al. Osteochondral lesions of the talus Few patients require surgery. Acta Orthop 2018;89(4):462–7.

20. Klammer G, Maquieira GJ, Spahn S, et al. Natural history of nonoperatively treated osteochondral lesions of the talus. Foot Ankle Int 2015;36(1):24–31.

21. van Dijk CN, Verhagen RAW, Tol JL. Arthroscopy for problems after ankle fracture. J Bone Joint Surg Br 1997;79-B(2):280–4.

22. Zengerink M, Struijs PAA, Tol JLC, et al. Treatment of osteochondral lesions of the talus: a systematic review. Knee Surg Sports Traumatol Arthrosc 2010;18(2): 238–46.

23. Rothrauff BB, Murawski CD, Angthong C, et al. Scaffold-based therapies: proceedings of the international consensus meeting on cartilage repair of the ankle. Foot Ankle Int 2018;39(1_suppl):41S–7S.

24. Ramponi L, Yasui Y, Murawski CD, et al. Lesion size is a predictor of clinical outcomes after bone marrow stimulation for osteochondral lesions of the talus: a systematic review. Am J Sports Med 2017;45(7):1698–705.

25. Hannon CP, Bayer S, Murawski CD, et al. Debridement, curettage, and bone marrow stimulation: proceedings of the international consensus meeting on cartilage repair of the ankle. Foot Ankle Int 2018;39(1_suppl):16S–22S.

26. O'Driscoll SW. The healing and regeneration of articular cartilage. J Bone Joint Surg Am 1998;80(12):1795–812.

27. Toale J, Shimozono Y, Mulvin C, et al. Midterm outcomes of bone marrow stimulation for primary osteochondral lesions of the talus: a systematic review. Orthop J Sports Med 2019;7(10):1–8.

28. Steman JAH, Dahmen J, Lambers KTA, et al. Return to sports after surgical treatment of osteochondral defects of the talus: a systematic review of 2347 cases. Orthop J Sports Med 2019;7(10):1–15.

29. Hurley ET, Shimozono Y, McGoldrick NP, et al. High reported rate of return to play following bone marrow stimulation for osteochondral lesions of the talus. Knee Surg Sports Traumatol Arthrosc 2019;27(9):2721–30.

30. van Bergen CJA, Kox LS, Maas M, et al. Arthroscopic treatment of osteochondral defects of the talus: outcomes at eight to twenty years of follow-up. J Bone Joint Surg Am 2013;95(6):519–25.

31. Ferkel RD, Zanotti RM, Komenda GA, et al. Arthroscopic treatment of chronic osteochondral lesions of the talus: long-term results. Am J Sports Med 2008;36(9): 1750–62.

32. Lynn AK, Brooks RA, Bonfield W, et al. Repair of defects in articular joints. Prospects for material-based solutions in tissue engineering. J Bone Joint Surg Br 2004;86(8):1093–9.

33. Savva N, Jabur M, Davies M, et al. Osteochondral lesions of the talus: results of repeat arthroscopic debridement. Foot Ankle Int 2007;28(6):669–73.

34. Reilingh ML, Lambers KTA, Dahmen J, et al. The subchondral bone healing after fixation of an osteochondral talar defect is superior in comparison with microfracture. Knee Surg Sports Traumatol Arthrosc 2018;26(3):2177–82.

35. Reilingh ML, van Bergen CJA, Blankevoort L, et al. Computed tomography analysis of osteochondral defects of the talus after arthroscopic debridement and microfracture. Knee Surg Sports Traumatol Arthrosc 2016;24(4):1286–92.

36. Robinson DE, Winson IG, Harries WJ, et al. Arthroscopic treatment of osteochondral lesions of the talus. J Bone Joint Surg Br 2003;85(7):989–93.

37. Delco ML, Goodale M, Talts JF, et al. Integrin α10β1high mesenchymal stem cells mitigate the progression of osteoarthritis in an equine talar impact model. Am J Sports Med 2019;48(3):612–23.

38. Guney A, Akar M, Karaman I, et al. Clinical outcomes of platelet rich plasma (PRP) as an adjunct to microfracture surgery in osteochondral lesions of the talus. Knee Surg Sports Traumatol Arthrosc 2015;23(8):2384–9.

39. Kim YS, Park EH, Kim YC, et al. Clinical outcomes of mesenchymal stem cell injection with arthroscopic treatment in older patients with osteochondral lesions of the talus. Am J Sports Med 2013;41(5):1090–9.

40. Reilingh ML, Murawski CD, DiGiovanni CW, et al. Fixation techniques: proceedings of the international consensus meeting on cartilage repair of the ankle. Foot Ankle Int 2018;39(1_suppl):23S–7S.

41. Lambers KTA, Dahmen J, Reilingh ML, et al. Arthroscopic lift, drill, fill and fix (LDFF) is an effective treatment option for primary talar osteochondral defects. Knee Surg Sports Traumatol Arthrosc 2019;28(1):141–7.

42. Kumai T, Takakura Y, Kitada C, et al. Fixation of osteochondral lesions of the talus using cortical bone pegs. J Bone Joint Surg Br 2002;84(3):369–74.

43. Schuh A, Salminen S, Zeiler G, et al. Ergebnisse der refixation der osteochondrosis dissecans des talus mit kirschnerdrähten. Zentralbl Chir 2004;129(6):470–5.

44. Nakasa T, Ikuta Y, Tsuyuguchi Y, et al. MRI tracking of the effect of bioabsorbable pins on bone marrow edema after fixation of the osteochondral fragment in the talus. Foot Ankle Int 2019;40(3):323–9.

45. Nakasa T, Adachi N, Kato T, et al. Appearance of subchondral bone in computed tomography is related to cartilage damage in osteochondral lesions of the talar dome. Foot Ankle Int 2014;35(6):600–6.

46. Haraguchi N, Shiratsuchi T, Ota K, et al. Fixation of the osteochondral talar fragment yields good results regardless of lesion size or chronicity. Knee Surg Sports Traumatol Arthrosc 2020;28(1):291–7.

47. Colin F, Gaudot F, Odri G, et al. Supramalleolar osteotomy: techniques, indications and outcomes in a series of 83 cases. Orthop Traumatol Surg Res 2014; 100(4):413–8.

48. Krähenbühl N, Zwicky L, Bolliger L, et al. Mid- to long-term results of supramalleolar osteotomy. Foot Ankle Int 2017;38(2):124–32.

49. Kim HN, Kim GL, Park JY, et al. Fixation of a posteromedial osteochondral lesion of the talus using a three-portal posterior arthroscopic technique. J Foot Ankle Surg 2013;52(3):402–5.

50. Smyth NA, Murawski CD, Adams SB, et al. Osteochondral allograft: proceedings of the international consensus meeting on cartilage repair of the ankle. Foot Ankle Int 2018;39(1_suppl):35S–40S.

51. Hurley ET, Murawski CD, Paul J, et al. Osteochondral autograft: proceedings of the international consensus meeting on cartilage repair of the ankle. Foot Ankle Int 2018;39(1_suppl):28S–34S.
52. Paul J, Sagstetter A, Kriner M, et al. Donor-site morbidity after osteochondral autologous transplantation for lesions of the talus. J Bone Joint Surg Am 2009; 91(7):1683–8.
53. Shimozono Y, Hurley ET, Nguyen JT, et al. Allograft compared with autograft in osteochondral transplantation for the treatment of osteochondral lesions of the Talus. J Bone Joint Surg Am 2018;100(21):1838–44.
54. Shimozono Y, Donders JCE, Yasui Y, et al. Effect of the containment type on clinical outcomes in osteochondral lesions of the talus treated with autologous osteochondral transplantation. Am J Sports Med 2018;46(9):2096–102.
55. Maia FR, Carvalho MR, Oliveira JM, et al. Tissue engineering strategies for osteochondral repair. Adv Exp Med Biol 2018;1059:353–71.
56. Mendes LF, Katagiri H, Tam WL, et al. Advancing osteochondral tissue engineering: bone morphogenetic protein, transforming growth factor, and fibroblast growth factor signaling drive ordered differentiation of periosteal cells resulting in stable cartilage and bone formation in vivo. Stem Cell Res Ther 2018;9(1):42.
57. Hu Y, Guo Q, Jiao C, et al. Treatment of large cystic medial osteochondral lesions of the talus with autologous osteoperiosteal cylinder grafts. Arthroscopy 2013; 29(8):1372–9.
58. Sung MS, Jeong CH, Lim YS, et al. Periosteal autograft for articular cartilage defects in dogs: MR imaging and ultrasonography of the repair process. Acta Radiol 2011;52(2):181–90.
59. Usuelli FG, D'Ambrosi R, Maccario C, et al. All-arthroscopic AMIC® (AT-AMIC®) technique with autologous bone graft for talar osteochondral defects: clinical and radiological results. Knee Surg Sports Traumatol Arthrosc 2018;26(3):875–81.
60. Miller JR, Dunn KW. Subchondroplasty of the ankle: a novel technique. Foot Ankle Online J 2015;8(1):7.
61. McWilliams GD, Yao L, Simonet LB, et al. Subchondroplasty of the ankle and hindfoot for treatment of osteochondral lesions and stress fractures: initial imaging experience. Foot Ankle Spec 2019;13(4):306–14.
62. Hanselman A, Cody E, Easley M, et al. Iatrogenic avascular necrosis of the talus following subchondroplasty [abstract]. AOFAS Annual Meeting 2019. Foot Ankle Orthop 2019;4(4).

Recognition of Failure Modes of Lateral Ankle Ligament Reconstruction
Revision and Salvage Options

Fred T. Finney, MD[a], Todd A. Irwin, MD[b],*

KEYWORDS

- Ankle instability • Lateral ankle ligaments • Surgical treatment
- Failed surgical stabilization • Revision ankle stabilization

KEY POINTS

- Primary lateral ankle ligament reconstruction has a high success rate, but failures may lead to recurrent instability.
- Patients with recurrent ankle instability following a stabilization procedure should be carefully evaluated to determine the cause of failure.
- A common underlying reason for failure of lateral ankle ligament reconstruction is cavovarus foot deformity, which must be addressed at the time of revision surgery.
- Anatomic and nonanatomic lateral ligament reconstructions have been described.
- The authors' preferred technique uses a semitendinosus allograft tendon to create an anatomic reconstruction of the anterior talofibular ligament and calcaneofibular ligament.

INTRODUCTION

Ankle sprain is one of the most common athletic injuries across all sports, and 85% of these injuries involve the lateral ankle ligament complex.[1–4] Most ankle sprains are successfully treated nonoperatively with a period of immobilization followed by functional bracing and physical therapy focused on proprioceptive training and kinetic chain strengthening.[1,5,6] However, lateral ankle instability may persist in 10% to 20% of cases following a sprain.[7] Instability may be mechanical, where laxity of the tibiotalar joint is demonstrable on physical examination, or functional, in which patients report a subjective feeling of instability. In both instances, lateral ankle instability may prevent an athlete from performing at the highest level, and surgical consideration is warranted. Primary surgical treatment options for lateral ankle instability are

[a] Peachtree Orthopedics, 3200 Downwood Circle NW, Suite 700, Atlanta, GA 30327, USA;
[b] OrthoCarolina Foot and Ankle Institute, Atrium Health Musculoskeletal Institute, 2001 Vail Avenue, Suite 200B, Charlotte, NC 28207, USA
* Corresponding author.
E-mail address: todd.irwin@orthocarolina.com

Foot Ankle Clin N Am 26 (2021) 137–153
https://doi.org/10.1016/j.fcl.2020.10.005
1083-7515/21/© 2020 Elsevier Inc. All rights reserved.

discussed elsewhere in this issue, including both open and minimally invasive proced-ures as well as arthroscopic techniques. The most common primary procedure con-tinues to be the modified Brostrom direct anatomic reconstruction.[8]

Failure rates of primary lateral ankle reconstructions range from 2% to 18% and may lead to recurrent instability.[9] Early recurrence of instability is most often caused by inadequate reconstruction of the anatomic constraints or reinjury, where an athlete sustains an ankle inversion injury leading to retearing of the lateral ankle ligament com-plex.[10] Two studies report a 6% failure rate after modified Brostrom procedures, with each failure secondary to repeat injury during athletic activity.[11,12] Late recurrence is often caused by chronic, repetitive minor trauma.[13] In both instances, consideration must be given to predisposing biological or mechanical factors for failure.

Biological factors for failure may include generalized joint hypermobility and con-nective tissue disorders, such as Ehlers-Danlos or Marfan syndrome.[6,10,13] For hyper-mobile individuals, ankle joint hypermobility has been reported as high as 93%, but recent studies have found no increased risk of ankle injury in athletes with generalized joint hypermobility.[14–16] Although little has been reported on failures of lateral ankle lig-ament reconstruction, generalized joint hypermobility has been associated with failure of lateral ligament repairs in at least 1 study.[17] For these patients, the quality of the re-sidual ligaments and soft tissues may be inadequate for successful repair and treat-ment of instability.

The mechanical axis of the ankle and hindfoot may also be a predisposing factor to primary ankle instability as well as failure of lateral ligament reconstruction. Varus alignment of the tibiotalar joint and/or cavovarus deformity of the foot medialize the weight-bearing axis in relation to the ankle, which results in higher stresses on the lateral ankle ligament complex.[10] If the underlying mechanical deformity is not addressed, athletes may be at increased risk of reinjury and recurrent instability following primary lateral ligament repair.[10,13,18,19]

CLINICAL EVALUATION

A detailed history is the first step in evaluation of a patient who has undergone a lateral ankle stabilization procedure and presents with a complaint of recurrent instability. First, it is important to understand what symptoms the patient experienced before the initial procedure and whether or not the instability improved after surgery and appropriate postoperative rehabilitation. The operative report of the primary proced-ure should be reviewed. The surgeon should determine whether the recurrent insta-bility is the result of insufficient stabilization/repair at the time of surgery; an acute traumatic event; or chronic, repetitive minor trauma. A family history of hypermobility disorders should be further investigated. In addition, history should be obtained regarding the location of pain and associated symptoms to identify other possible concomitant foot and ankle disorder. Inquiring about nonoperative treatment since the recurrence of symptoms, including physical therapy and bracing, may also be helpful in developing a treatment plan.

Physical examination begins with inspection of the patient's weight-bearing align-ment and evaluation of gait. Varus malalignment of the mechanical axis of the ankle and hindfoot can predispose patients to increased stress to the lateral ligament repair and repetitive injury if not addressed at the time of surgery. Coleman block testing may be useful in determining whether varus malalignment of the hindfoot is forefoot driven, caused by a plantarflexed first ray, as well as whether the deformity is fixed or flex-ible.[20] Range of motion of the ankle, hindfoot, and transverse tarsal joints should be evaluated and compared with the contralateral side. Limitations in range of motion may be related to a tarsal coalition, which may predispose the patient to repetitive injury and recurrent instability. In addition, pain or crepitus with tibiotalar range of motion may indicate intra-articular disorder such as an osteochondral lesion, loose body, or bony impingement lesions. Palpation of the ankle joint line, sinus tarsi, lateral ankle ligaments, deltoid ligament, and peroneal tendons should be performed. Although tenderness over the anterior talofibular ligament (ATFL) or calcaneofibular ligament (CFL) may be expected, other points of tenderness may indicate other associated disorders. Muscle strength testing should be assessed, including evaluation of the peroneal tendons, which act as dynamic lateral ankle stabilizers. In addition, ankle stability should be assessed manually with anterior drawer and talar tilt testing. More recently, the anterolateral drawer test has been described as being more sensitive to detecting subtle instability.[21] If there is any concern for generalized hypermobility, ligamentous laxity should be evaluated using the Beighton criteria.[22]

Radiographic evaluation begins with weight-bearing radiographs of the ankle, including anteroposterior (AP), mortise, and lateral views. Attention should be paid to the bony alignment of the ankle and hindfoot. In addition, the presence of hardware, bone tunnels, and/or suture anchors should be noted. Further evaluation may include weight-bearing AP and oblique views of the foot, anterior drawer and talar tilt stress views, contralateral comparison views, and/or Saltzman hindfoot alignment views.[23] Radiographic stress testing is controversial because many surgeons think that the diagnosis of both primary and recurrent ankle instability is best determined clinically. For surgeons who rely on or use radiographic stress testing, anterior drawer stress testing should be measured on the lateral radiograph. Anterior translation of 5 mm greater than the contralateral side or an absolute value greater than 9 mm indicates instability.[24] A talar tilt stress test is measured on the mortise view and considered positive when the talar tilt angle is 5° greater than the contralateral side or an absolute value greater than 10°.[24] Less commonly, subtalar stress radiographs may be obtained to evaluate subtalar instability when a patient has recurrent instability with normal talar tilt values on stress radiographs. These images are obtained with the ankle in dorsiflexion and 30° of internal rotation and the x-ray tube angled 45° caudocephalad. With inversion stressing, medial displacement of the calcaneus on the talus by more than 5 mm indicates a positive test. However, it is the authors' opinion that this test is difficult to interpret, with limited reproducibility. In patients in whom subtalar instability is suspected, reconstructive efforts should limit subtalar motion.[24,25] This limitation would typically be achieved by either a nonanatomic reconstruction or anatomic allograft reconstruction, which would create a ligamentous strut crossing the lateral subtalar joint as part of the reconstruction. Further details regarding both of these procedures are discussed later.

MRI is primarily used for evaluating osteochondral lesions or other suspected intra-articular disorders. It is also helpful in assessing for surrounding soft tissue disorders such as peroneal tendon tears or tenosynovitis, or deltoid ligament injury. However, MRI is less useful in evaluating the lateral ankle ligament complex following a reconstruction because of chronic postsurgical changes and possibly metallic suture anchors creating image artifact. Computed tomography scans may help with preoperative planning if prior bone tunnels were performed during the initial reconstruction.

SURGICAL TECHNIQUES/OPTIONS

The surgical plan then needs to be designed to address both the associated deformity, if present, as well as the ligament instability. Although not every patient with recurrent instability requires deformity correction, it is important to recognize and potentially correct any associated deformity concurrent with the revision ligament reconstruction. The surgeon should also consider location of previous incisions, presence of implants, and possible bone tunnels during the preoperative planning stage. Multiple options and considerations are outlined later regarding these concepts.

Deformity Correction

The most common underlying reason for failure of lateral ankle ligament reconstruction from a deformity standpoint is the cavovarus foot deformity. As noted earlier, the components of the cavovarus foot include a plantarflexed first ray and hindfoot varus. Also prevalent, but less common, are supramalleolar deformities of the tibia and significant midfoot cavus deformities. These types of deformities lead to overload of the lateral column of the foot and excess stress on the lateral ankle. If these deformities go unrecognized during the initial lateral ligament reconstruction, failure is more likely to occur. Not every cavovarus deformity requires surgical correction during the initial procedure, but, in the revision setting, deformity correction should be strongly considered. The patient's athletic status should also be taken into account. In high-level and elite athletes, the decision to perform deformity correction with osteotomies can be difficult given the increased time to recovery and potential for increased complications. In addition, osteotomies that create asymmetry compared with the opposite side may have an effect on the athlete's ability to perform because of the biomechanical change in alignment. No studies have shown what effect these osteotomies may have on the elite athletes' ability to return to play, but, if the persistent lateral ankle instability is preventing high-level performance, this may be the athlete's only way to achieve stability. Although there are no definitive rules as to when deformity correction should be undertaken in athletes, some general considerations include when there is underlying significant asymmetry in the deformity (ie, moderate to severe hindfoot varus or plantarflexed first ray), presence of other foot or ankle disorder that may be caused by the deformity (eg, stress fractures), or multiple previous failures.

Cavovarus Foot

In the setting of a flexible, forefoot-driven cavovarus deformity as confirmed by the Coleman block test,[20,26] a dorsiflexion first metatarsal osteotomy is indicated. This procedure can be performed in isolation or concurrent with other osteotomies or procedures. If the deformity is not flexible, or there is residual hindfoot varus on Coleman block, then adding a lateralizing calcaneal osteotomy is indicated. Multiple options exist for this procedure, including the Dwyer closing wedge osteotomy, the Z closing wedge osteotomy, or a lateral displacement calcaneal osteotomy.[27] Newer techniques include performing the lateral displacement calcaneal osteotomy through a minimally invasive approach, which may be advantageous for athletes because of less soft tissue dissection and disruption.[28]

Varus supramalleolar tibial deformities may also contribute to recurrent lateral ankle ligament instability. In this situation, the surgeon should consider addressing this deformity with a supramalleolar tibial osteotomy. Options include a medial opening wedge osteotomy, lateral closing wedge osteotomy, or a dome osteotomy.[29]

REVISION LATERAL ANKLE LIGAMENT RECONSTRUCTION

Techniques for revision lateral ankle ligament reconstruction can be grouped into 2 categories: nonanatomic reconstruction, and anatomic reconstruction. The nonanatomic procedures have mostly fallen out of favor because of the significant restriction of the subtalar joint that results; however, some modifications are still used, especially if significant subtalar instability is suspected. In addition, improvement in both technique and implant technology has allowed anatomic reconstructions to be more widely adopted.

Nonanatomic Reconstruction

Historically, several procedures have been described using the peroneus brevis tendon to either stabilize the lateral ankle or try to reconstruct the lateral ankle ligaments. The Watson-Jones procedure involved routing the cut peroneus brevis tendon from posterior to anterior through the fibula and then into the neck of the talus, leaving its distal attachment.[30] The Evans procedure routes the peroneus brevis tendon through the fibula from anterior to posterior in an oblique fashion and then sutured back to itself proximally, again leaving its distal attachment on the base of the fifth metatarsal.[31] The Chrisman-Snook[32] procedure involves taking a split peroneus brevis graft and routing it from the neck of the talus, through the fibula anterior to posterior, then inferior to the calcaneus.

Although most of these procedures have been abandoned, some modifications are still used in certain clinical situations. The modified Brostrom-Evans procedure involves performing a standard Brostrom procedure with vest-over-pants reconstruction of the ATFL, then adding a transfer of the anterior one-third of the peroneus brevis tendon into the distal fibula at an oblique angle and securing with an interference screw.[33,34] (**Fig. 1**). The Evans portion of the procedure (peroneus brevis transfer) is meant to provide more robust control of the coronal plane instability present. Indications for this procedure include laborers, patients with high body mass index, subtalar instability, and some athletes (typically larger athletes with specific athletic requirements, such as football lineman). Hsu and colleagues[33] reported on 19 patients with average 8.7-year follow-up, showing good outcome and pain scores and retained peroneal function as measured by eversion strength and range of motion compared with the opposite side. However, a 41% decrease in ankle inversion range of motion compared with the nonoperative extremity was seen.[33] It should be noted that, although most of these procedures can be used in the revision setting, the published reports were typically used in the primary setting.

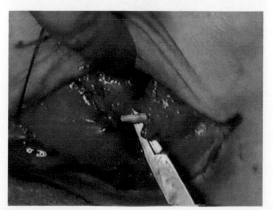

Fig. 1. Clinical picture of the Brostrom-Evans procedure showing the transfer of the anterior one-third of the peroneus brevis tendon into the fibula.

Anatomic Reconstruction

As noted earlier, the modified Brostrom-Gould procedure is typically performed for primary lateral ankle ligament reconstruction.[8] Some recent modifications and implant advancements may allow using this procedure for revision surgery.

Suture-Tape Augmentation

Adding a suture-tape augmentation to the typical Brostrom reconstruction is one technique to potentially strengthen the reconstruction as well as to protect the ligaments to allow early rehabilitation. This technique has become popular in recent years in certain clinical scenarios for primary lateral ankle ligament reconstruction, including ligamentous laxity and in the athletic population when surgeons want to accelerate rehabilitation. This procedure can also be considered in the revision setting if adequate soft tissue remains for a revision Brostrom reconstruction. It is nearly impossible to determine preoperatively whether adequate soft tissue will be present during the revision surgery. If the quality and excursion of the scar tissue present as a result of the initial surgery allows a stable reconstruction, then proceeding with the revision Brostrom and adding suture-tape augmentation is reasonable. If the quality of the tissue is poor or absent, then an alternative procedure should be chosen.

Suture-tape augmentation involves securing the suture-tape implant first into the talar neck at the footprint of the ATFL using an anchor. The standard vest-over-pants Brostrom reconstruction is performed and the suture-tape implant is passed over the top of the native ligament. Then the suture tape is secured into the fibula again with an anchor at appropriate tension (**Fig. 2**). There should be 1 to 2 mm of laxity in the implant to avoid overtightening and allow physiologic motion of the ankle ligaments.[4]

Coetzee and colleagues[4] reported on 81 patients treated with Brostrom and suture-tape augmentation at median follow-up 11.5 months postoperatively. In addition to

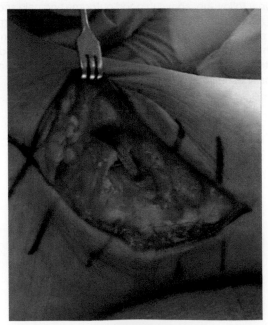

Fig. 2. Clinical picture showing the suture-tape augmentation of a Brostrom reconstruction. (*Courtesy of* J. K. Ellington, MD, Charlotte, NC.)

high clinical outcome and satisfaction scores, multiple functional tests were performed. Single-leg hop test revealed 86.4% of patients returned to normal or near-normal function and mean return to sport was 84.1 days.[4] Cho and colleagues[35] specifically investigated suture-tape augmentation in the revision setting. Twenty-four patients were evaluated after failing a standard Brostrom procedure. Revision Brostrom augmented with suture tape was performed with mean follow-up 38.5 months. Functional outcome scores improved significantly, and side-to-side stress radiograph comparison showed no significant difference. One patient failed and required revision to an allograft reconstruction.

Anatomic Reconstruction with Autograft/Allograft Tendon

Using either autograft or allograft tendon to replace the native ATFL and CFL is another technique frequently used to reconstruct the lateral ankle ligaments. Several different techniques have been described. The most commonly reported techniques involve hamstring tendons inserted with tenodesis screws in an anatomic or near-anatomic orientation. Gracilis tendon harvest from the proximal tibia is the most common autograft used.[36] However, using allograft tendon, typically either gracilis or semitendinosus, has become more popular and several studies have proved its efficacy.[37–40]

Coughlin and colleagues[36] reported on 28 patients who underwent a direct ATFL repair augmented with a free gracilis autograft inserted in an anatomic orientation. Although there were no revision cases in this cohort, all 28 patients reported good or excellent clinical outcome and satisfaction scores, and preoperative and postoperative stress radiographs showed significantly improved stability. Miller and colleagues[39] described a near-anatomic technique using semitendinosus allograft that was passed from the neck of the talus posteriorly through the fibula and then inferiorly into the calcaneus. Twelve of the 28 patients in this study were revisions, with 9 having prior Brostrom type reconstructions and 3 having prior nonanatomic split peroneus brevis reconstructions. At an average 32-month follow-up, pain and satisfaction scores were significantly improved, 3 patients had mild persistent instability, and no patients required revision surgery. Dierckman and Ferkel[40] described using semitendinosus allograft in an orientation that more closely replicated the anatomic position of the ATFL and CFL. In their cohort of 31 patients with mean follow-up of 38 months, 100% were completely satisfied with the procedure, pain and outcome scores significantly improved, and stress radiographs showed significantly improved stability. Six patients in this group had failed prior lateral ankle ligament reconstruction (5 Brostroms, 1 Watson-Jones).

AUTHORS' PREFERRED TECHNIQUE
Anatomic Reconstruction with Semitendinosus Allograft and Interference Screws

When the decision to proceed with revision lateral ankle ligament reconstruction has been made, the surgeon must also consider whether ankle arthroscopy and cavovarus reconstruction also need to be performed. Ankle arthroscopy should be performed if any osteochondral lesions need to be addressed at the time of the surgery, or if there are bony impingement lesions that are contributing to pain and would not be accessible from the surgical dissection (ie, anteromedial ankle joint). Ankle joint pain in addition to the ligament instability, in particular with anteromedial tenderness to palpation, triggers a low threshold to perform ankle arthroscopy at the beginning of the procedure.

If cavovarus reconstruction is required, this is typically done after the ankle arthroscopy but before the lateral ligament reconstruction. Osteotomies are typically performed sequentially from proximal to distal so that the deformity correction can be evaluated after each step. For example, if a supramalleolar osteotomy gives enough coronal plane correction, then a lateralizing calcaneal osteotomy may not be needed. Dorsiflexion first metatarsal osteotomy is typically performed after the lateralizing calcaneal osteotomy, and is sometimes the only osteotomy that is required based on preoperative planning. One technical issue to consider during the lateralizing calcaneal osteotomy is the location of screw fixation. Because the CFL arm of the allograft reconstruction will require drilling into the calcaneus and placing a tenodesis screw, placement of screws for the osteotomy should leave enough room for this step of the procedure.

Surgical Technique

- The patient is positioned supine with a bump under the ipsilateral hip, making sure the leg is internally rotated to allow adequate access to the lateral ankle. Curvilinear incision is made overlying the posterior one-third of the distal fibula and carrying this distally along the inferior portion of the sinus tarsi. The incision may have to be modified based on presence of previous incisions and timing since the previous surgery. Dissection should allow exposure of the entire distal fibula and ankle capsule, the peroneal tendon sheath, and the inferior extensor retinaculum (**Fig. 3**).
- The ankle capsule, ATFL, and CFL are incised along the anterior and distal border of the fibula, taking care to avoid damaging the peroneal tendons. The peroneal

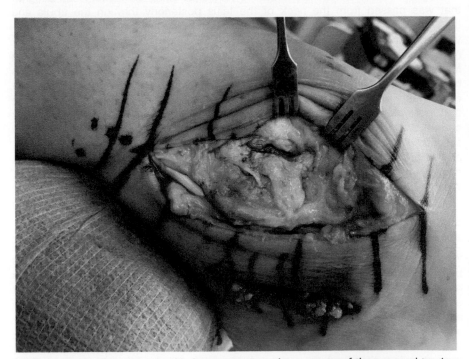

Fig. 3. Exposure of the lateral ankle ligaments. Note the exposure of the peroneal tendons proximally, and the incision posteriorly for the lateralizing calcaneal osteotomy.

tendon sheath needs to be opened distally to allow inferior retraction. An incision should also be made in the peroneal tendon sheath proximal to the superior peroneal retinaculum (SPR) to allow for manipulation of the allograft during placement. The SPR should be preserved.

- The capsule and periosteum of the distal fibula is slightly elevated to expose the anatomic footprint of the ATFL and CFL insertion. The capsule and scar tissue should be dissected distally to expose the talar neck just distal to the articular surface. The peroneal tendons should be retracted inferiorly and the periosteum of the lateral calcaneus can be elevated at the site of the CFL insertion.
- The semitendinosus allograft should be thawed. Once thawed, tag sutures should be placed on either end using #1 or #2 nonabsorbable suture. Alternatively, presutured and appropriately sized tendons are commercially available (**Fig. 4**). Some surgeons advocate pretensioning of the allograft before implantation as supported by described techniques for anterior cruciate ligament reconstruction.[41] However, no studies have evaluated the necessity of pretensioning for lateral ankle ligament reconstruction, and the authors have used both techniques (pretension, and no pretension) and anecdotally have found no difference in clinical results.
- The allograft is initially placed at the ATFL insertion site on the talus. A beath pin is placed just distal to the lateral talus articular cartilage at the neck-body junction and carried through the medial side. Based on the size of the graft, an appropriately sized hole is reamed into the talus but not through the far cortex. The beath pin is used to deliver 1 end of the allograft into the reamed hole in the talar neck. The suture is pulled medially, docking the allograft into the base of the reamed hole, and an appropriately sized interference screw is placed (**Fig. 5**).

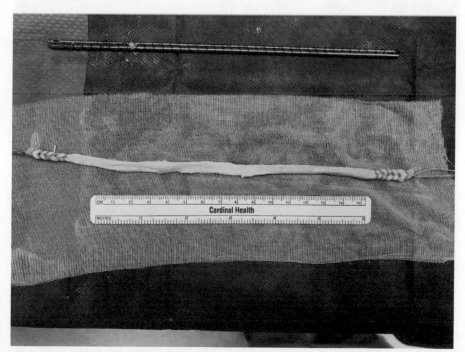

Fig. 4. Presutured semitendinosus allograft with tag sutures on either end.

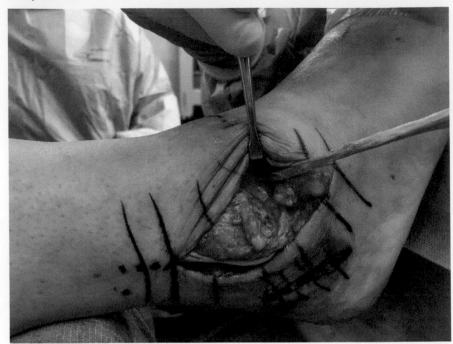

Fig. 5. Initial docking of the allograft into the lateral talus neck-body junction with interference screw.

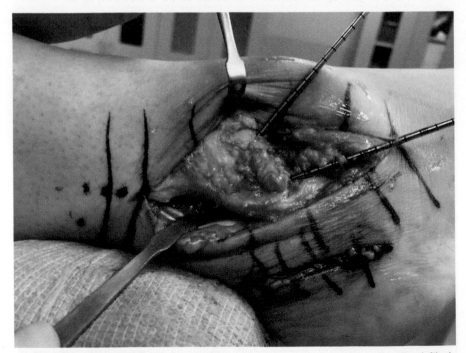

Fig. 6. Beath pin placement at the insertion site of the ATFL and CFL in the distal fibula. Note the Hohmann retractor protecting the peroneal tendons, and the bridge of bone between the 2 pins posteriorly.

- The beath pin is then passed into the fibula at an oblique angle, starting at the ATFL insertion site on the anterior distal fibula and aiming proximally. A second beath pin can then be passed from the insertion site of the CFL on the anterior aspect of the distal tip of the fibula, aiming to exit the posterior fibula just distal to the first beath pin. It is important to protect the peroneal tendons with a Hohmann retractor while passing the pins and reaming (**Fig. 6**).
- Both pins can then be reamed with an appropriately sized reamer (typically around 5 mm, but this may depend on the size of the graft chosen). The authors prefer to leave a bridge of bone posteriorly between the reamed holes as opposed to a sharp edge of bone that the allograft will wrap around.
- The beath pin can then be inserted in the calcaneus, posterior and inferior to the second reamed hole in the fibula, at the insertion site of the CFL. The peroneal tendons are aggressively retracted inferiorly to access this site. The pin is aimed posteriorly and inferiorly and exits out the medial side of the heel. If screws had been placed for a calcaneal osteotomy previously, it is important to try to avoid

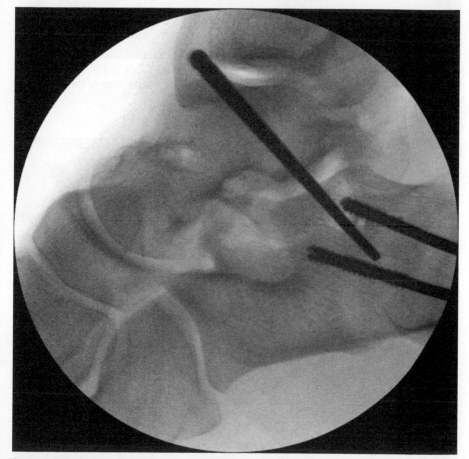

Fig. 7. Intraoperative fluoroscopic radiograph showing the position of the beath pin for the calcaneal interference screw placed between the 2 previously placed screws for the lateralizing calcaneal osteotomy.

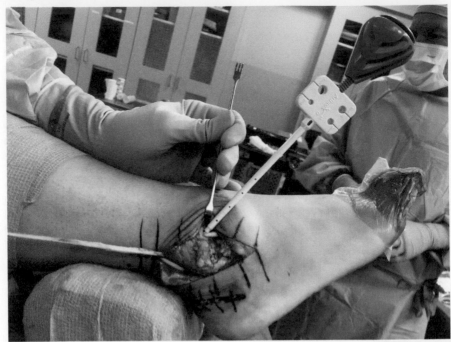

Fig. 8. After the allograft is delivered into the superior reamed hole of the fibula, the tension is set manually and an interference screw is placed. Note the position of the bump, and the posterior translation of the ankle.

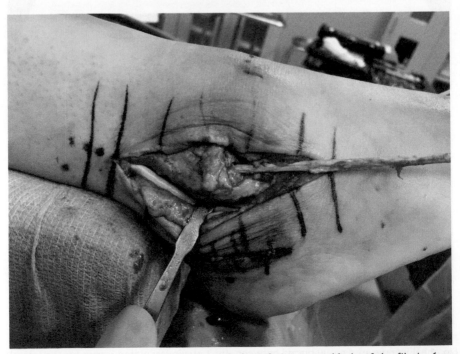

Fig. 9. The allograft is delivered back through the inferior reamed hole of the fibula, from posterior to anterior.

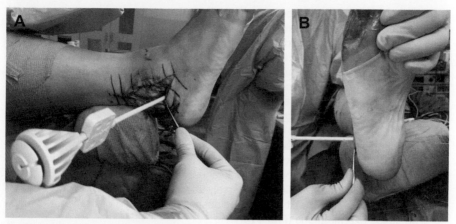

Fig. 10. (*A, B*) The final interference screw is placed into the calcaneus while pulling tension on the graft from the medial side.

these screws with the beath pin. Fluoroscopy may need to be used. An appropriately sized hole is then reamed through the entire calcaneus (**Fig. 7**).

- The free allograft end is then passed into the superior reamed hole in the fibula using a suture passer. The authors prefer to independently tension this limb of the graft with a manual pull while also posteriorly translating the talus. An

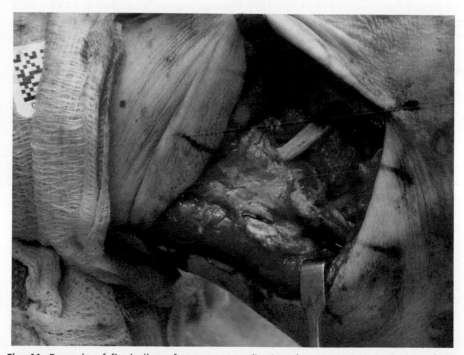

Fig. 11. Example of final allograft construct replicating the anatomic orientation of the ATFL and CFL.

appropriately sized interference screw is then placed into the fibula, thereby setting the tension of the reconstructed ATFL (**Fig. 8**).

- The allograft is then passed from posterior to anterior through the inferior reamed hole in the fibula (**Fig. 9**). It is finally passed into the reamed hole in the calcaneus using the beath pin, making sure the graft is deep to the peroneal tendons. With the foot held in a neutral to everted position, the tag sutures are manually pulled to tension the graft and the final interference screw is placed into the calcaneus (**Fig. 10**A,B). Because the bone in the calcaneal tuberosity is soft, the interference screw is typically press fit by sizing it 0.5 to 1 mm larger than the reamed hole. Care should be taken to ensure appropriate length of the allograft, because excess graft may be pulled into the medial soft tissues of the heel, which could prevent appropriate tension to the calcaneal limb of the graft.
- Final construct should replicate as closely as possible the anatomic orientation of the ATFL and CFL. Stability should be assessed with anterior drawer and inversion stress examinations (**Fig. 11**).

Aftercare

The patient is immobilized in a short-leg non–weight-bearing splint with the foot in slight eversion for the initial 2 weeks. For allograft reconstruction, the authors prefer cast immobilization for the following 4 weeks. Weight-bearing status during these 4 weeks is determined by the concomitant procedures. An isolated allograft ligament reconstruction can be weight bearing as tolerated in the cast. When osteotomies are performed for cavovarus reconstruction, non–weight bearing is preferred until 6 weeks nonoperatively. The patient is then transitioned to a tall walking boot until 10 to 12 weeks postoperatively. Ankle lace-up brace is used once out of the boot, which the patient can wean out of as tolerated. Physical therapy is initiated at 6 to 8 weeks postoperatively, with restrictions of no passive inversion greater than 10° until 10 weeks postoperatively.

SUMMARY

Revision of a failed lateral ankle stabilization procedure can be challenging, in particular when considering a high-level athlete and the associated demands that are placed on the lower extremities and the lateral ligaments specifically. There is a paucity of literature regarding revision lateral ankle ligament procedures and outcomes. Mechanisms of failure may include biological factors or mechanical factors. It is essential to address the underlying cause of failure with any revision procedure. A common underlying reason for failure of lateral ankle ligament reconstruction is cavovarus foot deformity, which may be treated with a dorsiflexion osteotomy of the first ray or a lateralizing calcaneal osteotomy to prevent repetitive stresses on the lateral ligament reconstruction. No studies have shown what effect these osteotomies may have on the ability of elite athletes to return to play. The modified Brostrom-Gould procedure is typically performed for primary lateral ankle ligament reconstruction, but it may be used in revision stabilization procedures, often with a suture-tape augmentation. Nonanatomic reconstructions are primarily based on rerouting the peroneus brevis tendon, which may limit subtalar motion. However, anatomic reconstructions of the ATFL and CFL using tendon autograft or allograft have gained more favor.

The authors' preferred technique uses a semitendinosus allograft and interference screw fixation to perform an anatomic reconstruction of the ATFL and CFL. This technique minimizes the donor site morbidity associated with autograft harvest, restores the anatomic restraints of the ATFL and CFL without limiting subtalar motion, and provides a robust tissue reconstruction in a revision setting. Further studies are needed to provide evidence of the optimum stabilization procedure in the revision setting.

DISCLOSURE

The authors have nothing to disclose.

REFERENCES

1. Maffulli N, Ferran NA. Management of acute and chronic ankle instability. J Am Acad Orthop Surg 2008;16(10):608–15.
2. Beynnon BD, Murphy DF, Alosa DM. Predictive factors for lateral ankle sprains: a literature review. J Athl Train 2002;37(4):376–80.
3. Roos KG, Kerr ZY, Mauntel TC, et al. The epidemiology of lateral ligament complex ankle sprains in national collegiate athletic association sports. Am J Sports Med 2017;45(1):201–9.
4. Coetzee JC, Ellington JK, Ronan JA, et al. Functional results of open broström ankle ligament repair augmented with a suture tape. Foot Ankle Int 2018;39(3): 304–10.
5. van den Bekerom MPJ, Kerkhoffs GMMJ, McCollum GA, et al. Management of acute lateral ankle ligament injury in the athlete. Knee Surg Sports Traumatol Arthrosc 2013;21(6):1390–5.
6. Schenck RC, Coughlin MJ. Lateral ankle instability and revision surgery alternatives in the athlete. Foot Ankle Clin 2009;14(2):205–14.
7. de Vries JS, Krips R, Sierevelt IN, et al. Interventions for treating chronic ankle instability. Cochrane Database Syst Rev 2011;8:CD004124.
8. Gould N, Seligson D, Gassman J. Early and late repair of lateral ligament of the ankle. Foot Ankle 1980;1(2):84–9.
9. Sammarco GJ, Carrasquillo HA. Surgical revision after failed lateral ankle reconstruction. Foot Ankle Int 1995;16(12):748–53.
10. Sammarco VJ. Complications of lateral ankle ligament reconstruction. Clin Orthop 2001;391:123–32.
11. Petrera M, Dwyer T, Theodoropoulos JS, et al. Short- to medium-term outcomes after a modified broström repair for lateral ankle instability with immediate postoperative weightbearing. Am J Sports Med 2014;42(7):1542–8.
12. Li X, Killie H, Guerrero P, et al. Anatomical reconstruction for chronic lateral ankle instability in the high-demand athlete: functional outcomes after the modified Broström repair using suture anchors. Am J Sports Med 2009;37(3):488–94.
13. O'Neil JT, Guyton GP. Revision of surgical lateral ankle ligament stabilization. Foot Ankle Clin 2018;23(4):605–24.
14. Kamanli A, Sahin S, Ozgocmen S, et al. Relationship between foot angles and hypermobility scores and assessment of foot types in hypermobile individuals. Foot Ankle Int 2004;25(2):101–6.
15. Pacey V, Nicholson LL, Adams RD, et al. Generalized joint hypermobility and risk of lower limb joint injury during sport: a systematic review with meta-analysis. Am J Sports Med 2010;38(7):1487–97.
16. Blokland D, Thijs KM, Backx FJG, et al. No effect of generalized joint hypermobility on injury risk in elite female soccer players: a prospective cohort study. Am J Sports Med 2017;45(2):286–93.
17. Karlsson J, Bergsten T, Lansinger O, et al. Reconstruction of the lateral ligaments of the ankle for chronic lateral instability. J Bone Joint Surg Am 1988;70(4):581–8.

18. Broström L. Sprained ankles. V. Treatment and prognosis in recent ligament ruptures. Acta Chir Scand 1966;132(5):537–50.

19. Brunner R, Gaechter A. Repair of fibular ligaments: comparison of reconstructive techniques using plantaris and peroneal tendons. Foot Ankle 1991;11(6):359–67.

20. Younger ASE, Hansen ST. Adult cavovarus foot. J Am Acad Orthop Surg 2005; 13(5):302–15.

21. Miller AG, Myers SH, Parks BG, et al. Anterolateral drawer versus anterior drawer test for ankle instability: a biomechanical model. Foot Ankle Int 2016;37(4): 407–10.

22. Remvig L, Jensen DV, Ward RC. Are diagnostic criteria for general joint hypermobility and benign joint hypermobility syndrome based on reproducible and valid tests? A review of the literature. J Rheumatol 2007;34(4):798–803.

23. Saltzman CL, el-Khoury GY. The hindfoot alignment view. Foot Ankle Int 1995; 16(9):572–6.

24. Colville MR. Surgical treatment of the unstable ankle. J Am Acad Orthop Surg 1998;6(6):368–77.

25. Thermann H, Zwipp H, Tscherne H. Treatment algorithm of chronic ankle and subtalar instability. Foot Ankle Int 1997;18(3):163–9.

26. Coleman SS, Chesnut WJ. A simple test for hindfoot flexibility in the cavovarus foot. Clin Orthop 1977;123:60–2.

27. Cody EA, Kraszewski AP, Conti MS, et al. Lateralizing calcaneal osteotomies and their effect on calcaneal alignment: a three-dimensional digital model analysis. Foot Ankle Int 2018;39(8):970–7.

28. Gutteck N, Zeh A, Wohlrab D, et al. Comparative results of percutaneous calcaneal osteotomy in correction of hindfoot deformities. Foot Ankle Int 2019;40(3): 276–81.

29. Hintermann B, Knupp M, Barg A. Supramalleolar osteotomies for the treatment of ankle arthritis. J Am Acad Orthop Surg 2016;24(7):424–32.

30. Watson-Jones R. Fractures and Joint Injuries. Edinburgh: Livingstone, LTD; 1955.

31. Evans DL. Recurrent instability of the ankle; a method of surgical treatment. Proc R Soc Med 1953;46(5):343–4.

32. Chrisman OD, Snook GA. Reconstruction of lateral ligament tears of the ankle. An experimental study and clinical evaluation of seven patients treated by a new modification of the Elmslie procedure. J Bone Joint Surg Am 1969;51(5):904–12.

33. Hsu AR, Ardoin GT, Davis WH, et al. Intermediate and long-term outcomes of the modified brostrom-evans procedure for lateral ankle ligament reconstruction. Foot Ankle Spec 2016;9(2):131–9.

34. Girard P, Anderson RB, Davis WH, et al. Clinical evaluation of the modified Brostrom-Evans procedure to restore ankle stability. Foot Ankle Int 1999;20(4): 246–52.

35. Cho BK, Kim YM, Choi SM, et al. Revision anatomical reconstruction of the lateral ligaments of the ankle augmented with suture tape for patients with a failed Broström procedure. Bone Joint J 2017;99-B(9):1183–9.

36. Coughlin MJ, Schenck RC, Grebing BR, et al. Comprehensive reconstruction of the lateral ankle for chronic instability using a free gracilis graft. Foot Ankle Int 2004;25(4):231–41.

37. Jung H-G, Shin M-H, Park J-T, et al. Anatomical reconstruction of lateral ankle ligaments using free tendon allografts and biotenodesis screws. Foot Ankle Int 2015;36(9):1064–71.

38. Jung H-G, Kim T-H, Park J-Y, et al. Anatomic reconstruction of the anterior talofib-ular and calcaneofibular ligaments using a semitendinosus tendon allograft and interference screws. Knee Surg Sports Traumatol Arthrosc 2012;20(8):1432–7.
39. Miller AG, Raikin SM, Ahmad J. Near-anatomic allograft tenodesis of chronic lateral ankle instability. Foot Ankle Int 2013;34(11):1501–7.
40. Dierckman BD, Ferkel RD. Anatomic reconstruction with a semitendinosus allo-graft for chronic lateral ankle instability. Am J Sports Med 2015;43(8):1941–50.
41. Heis FT, Paulos LE. Tensioning of the anterior cruciate ligament graft. Orthop Clin North Am 2002;33(4):697–700.

Anterior and Posterior Ankle Impingement Syndromes
Arthroscopic and Endoscopic Anatomy and Approaches to Treatment

Caio Nery, MD, PHD[a,1], Daniel Baumfeld, MD, PHD[b,*]

KEYWORDS

- Ankle pain • Anterolateral impingement • Posterior impingement • Arthroscopy
- Endoscopy

KEY POINTS

- Impingement is a clinical syndrome of end-range joint pain or motion restriction caused by the direct mechanical impact of bone or soft tissues.

- Imaging studies can show osseous and soft tissue diseases and anatomic variations that can help diagnose and treat impingement syndromes.

- Soft tissue impingement occurs more frequently on the lateral side as a consequence of synovial scarring, inflammation, and hypertrophy in the anterolateral recess of the tibiotalar joint.

- Advantages of arthroscopic treatment over open arthrotomy include reduced recovery time and earlier return to sports activities.

INTRODUCTION

Ankle impingement syndrome refers to a chronic painful mechanical limitation of the ankle caused by soft tissue or osseous abnormalities.[1] Posttraumatic synovitis, intra-articular fibrous bands/scar tissue, capsular scarring, or developmental and acquired bony spurs or prominences are the most common causes.[2] A single traumatic event or repetitive microtrauma can be the cause of this syndrome.[1] Impingement at the tibiotalar joint can be subdivided into anterior, anterolateral, anteromedial, posterior, or posteromedial, although the anterolateral soft tissue impingement is the most

[a] UNIFESP - Federal University of São Paulo, Brazil; [b] UFMG - Federal University of Minas Gerais, Brazil
[1] Present address: Av. Rouxinol, 404 - #21, Moema, São Paulo, São Paulo CEP 04516-000, Brazil.
* Corresponding author. Rua Eng. Albert Charle, 30 - #701, Luxemburgo, Belo Horizonte, Minas Gerais CEP 30380-530, Brazil.
E-mail address: danielbaumfeld@gmail.com

Foot Ankle Clin N Am 26 (2021) 155–172
https://doi.org/10.1016/j.fcl.2020.07.002
1083-7515/21/© 2020 Elsevier Inc. All rights reserved.

commonly encountered. Although ankle impingement is largely a clinical diagnosis, imaging is often used to evaluate suspected ankle impingement to confirm the presence of typical changes and as a tool for preoperative planning. Imaging also can help differentiate impingement from alternative diagnoses that may have overlapping clinical presentations,[3] such as osteochondral lesion, synovitis, loose bodies, and/or bone bruises. Currently, the preferred surgical approach to this pathology is with arthroscopic/endoscopic assistance, which provides a highly accurate means of locating and treating intra-articular abnormality.[3,4]

ANTEROLATERAL ANKLE IMPINGEMENT

Anterolateral ankle impingement (ALAI) is the result of mechanical factors, traction, trauma, recurrent microtrauma, and/or chronic ankle instability.[5] Symptoms are believed to result from the entrapment of hypertrophic soft tissues or torn and inflamed ligaments in the lateral gutter and anterolateral ankle joint.[4] Several types of soft tissue impingement have been reported, including a "meniscoid" lesion, impinging fascicle of the anterior inferior tibiofibular ligament, and hypertrophied synovium.[6]

Patients are typically young, athletic, and present with chronic ankle pain, limited dorsiflexion, and swelling, thereby reducing activity. The patient may have a history of recurrent ankle inversion injuries.[4,7] Anterolateral impingement can be differentiated from anteromedial impingement (AMAI) by the location of tenderness, which is elicited at the joint line lateral to the peroneus tertius. Forced hyperdorsiflexion may induce pain, but false negatives can occur[1,8] Transient inflammatory process, caused by trauma or any other unspecific condition, can produce temporary symptoms that mimic anterolateral or anteromedial ankle impingement. The normal soft tissue mass found in the anterior compartment of the ankle joint is compressed by the bony borders beyond 15° of dorsiflexion.[1] This compression is well tolerated and pain free for most people, but sometimes can be referred as a discomfort or a light pain and may be confused with some pathologic cause of the anterior ankle impingement.

IMAGING STUDIES

Conventional radiographs are performed in the setting of subacute or chronic anterolateral ankle pain to assess for evidence of a possible previous fracture and subsequent complication (eg, joint degeneration).[4] Radiographs allow for the assessment of both talar and tibial osteophytes, as well as the tibiotalar joint space[5]; however, radiographs are unable to assess soft tissue pathology. MRI can be useful to determine the presence of soft tissue pathology that may be causing ALAI. Furthermore, MRI allows the physician to rule out other potential differential diagnoses, including osteochondral lesions, loose bodies, and stress fractures (**Fig. 1**). Conventional axial T1-weighted images are useful for assessing scarring in the anterolateral gutter, as well as hypertrophy of the synovial tissue.[4,7,9]

The literature assessing the efficacy of standard MRI to detect anterolateral soft tissue pathology has shown a wide range of sensitivity (39%–100%) and specificity (50%–100%).[4,9,10] In a paper describing the use of MRI for diagnosis of ALAI, Ferkel and colleagues[11] determined that MRI has a sensitivity of 83.3% and specificity of 78.6% (**Fig. 2**). In our daily practice managing athletes, we always start with a clinical, radiographic, and ultrasonographic diagnosis. If there are no chondral injuries or major joint instability, local anesthetic or corticosteroid infiltrations are used as the first therapeutic line, especially during the sports season. Thus, the definitive therapy through arthroscopy or conventional surgery for mild cases can be postponed to the off

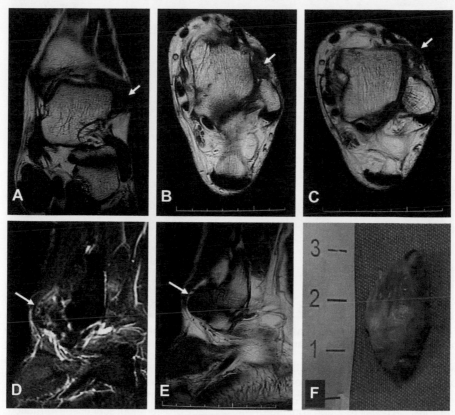

Fig. 1. (*A*) MRI coronal ankle view, (*B*, *C*) MRI transversal ankle views, and (*D*, *E*) MRI sagittal ankle views of a patient complaining of anterolateral impingement. The arrows point to the mass of soft tissues responsible for the patient's complaint. (*F*). The fibrous mass after surgical resection.

season. When lateral impingement does not improve with local management, MRI is our best option to decide the next step of diagnosis and treatment.

ANTEROMEDIAL ANKLE IMPINGEMENT

The clinical entity of AMAI, as with anterolateral impingement, is subsequent to repeated microtrauma followed by synovitis and capsular thickening. In addition, bony injury and cartilage damage may result in anteromedial spurs with associated capsular and synovial thickening. The exact mechanism responsible for anteromedial impingement is not fully understood.[7,12,13]

Different theories regarding the etiology of anteromedial impingement exist.[6] Traction to the anterior ankle capsule during forced plantar flexion in athletes (eg, soccer players) is no longer an accepted hypothesis. The anterior joint capsule is attached more proximally to the site than where the tibial spurs originate, and the osteophytes are found within the confines of the anterior joint capsule. One of the explanations for spur formation is direct mechanical trauma or recurrent microtrauma associated with impingement of the anterior articular border of the tibia and the talar neck during forced dorsiflexion.[1] In soccer players, spur formation is related to recurrent ball impact on the anteromedial side of the cartilaginous rim of the ankle.[10] Chronic ankle instability is also associated

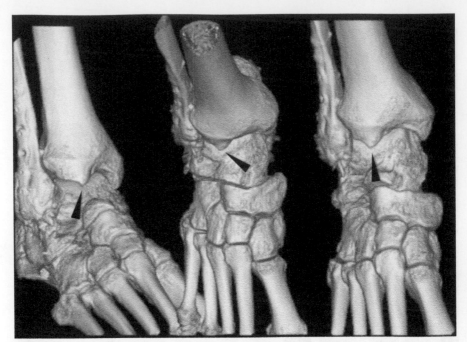

Fig. 2. Three-dimensional reconstruction of anterolateral ankle impingement. The arrowheads point to protrusion on the lateral portion of the anterior margin of the tibia.

with osteophyte formation in the medial ankle compartment.[14] Osteophytes in AMAI originate at the non–weight-bearing cartilage rim along the distal tibia, which extends up to 3 mm proximal to the joint line. Damage to this rim occurs in most supination traumas.[15] A repair reaction is initiated, with cartilage proliferation, scar tissue formation, and calcification. This reaction is further enhanced not only by ankle sprains due to chronic instability, but also by forced dorsiflexion.[13] The pain in anterior ankle impingement is likely caused by the inflamed soft tissue along the anterior tibiotalar joint line, which is compressed by the talar and tibial osteophytes during forced dorsiflexion.[4,8]

IMAGING STUDIES

Similar to the diagnosis of ALAI, diagnostic imaging for AMAI should begin with routine weight-bearing radiographs in anteroposterior (AP) and lateral directions associated with an oblique AMAI radiograph. The oblique AMAI view has been reported to detect anteromedial osteophytes that were not present on lateral radiograph with 96% sensitivity for detecting tibial osteophytes and 67% sensitivity for talar osteophytes.[6,16] The combination of forced passive dorsiflexion and forced passive plantarflexion may be useful to increase the diagnostic accuracy of conventional radiographic views.

Similar to ALAI, swelling and inflammation of the soft tissues along the joint are best assessed via MRI in patients with suspicion of AMAI. Anterior deltoid thickening, synovitis, and ossifications also can be distinguished with this modality. MRI also has the capacity to rule out differential soft tissue diagnoses, including osteochondral lesions, loose bodies, and stress fractures[9,15,17] **(Fig. 3)**.

ANTERIOR ANKLE IMPINGEMENT

Anterior ankle impingement refers to disease at the central anterior aspect of the ankle, either anterolateral or anteromedial, resulting in impingement symptoms.

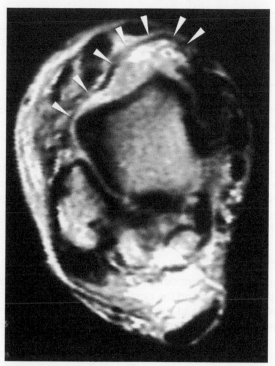

Fig. 3. MRI (transverse plane) of the ankle with anteromedial ankle impingement. The arrowheads point to extensive ossification in the anterior margin of the tibia responsible for the symptoms.

Anterior impingement is less common than anterolateral or anteromedial impingement. Anterior impingement most commonly relates to bone spurs of the anterior tibial plafond and is typically seen in athletes who subject their ankles to repetitive, forced dorsiflexion. Repeated direct microtrauma can lead to bone spur formation. Spurs less commonly form in the superior recess of the talus and are frequently asymptomatic.[4,5,10] It is believed that irritation of the anterior capsule and associated synovitis may be the cause of pain.[4] Acute hyperdorsiflexion injuries also may result in anterior impingement symptoms as a result of capsular and pericapsular scar. In a cadaveric investigation of 670 ankle specimens from 344 individuals, Talbot and colleagues,[18] looking for a large population and the individual contributions of the talus and tibia to osseous impingement, found only 21% (n = 72) of specimens with bone spurs. Impingement was seen on the talus only in 61%, on the tibia only in 14%, and on both the tibia and talus in 26%. They concluded that spurs were predominately located on the anterolateral talus (78%) and the anterolateral portion of the distal tibial margin (80%).[18] This information can help surgeons during surgical approaches to this pathology.

Another type of anterior impingement is the so-called "cam-type impingement of the ankle," similar to what has been described in the hip femoral neck. In this situation, the sagittal contour of the talar dome forms a noncircular arc with an anterior flattening that causes loss of the normal concavity of the talar neck and pathologic contact with the anterior aspect of the tibial plafond in dorsiflexion, and abnormal loading of the talar dome cartilage. This anatomic relationship also could lead to the formation of reactive osteophytes and soft tissue hypertrophy but specifically differs from usual anterior impingement syndrome in that there appears to be an underlying anatomic bony deformity of the talar body-neck junction. Surgeons must pay attention to this type of anterior translation of the talus because it may alter the results of anterior impingement treatment.[19]

IMAGING STUDIES

Bony spur formation at the anterior margin of the tibial plafond and dorsal talar neck is usually shown on plain radiographs or MR imaging and described for ALAI and AMAI. In this type of impingement, arthrofibrosis may occasionally be involved in the midline joint and cause impingement symptoms[4,10] (**Fig. 4**). The radiographic views in maximum dorsiflexion and plantar flexion help to recognize the contours of the anterior margin of the tibia and neck of the talus. Although the symptoms are not directly related to the contact or the size of the marginal osteophytes in these regions, these radiological views are extremely useful in the decision-making process of the anterior impingement of the ankle.

POSTERIOR ANKLE IMPINGEMENT

Posterior impingement arises from compression of the soft tissues between the posterior process of the calcaneus and the posterior tibial border on plantar flexion of the ankle.[6,12,20] Hamilton[21] was one of the first one to describe pain "in the back of the ankle" as a common complaint in dancers and athletes who perform in the plantarflexion position.

The soft tissues compressed include the tibiotalar capsule, posterior talofibular, intermalleolar, and tibiofibular ligaments. The flexor hallucis longus (FHL) and the lateral posterior process of the talus are also important because additional bony impingement with these structures can occur as a consequence of prominent "os trigonum"[22,23] (**Fig. 5**).

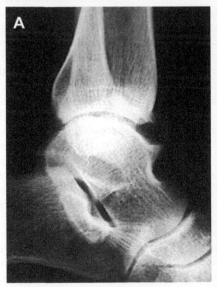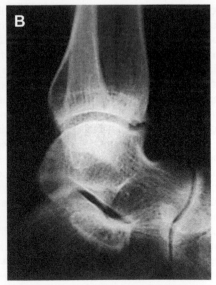

Fig. 4. (*A*) Plain lateral radiograph of the ankle in slight plantar flexion of a patient with anterior ankle impingement. (*B*) Plain lateral radiograph of the ankle in full dorsiflexion demonstrating the "contact" between the tibial and talar bone spurs.

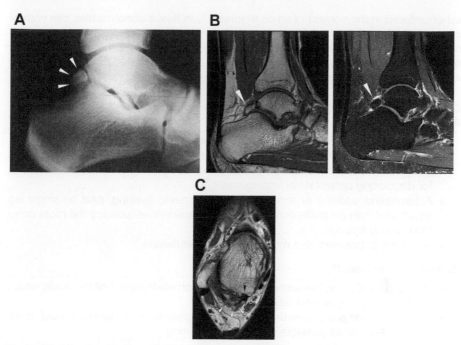

Fig. 5. (*A*) "Os trigonum" syndrome. (*B*) Sagittal MRI (T1 and T2) images. The arrowheads point to the "os trigonum." (*C*) T1 cross-section. White arrowheads point to os trigonum; the black arrowhead points at the FHL tendon and the dashed line circumscribes the navicular bundle.

The lateral process of the talus initially forms as a secondary ossification center between the ages of 7 to 13 years and usually fuses with the main body of the talus within 1 year.[7,8,22] If there is a failure of fusion, the ossicle is known as an os trigonum and articulates with the talus via a synchondrosis (incidence 7%–14%).[24] If the lateral talar process is unusually large or prominent, it is termed as Stieda process.

The posterior ankle impingement can develop after a significant acute injury, such as avulsion of the posterior talofibular ligament, talar fracture, or fracture of the os trigonum[25]; however, this is relatively rare, and the syndrome usually arises insidiously in predisposed athletes. It is believed that repetitive forced plantar flexion of the foot results in chronic injury to the posterior osseous and soft tissues.[22] Ballet dancers are especially prone to this injury, as the ankle is commonly at the extremes of its full range of movement and is maintained in these positions for relatively prolonged periods.[25,26]

Professional soccer players are also at increased risk because ball kicking leads to repeated sudden forced plantar flexion.[23]

IMAGING STUDIES

Conventional radiographs can demonstrate an os trigonum or a Stieda process; however, these findings are commonly seen in asymptomatic individuals.[4,9] MRI is the optimal modality, as it can define osseous and nonosseous abnormalities. Osseous findings associated with posterior impingement include bone marrow edema pattern within a Stieda process or os trigonum and the adjacent talus and/or fluid signal at the synchondrosis in the context of an os trigonum. Soft tissue abnormalities can consist of prominent fluid distending the posterior joint recess, posterior ganglia, posterior synovial thickening, edemalike signal within the surrounding soft tissues, and FHL tenosynovitis. MRI also allows accurate assessment of the remainder of the tibiotalar joint and surrounding tendons, which can aid treatment and surgical planning.[27]

COMMON CLINICAL PRESENTATION
Anterior Impingement

- Production or aggravation of pain when an examiner attempts to pinch hypertrophied synovium between the talus and tibia (the positive impingement sign) has been reported to be both sensitive and specific (94.8% and 88.0%, respectively) for diagnosing anterolateral impingement.[10]
- Anterolateral, anterior or anteromedial tenderness, swelling, pain on single leg squat, and pain on ankle dorsiflexion and eversion/inversion are the most common clinical findings.
- Snapping or popping also may occur with dorsiflexion.

Posterior Impingement[8]

- Pain and swelling at the posterolateral/posteromedial aspect of the ankle, which is exacerbated by plantar flexion
- Pain with passive or active movement of the great toe (FHL tenosynovitis); there may be associated palpable crepitus or triggering

APPROACHES TO TREATMENT

The initial treatment of choice for anterior impingement is generally conservative.[28] Potential options include rest, physical therapy, ankle bracing or taping, shoe modification, and local injection, discussed later in this article.

Frequently, conservative treatment fails, and surgery is recommended. Open surgical techniques have been used with moderate success, but current guidelines consider arthroscopy as the ideal surgical approach with its high safety and low complication rates (approximately 4%).[13] A recent meta-analysis of arthroscopic treatment for anterolateral impingement showed patient satisfaction ranging from 76% to 100%.[1,10,13] When comparing open with endoscopy treatment, no changes were found in patient satisfaction; however, it should be noted that patients with endoscopy treatment had fewer complications (15.9% vs 7.3%) and, in particular, fewer major complications (13.8% vs 5.4%).[12,29] Most patients returned to full activity on average within 8 or 16 weeks with endoscopic and open surgical technique, respectively.

ARTHROSCOPIC ANATOMY OF THE ANTERIOR ANKLE JOINT

Arthroscopy of the ankle joint provides a highly accurate means of locating and treating intra-articular abnormalities. Important anatomic reference point of the anterior ankle joint helps to understand and treat anterior ankle impingement[30,31] (**Fig. 6**).

1. Capsule attaches on the tibia at an average of 6 mm proximal to the joint level. The location of tibial spurs is reported to be at the joint level, and always within the confines of the joint capsule.
2. On the talar side, the capsule attaches likewise approximately 3 mm from the distal cartilage border. The typical osteophytes are found proximal to the notch of the talar neck.

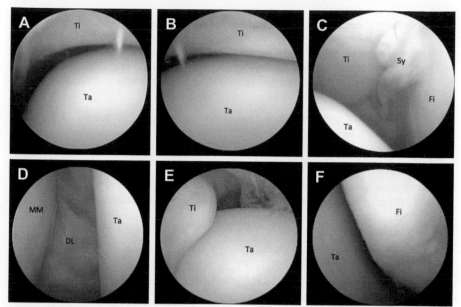

Fig. 6. Arthroscopic anterior points of reference for the ankle. (*A*) Medial "shoulder" of the talus. (*B*) Anterior margin of the tibia and the articular surface of the talus body. (*C*) The lateral "corner" of the ankle with the lateral "shoulder" of the talus, the lateral end of the tibial margin, and normal synovial tissue at the inferior tibiofibular recess. (*D*) The medial gutter with normal deep deltoid ligament fibers. (*E*) The anterior "curved" margin of the tibia over the tibial articular surface of the talus. (*F*) The lateral gutter showing the lateral surface of the talus and the anterior margin of the distal fibula. DL, deltoid ligament; Fi, fibula; MM, medial malleolus; Sy, synovial; Ta, talus; Ti, tibia.

3. The distance of capsular attachment to the most frequent location of bony spurs is relatively large in patients with bony impingement.[32] The tibial and talar spurs typically do not overlap each other.
4. Soft tissue impingement occurs more frequently on the lateral side as a consequence of synovial scarring, inflammation, and hypertrophy in the anterolateral recess of the tibiotalar joint.
5. Hypertrophy of the inferior portion of the anterior tibiofibular ligament must be checked and occasionally lateral osseous spur.
6. Anteromedial "meniscoid" lesion may cause impingement and is frequently associated with arthrofibrosis.[7]

ARTHROSCOPIC TREATMENT FOR ANTERIOR ANKLE JOINT

Creation of arthroscopic portals is not be discussed in detail in this article, as ankle arthroscopic portals are performed following a well-established protocol that ensures portals to be made within "safety areas." Numerous important structures cross the ankle joint, and anterior arthroscopic ankle portals must be performed in such a way that injury to these structures is prevented.

Portals can be performed with ankle distraction or dorsiflexion. There are advantages and disadvantages of each approach.

- Anteromedial portal: created at the level of the tibiotalar joint just medial to the tibialis anterior tendon, within a safety area for the saphenous nerve and greater saphenous vein.

- Anterolateral portal: created at the level of the tibiotalar joint lateral or medial to the superficial peroneal nerve, which is usually previously marked and identified with an ankle inversion and the fourth toe sign.[28] As the nerve moves laterally from ankle inversion to neutral position, the safety area to create the anterolateral portal is medial to the superficial peroneal nerve and lateral to the peroneus tertius tendon.

A 4-mm 30° angle arthroscope or an 11-cm length 2.7-mm scope with a high-volume sheath (4.6 mm) can be used.

After the portals are made, the surgeon can identify numerous different structures that can lead to an anterior ankle impingement.

- Bone structures: anteromedial/central/lateral bone spurs and talus bone spur
- Hypertrophy of the inferior portion of the anterior tibiofibular ligament
- Synovitis
- Arthrofibrosis
- Loose bodies
- Meniscoid lesions

Arthroscopic debridement is performed, for both soft tissue and bony impingement, with the ankle in the dorsiflexed position. The joint line of the anterior tibia is identified by shaving away the tissue just superior to the osteophytes.[1,33,34] A small osteotome and/or shaver burr system is subsequently used to remove the osteophytes. If there are osteophytes or ossicles at the tip of the medial malleolus, the medial malleolus is shaved generously after resection of the osteophyte, both medial and lateral gutters must also be cleaned[6] (**Fig. 7**).

The resection of the anterior osteophytes and the hypertrophic and inflamed synovial tissue that produces the painful condition in the anterior impingement of the ankle is quite effective in controlling symptoms. In patients with no ankle arthritic changes, the success rate of this procedure is close to 100%.

The recurrence of the anterior osteophytes can be observed in almost one-third of the patients treated arthroscopically, but the symptoms are not directly related to this recurrence, but to the presence of soft tissues in the anterior compartment of the ankle, capable of undergoing impingement. In patients with ankle osteoarthritis, the recurrence of previous osteophytes, and also of symptoms, is much higher after arthroscopic resection, reaching 70% of cases.[19]

It is believed that the main determinant of the formation of new anterior osteophytes is the chronic instability of the ankle, which can assume different degrees and combinations as we know at the present time. For this reason, it is suggested to carefully evaluate the ankle as a whole before attempting to resolve the anterior impingement alone, because it may be necessary to treat joint instability concomitantly.

SPECIFIC CONDITION REGARDING ANTERIOR ANKLE IMPINGEMENT SYNDROME

Approaches described previously are the usual treatment that surgeons can follow to manage this pathology, but there are special presentations in daily practice that make the decision hard and, in many times, different from usual. Athletes during the season can be managed with nonvalidated biological treatments such as platelet-rich plasma (PRP) or platelet-rich fibrin (PRF), with injection solution of homeopathic combination drugs or even with lidocaine to allow them to participate during training of official games. During the season, we usually start with lidocaine and or homeopathic injection; if this option presents with a relative good result that allows the athlete to play, 10 days later a PRP or PRF injection is planned. Another possibility that may help is

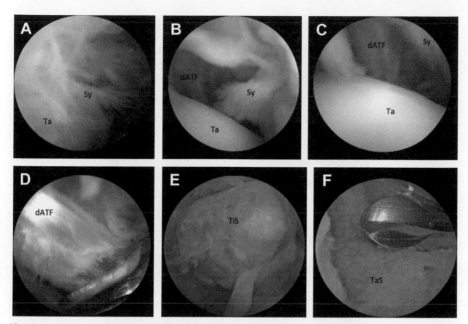

Fig. 7. Anterior arthroscopy. (*A*) Acute hypertrophic synovial occupying the anterolateral space of the ankle. (*B*) Anterolateral ankle impingement caused by fibrous tissue, hypertrophic synovial tissue, and by the cartilage erosion by the distal fascicle of the anterior tibiofibular ligament. (*C*) The same patient shown in **Fig. 6**B after removal of the scar tissue and hypertrophic synovial. (*D*) Removing the distal fascicle if the anterior tibiofibular ligament. (*E*) Anterior impingement of the ankle caused by the spur at the anterior margin of the distal tibia. (*F*) Removing the dorsal spur from the dorsal surface of the talar neck with the help of an arthroscopic bur. dATF, distal anterior tibiofibular ligament; Sy, synovial; Ta, talus; TaS, dorsal talar spur; TiS, anterior tibial spur.

percutaneous electrolysis therapy. This treatment involves applying a modulated direct electrical current directly to damaged soft tissue via an acupuncture needle, which may induce tissue recovery; shock wave therapy is another possibility that can be used. Both of these modalities intend to stimulate fast soft tissue healing and pain relief, but until now, they do not have prospective studies to prove this improvement.

Normally the decision to move on the treatment to surgery is discussed with the team executive, coaches, and the athlete. Only in cases of persistent pain, loose bodies, and progressive incapability to perform at a high level is the medical decision superior to the staff desire.

A controversial type of anterior ankle impingement is called the "cam-type" and is characterized by a noncircular arc of the sagittal contour of the talar dome (flattened talar dome) or a thicker talar neck, especially at its body junction (**Fig. 8**). This condition, which can result from repetitive trauma, creates the cam impingement effect that can be summarized as a pathologic contact between the talus and the anterior border of the tibia during dorsiflexion with a marked impairment of the ankle function. In a large series of patients, a positive correlation with cavo-varus foot type was observed.[35]

It can be sensed that the exaggerated contact between the anterior portion of the tibia and the flat, protruding surface of the talar neck increases the pressure exerted on the distal tibia articular cartilage, causing its early degeneration.

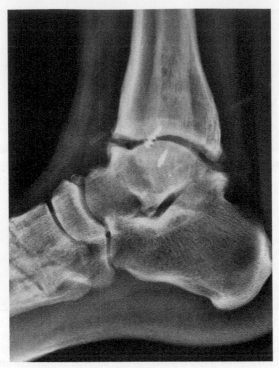

Fig. 8. The "cam-type" anterior ankle impingement.

Surgical removal of the protrusion responsible for the cam effect can be beneficial, but there is no evidence in the current literature that this occurs.

ENDOSCOPIC ANATOMY OF THE POSTERIOR ANKLE

The endoscopic approach for diagnosis and treatment of posterior ankle pathology has been proven to be an effective and safe procedure for bony posterior ankle impingement due to different causes. The knowledge of particular anatomy of the posterior ankle joint is imperative to achieve good results and perform a safe procedure. There are some particular anatomic issues of the posterior ankle joint that may help.[36,37]

1. The synchondrosis of the os trigonum may vary in orientation from coronal to oblique sagittal plane.
2. There are unusual muscles that can cause posterior ankle impingement; these include the peroneus quartus, flexor accessories digitorum longus, accessory soleus, peroneus-calcaneus internus muscle, tibiocalcaneal internus, and low-lying FHL muscle belly. All of these can be identified by arthroscopic procedures.
3. The deep transverse ligament of the posterior inferior tibiofibular ligament is considered a true labrum of the posterior ankle joint and has been implicated in posterior ankle impingement.
4. A tight and thickened crural fascia can hinder the free movement of instruments. It can be helpful to enlarge the portals deep in the fascia by means of a punch or shaver.

ENDOSCOPIC TREATMENT OF THE POSTERIOR ANKLE IMPINGEMENT

When addressing posterior ankle impingement, hindfoot endoscopic portals with the patient in the prone position is recommended.[38]

- The classic hindfoot endoscopic portals (posterolateral and posteromedial) located at the junction of the tip of the lateral malleolus and the medial and lateral borders of the calcaneal tendon.

Creation of these portals does not have a risk for injuries when performed close to the Achilles tendon; however, the creation of a working area during hindfoot endoscopy has a high potential risk of injury to the posterior neurovascular structures. A systematic technique when creating this space and working lateral to the FHL tendon are both recommended to avoid complications.

The initial posterior ankle debridement is often done in a blind fashion. Once the bone can be visualized, the arthroscope and shaver can be advanced medially to identify the FHL tendon. There is often a large amount of fibrous soft tissue and capsule that make initial visualization difficult. The key is to be patient with shaver dissection and to always be aware of instrument position in the posterior ankle, especially in relation to the FHL tendon. The safe initial working zone is midline to lateral to avoid the tendon and deeper rather than superficial to avoid the Achilles tendon. After the fatty tissue overlying the posterior ankle capsule lateral from the FHL tendon is resected, the possible posterior anatomic structures (**Fig. 9**) causing impingement can be identified.[6,13]

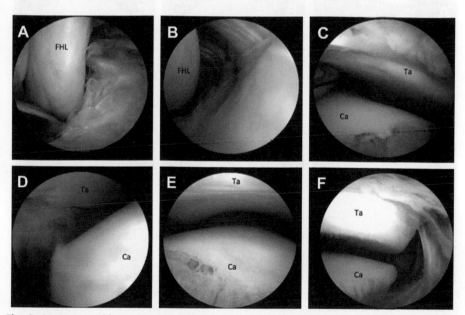

Fig. 9. Posterior ankle endoscopy. (*A*) The most important safety and reference point for posterior ankle arthroscopy is the FHL. The tibial nerve bundle beam is 2 mm from this reference point in the medial direction. (*B*) FHL can be arthroscopically evaluated distally within its own sheath. (*C*) The central portion of the subtalar joint. (*D*) The medial "shoulder" of the calcaneus at the subtalar joint. (*E*) The concavity of the talar articular surface and the convexity of the calcaneal articular surface at the subtalar joint. (*F*) The lateral "shoulder" of the calcaneus at the subtalar joint. Ca, calcaneus; FHL, flexor hallucis longus; Ta, talus.

- Hypertrophic posterior joint capsule
- Synovitis
- Os trigonum
- Hypertrophic posterior talar process
- Entrapment of the FHL

A 4.0-mm aggressive soft tissue shaver is typically used for soft tissue debridement and a 3.5-mm or 4.0-mm barrel burr is typically used for bony resection. Synovectomy may be safely performed with the shaver and a radiofrequency ablation instrument. The surgeon should be careful with radiofrequency when working around the FHL tendon to avoid thermal injury to the tibial nerve and vascular structures. If there is also FHL tenosynovitis, or a distal insertion of the FHL muscle belly, then the shaver or a punch can be used to release the flexor retinaculum from the medial border of the talus and to resect the distal portion of the muscle belly. The FHL can be thoroughly debrided and a smooth excursion of the tendon can be directly verified with the arthroscope. Identifying the os trigonum or Stieda process before initiating burring is also an important recommendation[20,29] (**Fig. 10**).

SPECIFIC CONDITION REGARDING POSTERIOR IMPINGEMENT SYNDROME

As it was described to anterior ankle impingement, athletes who present posterior impingements also may present a special condition. The most common seen are

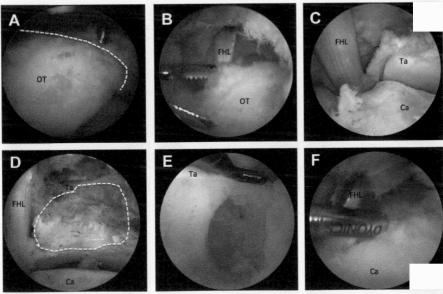

Fig. 10. Posterior ankle impingement: os trigonum syndrome. (*A*) Regularly the limits between the talus and the os trigonum are not so easy to find (*dotted line*). (*B*) After removal of the fibrous tissue (symphysis) or cartilage (synchondrosis) existing in the contact zone, the os trigonum can be removed. (*C*) After os trigonum removal, the FHL runs completely free. (*D*) The dotted white line delimits the area from which the os trigonum was removed. (*E*) Osteochondral lesions of the posterior aspect of the talus could be accessed from the posterior arthroscopy. (*F*) Symptoms of posterior impingement may be due to low FHL muscle belly implantation. These fibers can be removed with the aid of a soft tissue shaver. Ca, calcaneus; OT, os trigonum; Ta, talus.

management of a typical ballet dancer with posterior pain. How do we manage during the season? Inject or not? How often? This decision is the same based on anterior ankle impingement. Corticoid injections should be used as single shots or be avoided; first, they are considered doping in some sports, and second, they may lead to local consequences such as tendon ruptures, skin problems, and local adhesion.[39] During season, it is preferable to use shock wave therapies, injections with hyaluronic acid, PRP or PRF, and even homeopathic substances, such as Arnica Montana. The use of percutaneous electrolysis therapy or shock wave therapy also can be used as nonsurgical treatments.

SUMMARY

Based on most literature reviews, prognosis of anterior ankle impingement relates to the staging of osteoarthrosis (OA). Excellent results are obtained with arthroscopic debridement in almost 100% of patients without OA.[3,15] Success rates decline to 77% in patients with grade I OA and to 53% in case of grade II OA.[3,40] Associated syndesmotic lesions, cartilage damage, and repeated ankle inversion injuries after surgery have negative effects on clinical results during long-term follow-up.[1,3] Size and location of the osteophytes are not related to the outcome and pain score. Recurrence of an osteophyte projection can occur after debridement. Osteophytes recurred in two-thirds of the ankles with grade I OA, but no correlation was found between the recurrence of osteophytes and the symptoms. There was increased narrowing of the joint space in 47% of patients with grade II OA.[1,26] Bony impingement and soft tissue impingement have been distinguished, and the prognostic factors, including presence of anteromedial versus anterolateral osteophytes, that influence outcomes of ankle arthroscopy also have been reported. Numerous investigators have recently reported good to excellent results with arthroscopic debridement.[13,15,28] Success rates of approximately 67% to 88% were described for the arthroscopic debridement in different case series, including both bony and soft tissue anterior ankle impingement.[41] Advantages of arthroscopic treatment over open arthrotomy include reduced recovery time and earlier return to sports activities.[3,15,31] Complication rates from the arthroscopy are reported to be approximately 9% to 17% with difficulties such as neurovascular injury, reflex sympathetic dystrophy, instrument breakage, and painful scars.[31] The most common complication is injury to cutaneous nerves. Unusual complications, such as vascular injury, pseudoaneurysm formation of the dorsalis pedis artery, and extensor hallucis longus tendon rupture, following arthroscopic debridement for impingement syndrome have been reported.

Endoscopic management of posterior ankle impingement is associated with a low morbidity, a short recovery time, and provides good/excellent results at 2 years of follow-up in 80% of patients.[6,20,29,37] The theoretic advantages of posterior ankle arthroscopy include better visualization of the posterior ankle and subtalar joint, earlier return to activity due to less dissection and smaller incisions, and lower complication rates. The disadvantages are that this technique is complex and demanding with a steep initial learning curve and longer operating times. Comparing open and arthroscopic os trigonum excision, there was no significant difference in American Orthopedic Foot and Ankle Society and visual analog scale scores reported in the literature; however, the time for return to sports was almost 6 weeks earlier for the arthroscopic patients (6.0 vs 11.9 weeks).[23,29,36] The overall complication rate was reported to be 3.8% to 8.5% after posterior hindfoot endoscopy for posterior ankle impingement, FHL tenosynovitis, os trigonum syndrome, or a fractured Stieda process, whereas the rate of complications in open posterior hindfoot and ankle surgery for the same pathologies ranged from 10% to 24%.[42,47] The potential for nerve injury appears to be similar for both open and arthroscopic techniques. Ribbans and colleagues[48] compared open and arthroscopic debridement. Open cases had a 4.2% incidence of nerve injury and a wound complication and infection rate of 2.8%. Arthroscopic cases had a 3.7% incidence of nerve injury and 0.96% incidence of wound complication and infection rate. Although rare, injury to the tibial nerve and its branches for procedures around the posterior talar process has been reported.[20,29] This procedure has proven to be particularly effective in patients with overuse injuries that have frequent plantar flexion activities, such as dancers and soccer players. The main complication, sural nerve neuropraxia, can be minimized by correct portal placement and instrumentation.

In conclusion, correct diagnosis and treatment are essential to diagnose and treat anterior or posterior ankle impingent, especially in professional athletes. Arthroscopic treatment for both pathologies is minimally invasive and suitable for athletes and non-athletes who desire an early return to activity.

DISCLOSURE

D. Baumfeld: Arthrex, Consultant/Speaker; Geistlish, Speaker; Merck Sharp Dome, Speaker. C. Nery: Arthrex, Consultant/Speaker; Geistlish, Speaker; Wright Medical, Speaker.

REFERENCES

1. Lavery KP, McHale KJ, Rossy WH, et al. Ankle impingement. J Orthop Surg Res 2016;1–7. https://doi.org/10.1186/s13018-016-0430-x.
2. Tol JL, van Dijk CN. Anterior ankle impingement. Foot Ankle Clin N Am 2006; 11(2):297–310.
3. Ross K, Murawski CD, Smyth NA, et al. Current concepts review: arthroscopic treatment of anterior ankle impingement. Foot Ankle Surg 2017;23(1):1–8.
4. LiMarzi GM, Khan O, Shah Y, et al. Imaging manifestations of ankle impingement syndromes. Radiol Clin North Am 2018;56(6):893–916.
5. Robinson P. Impingement syndromes of the ankle. Eur Radiol 2007;17(12): 3056–65.
6. Niek van Dijk C. Anterior and posterior ankle impingement. Foot Ankle Clin N Am 2006;11(3):663–83.
7. Dimmick S, Linklater J. Ankle impingement syndromes. Radiol Clin North Am 2013;51(3):479–510.
8. Zbojniewicz AM. Impingement syndromes of the ankle and hindfoot. Pediatr Radiol 2019;1–11. https://doi.org/10.1007/s00247-019-04459-5.
9. Donovan A, Rosenberg ZS. MRI of ankle and lateral hindfoot impingement syndromes. AJR Am J Roentgenol 2010;195(3):595–604.
10. Hess GW. Ankle impingement syndromes: a review of etiology and related implications. Foot Ankle Spec 2011;4(5):290–7.
11. Ferkel RD, Tyorkin M, Applegate GR, et al. MRI evaluation of anterolateral soft tissue impingement of the ankle. Foot Ankle Int 2010;31(8):655–61.
12. Larciprete M, Giudice G, Balocco P, et al. [Ankle impingement syndrome]. Radiol Med 2000;99(6):415–9.
13. Buchhorn T, Koch M, Weber J, et al. [Ankle impingement. Indications and arthroscopic therapy]. Unfallchirurg 2016;119(2):115–9.
14. Strauss JE, Forsberg JA, Lippert FG III. Chronic lateral ankle instability and associated conditions: a rationale for treatment. Foot Ankle Int 2007;28(10):1041–4.

15. Vaseenon T, Amendola A. Update on anterior ankle impingement. Curr Rev Musculoskelet Med 2012;5(2):145–50.

16. Tol JL, Verhagen RAW, Krips R, et al. The anterior ankle impingement syndrome: diagnostic value of oblique radiographs. Foot Ankle Int 2004;25(2):63–8.

17. Cerezal L, Abascal F, Canga A, et al. MR imaging of ankle impingement syndromes. AJR Am J Roentgenol 1998;181(2):551–9.

18. Talbot CE, Knapik DM, Miskovsky SN. Prevalence and location of bone spurs in anterior ankle impingement: a cadaveric investigation. Clin Anat 2018;31(8): 1144–50.

19. Amendola A, Drew Newhoff, Vaseenon T, et al. Cam type impingement in the ankle. Iowa Orthop J 2012;32(1):1–8.

20. Heier KA, Hanson TW. Posterior ankle impingement syndrome. YOTSM 2017; 25(2):75–81.

21. Hamilton WG. Differential diagnosis and treatment of posterior ankle pain in dancers and equinus athletes. J Back Musculoskelet Rehabil 1995;5:201–7.

22. Hayashi D, Roemer FW, D'Hooghe P, et al. Posterior ankle impingement in athletes: Pathogenesis, imaging features and differential diagnoses. Eur J Radiol 2015;1–11. https://doi.org/10.1016/j.ejrad.2015.07.017.

23. Kudaş S, Dönmez G, Işık Ç, et al. Posterior ankle impingement syndrome in football players: case series of 26 elite athletes. Acta Orthop Traumatol Turc 2016; 50(6):649–54.

24. Zwiers R, Baltes TPA, Opdam KTM, et al. Prevalence of os trigonum on CT imaging. Foot Ankle Int 2018;39(3):338–42.

25. Spiga S, Vinci V, Tack S, et al. Diagnostic imaging of ankle impingement syndromes in athletes. Musculoskelet Surg 2013;97(Suppl 2):S145–53.

26. Hong C, Pearce C, Ballal M, et al. Management of sports injuries of the foot and ankle. Bone Joint J 2016;98(B):1–13.

27. Berman Z, Tafur M, Ahmed SS, et al. Ankle impingement syndromes: an imaging review. Br J Radiol 2017;90(1070):20160735.

28. Epstein DM, Black BS, Sherman SL. Anterior ankle arthroscopy. Foot Ankle Clin 2015;20(1):41–57.

29. Carreira DS, Vora AM, Hearne KL, et al. Outcome of arthroscopic treatment of posterior impingement of the ankle. Foot Ankle Int 2016;37(4):394–400.

30. Golanó P, Vega J, Pérez-Carro L, et al. Ankle anatomy for the arthroscopist. Part II: role of the ankle ligaments in soft tissue impingement. Foot Ankle Clin N Am 2006;11(2):275–96.

31. van Dijk CN, Vuurberg G, Amendola A, et al. Anterior ankle arthroscopy: state of the art. J ISAKOS 2016;1(2):105–15.

32. Golanó P, Vega J, Leeuw PAJ, et al. Anatomy of the ankle ligaments: a pictorial essay. Knee Surg Sports Traumatol Arthrosc 2016;24(4):944–56.

33. Hsu A, Lee S, Gross C, et al. Extended indications for foot and ankle arthroscopy. J Am Acad Orthop Surg 2014;(22):1–11.

34. Dalmau-Pastor M, Vega J, Malagelada F, et al. Surgical arthroscopic anatomy. In: Arthroscopy and endoscopy of the foot and ankle, vol. 21, 2nd edition. Singapore: Springer Singapore; 2019. p. 13–27. Principle and Practice.

35. Templeton-Ward O, Solan M. Posterior ankle and hind foot arthroscopy – How do you responsibly learn this new technique? Foot Ankle Surg 2014;20(4):229–30.

36. Lui TH. Arthroscopy and endoscopy of the foot and ankle: indications for new techniques. Arthroscopy 2007;23(8):889–902. https://doi.org/10.1016/j.arthro.2007.03.003.

37. Beimers L, Frey C, van Dijk CN. Arthroscopy of the posterior subtalar joint. Foot Ankle Clin N Am 2006;11(2):369–90.
38. Hamilton WG, Geppert MJ, Thompson FM. Pain in the posterior aspect of the ankle in dancers. differential diagnosis and operative treatment. J Bone Joint Surgery Am 1996;78:1–10.
39. Vogler HW, Stienstra JJ, Montgomery F, et al. Anterior ankle impingement arthropathy. The role of anterolateral arthrotomy and arthroscopy. Clin Podiatric Med Surg 1994;11(3):425–47.
40. Wang L, Gui J, Gao F, et al. Modified posterior portals for hindfoot arthroscopy. Arthroscopy 2007;23(10):1116–23.
41. Calder JD, Sexton SA, Pearce CJ. Return to training and playing after posterior ankle arthroscopy for posterior impingement in elite professional soccer. Am J Sports Med 2017;38(1):120–4.
42. Ribbans W, Ribbans H, Cruickshank J, et al. The management of posterior ankle impingement syndrome in sport: a review. Foot Ankle Surg 2014;1–10. https://doi.org/10.1016/j.fas.2014.08.006.

Epidemiology of Sports-Specific Foot and Ankle Injuries

Christopher W. Hodgkins, MD[a],*, Nicholas A. Wessling, MD[b]

KEYWORDS

• Epidemiology • Injury • Prevention • Sports • Cleat • Playing surface

KEY POINTS

- Epidemiology is the branch of medicine that deals with the incidence and distribution of disease and the possible control of disease.
- The aim of studying epidemiology in sports medicine is to identify injury patterns so as to potentially prevent such injuries.
- The role of the sports medicine team must be not only to treat injuries but also to prevent them, and this actually may contribute the most to the success of the entire team.
- This article aims to summarize the incidence of foot and ankle injuries in individual sports and discover potential injury prevention strategies.

INTRODUCTION

Epidemiology is the branch of medicine that deals with the incidence, distribution, and possible control of disease. In cases of sports injuries, that control is prevention. No doubt the readers, in particular those involved with professional sports teams, would agree that a physician who provides a service to sporting organizations who prevents injuries to their athletes is far more valuable than one who simply repairs them. Furthermore, data is knowledge and, through this, injury patterns and future performance can be estimated, allowing the physician to be a valuable resource when considering prospects for the team.

The aim of this article is to identify meaningful epidemiology of sports-specific foot and ankle injuries by major sporting arena, to educate how proactive injury prevention rather than reactive injury treatment is practiced. Epidemiology is addressed first, from the perspective of the sport, followed by specific foot and ankle injuries.

[a] Miami Orthopedics and Sports Medicine Institute, 1150 Campo Sano Avenue, Miami, FL 33146, USA; [b] Lenox Hill Hospital, 159 East 74th Street, 2nd Floor, New York, NY 10021, USA
* Corresponding author.
E-mail address: cwh@cwhmd.com

Foot Ankle Clin N Am 26 (2021) 173–185
https://doi.org/10.1016/j.fcl.2020.10.001
1083-7515/21/© 2020 Elsevier Inc. All rights reserved.

EPIDEMIOLOGY

Injury epidemiology relies on data. Meaningful epidemiology relies on large volumes of reliable data. Such data, historically, has been poorly recorded both by athletes and medical personnel. Meaningful injury data requires a consistent, uniform reporting and recording process across the broad world of organized sports to be reproducible. Realistically, this is possible only in larger individual sporting organizations but still relies on accurate reporting and detailed recording. Even with this achieved, the data must be in a format that can be audited easily, to allow useful examination for identifying patterns and trends.

When surveying what was most relevant to the reader, the authors examined the most popular sports worldwide. To their surprise, the list (**Table 1**) was not familiar. In order of worldwide popularity, the most pertinent epidemiologic work by each sport is presented and the most interesting and pragmatic information to help impart the changes necessary for injury prevention discussed.

Epidemiologic Data Based on Sport

Soccer

Soccer is the most popular worldwide sport and, therefore, many injuries arise during its participation.

Pfirrmann and colleagues[1] looked at injury incidence in male professional adult and elite youth soccer players and found approximately 70 injuries per 1000 hours of exposure in professional competitive matches.

O'Connor and James[2] produced an impactful and informative article examining the association of lower limb injury with boot cleat design and playing surface in elite soccer. It is important to point out to the international readership that when dealing with soccer (*football*, as Europeans call it), a cleat is a boot; to avoid confusion, referencing a boot under the title heading of soccer refers to a cleat. The investigators identified that 17% to 23% of all injuries in soccer were in the foot or ankle: 67% were sprains and caused at least 2 days of training missed, and 39% of total ankle injuries were noncontact and thus attributable to the boot/playing surface interaction. Modern boot design, aimed at increasing player speed and stamina, has led to lighter-

Table 1 Most popular sports worldwide	
Sport	**Estimated Fans**
Soccer	3.5 Billion
Cricket	2.5 Billion
Basketball	2.2 Billion
Field Hockey	2 Billion
Tennis	1 Billion
Volleyball	900 Million
Table Tennis	850 Million
Baseball	500 Million
American Football	410 Million
Rugby	410 Million

From Top 10 Most Popular Sports in the World [Updated 2020]. Sports Show website. Published October 3, 2020. Accessed October 9, 2020. https://sportsshow.net/top-10-most-popular-sports-in-the-world/: with permission.

weight, more minimalist, and thinner constructs that potentially put the metatarsals at greater risk of injury. They looked at the position of the studs in relation to the metatarsals and suggested more stud numbers, increased forefoot cushion, and stiff soled boots, with softer playing surfaces, were more protective for metatarsal injuries. They found, however, that many variables, particularly in the athlete's foot, make this more complex and not easy to standardize. More importantly, in soccer, the feel of the ball on the foot is important for skill and proprioception and thus has led to lighter weight and thinner materials, which also have decreased the stability of the boot.

Ekstrand and Nigg[3] found that 24% of lower extremity injuries in soccer were associated with the playing surface or shoe wear. Their article, however, was published 30 years ago.

Playing surfaces, even if natural grass, can vary significantly in original makeup and seasonal variability, depending on temperature/moisture, wear, and other factors.

Williams and colleagues[4] analyzed 20 cohort studies looking at injury rates on natural and modern synthetic turf. They presented strong evidence that there was only a trivial difference in injury incidence rates between the 2 surfaces but that turf did increase the risk of ankle injury in 8 of 14 cohorts and suggested that prospective standardized research was required to learn more.

In summary, there are significant differences in individual feet, shoes, and playing surfaces. The interaction of each one adds further complex variability and thus standardizing recommendations is difficult. Shoe type is athlete-specific, depending on foot type, position, preferences, and sponsors and must be matched to specific properties of the foot and playing surface. Playing surfaces are not standardized and also can vary, depending on weather and other extrinsic factors. Thus, choosing the right shoe for a specific surface is complex, and athletes should have a range of boots and understanding of the surface conditions for each game.

The authors have personal experience not only with recent and ongoing involvement with the medical care of collegiate-level (and above) soccer teams but also with collegiate-level participation, albeit somewhat removed now in the twilight stage of their sporting careers. From this experience, the authors suggest that such attention to individual athletes' foot makeup in relation to their cleat choice for the particular playing surface for each individual game is relatively lacking. Although it is understood that this area is complex and time consuming, it likely warrants more attention, time, and funding in an attempt to decrease the potential for injury. The authors expect the excellent research from the American National Football League (NFL) (discussed later) eventually will be disseminated to all other professional sports and lead to a decrease in foot and ankle injuries.

Cricket

Although cricket may not be a familiar sport to many in the United States, it is popular worldwide and is the second most popular spectator sport after soccer. Despite being noncontact, there are many injuries associated with running, throwing, batting, bowling, catching, and diving. Lower limb injuries account for approximately 50% of incidences, with hamstring strains (18%) the most common and ankle injuries representing 10%.[5] Posterior impingement is common in cricketers, usually affecting fast bowlers on the contralateral side of the bowling arm.

The author (CWH) has personal experience of collegiate-level participation in this summer sport, having grown up in a cricket-friendly country. Cricket traditionally has not been the most athletic of sports and although this sport is trending closer to the strength and conditioning standards of more traditional sports, there certainly is an element of epidemiology in this realm that results from under-preparation, both in long-term and short-term conditioning. Therefore, better acute and chronic approaches to fitness and injury prevention potentially could lead to the decreased incidence of injuries.

Basketball

Tummala and colleagues[6] reviewed 10 years of National College Athletic Association (NCAA) Injury Surveillance System (ISS) data. They found an overall incidence of 1.49 injuries per 1000 athletic exposures, with a higher rate of 2.51 in competition compared with practice. Ankle ligament sprain was the most common injury regardless of level of competition. Rebounding was the most common activity at the time of injury due to contact with another player. Guards were injured most commonly. Most ankle injuries were new injuries, were nonsurgical, and resulted in time missed less than 7 days. Screening of athletes for prior ankle injuries, proprioception defects, weak postural sway scores, history of ankle sprains, and prophylactic injury prevention programs can reduce the incidence of lower extremity injuries significantly. Following injury, a continued training program that involves neuromuscular performance is effective in decreasing ankle and knee sprains and low back pain. Bracing and taping also are supported to decrease the incidence of ankle sprains.

Taylor and colleagues[7] reported an overall incidence of 7 to 10 injuries per 1000 hours in their meta-analysis. More than 60% occurred in the lower extremity, with ankle sprains accounting for 25% of these. They also reported evidence supporting neuromuscular training to decrease ankle injuries and support bracing as a preventative measure without detriment.

Evidence supporting impactful and positive findings in injury prevention largely was from Riva and colleagues,[8] who conducted a 6-year prospective study looking at the effectiveness of proprioceptive training on the incidence of ankle, knee sprains, and low back pain. These injuries are thought to be higher in single-limb stance sports. Ankle sprains and low back pain showed significant reductions with proprioceptive training. Given ankle sprains are the most common injury in the National Basketball Association (NBA), this represents a major area for injury prevention and had been adopted by NBA teams at the time of publication of this article with positive effect.

The authors' experience echoes the literature in realizing the importance of such proprioception training for injury prevention.

Field hockey

Barboza and colleagues[9] reviewed pertinent literature in field hockey and found that the most common sites of injury were the lower limbs, knee, ankle, lower leg, and thigh. Contusions and hematomas were the most common injury type followed by abrasions, lacerations, sprains, and strains. Injury mechanisms, in order of frequency, which differ from some sports, were no contact, contact with the ball, contact with the stick, another player, and the ground. Given the high frequency of stick and ball contact injuries, more protective gear was recommended as a result of this study's findings, in particular shin, ankle, and mouth protection. The high rate of noncontact injuries in this study also prompted recommendations to introduce exercise programs aimed at injury prevention. This study highlights the effectiveness of such epidemiologic investigations, allowing identification of effective injury prevention tactics.

Volleyball

Baugh and colleagues[10] examined 2 years of men's and women's NCAA volleyball data. Injury rates were 4.69 for men and 7.07 for women per 1000 athletic events. The knee was injured most commonly without time lost from competition. Time loss to injuries more commonly were to ankle sprains. Although beyond the scope of this article, there were a notable number of concussions for a noncontact sport, most of which were due to ball contact.

Baseball

Dick and colleagues[11] looked at foot and ankle injuries in baseball. They reviewed 16 years of NCAA data and found an overall injury incidence of 5.78 per 1000 athlete-exposures, with ankle sprains accounting for 7% of these.

American football

Injury exposure risk in football is estimated at 35.9 injuries per 1000 exposures. This is the one of highest in studied collegiate sports. Foot and ankle injuries represent 15 per 10,000.[12]

The NFL, with the consent of the players through the collective bargaining agreement, implemented a uniform electronic health record that requires the documentation of specific information designed to identify potential risk factors and trends.

Kluczynski and colleagues[13] reviewed the literature surrounding involving NFL injuries. They found consistent support that lower extremity injuries were more common on artificial surfaces when compared with natural turf. The most commonly injured site was the knee, followed by hamstrings. Injuries were more common in the first 2 weeks of training camps, then games, and most common in defensive players. More than 70% of players had a history of lateral ankle sprains. Syndesmotic injuries were more common in special teams and offensive linemen. Isolated fibular fractures were found to require surgery in 50% of cases and allowed for faster return to play (RTP) when isolated, but when treated with surgery, even isolated fractures required a mean of 10 weeks to RTP.

They identified that Lisfranc sprains at the NFL Scouting Combine negatively affected draft position and player availability, particularly when more than 2 mm of Lisfranc diastasis existed.

Achilles rupture RTP numbers were 66% to 72% (up to 78% in a single surgeon's experience), with performance metrics decreased for 2 years to 3 years.

Jones fracture incidence at the NFL Scouting Combine was 2%. This was higher in athletes with long straight narrow fifth metatarsals and an adducted forefoot; 7% to 12% had nonunions after surgery compared with 20% without surgery. Operative treatment was successful at maximizing RTP when employed.

Beaulieu-Jones and colleagues[14] also looked at the epidemiology of injuries identified at the NFL Scouting Combine and their impact on performance in the NFL.

They analyzed more than 2000 athletes over 7 years who ultimately played 2 years in the NFL. The ankle was the most common site of injury at 52.7%, with running backs affected most commonly. Defensive players demonstrated a greater negative impact due to injury than offensive players. Low ankle sprain accounted for close to 60% of those injuries with high ankle sprains at 20%.

The principal finding of this study was that performance in the NFL is affected significantly by a history of prior injury. The number of games missed by an athlete in college was a reliable indicator of athletes ultimately being drafted into the NFL.

They also found that a trend in player position and certain injuries correlated with a significant drop in ultimate draft ranking.

This article might be a resource for team physicians examining NFL prospects based on their history of injury and position.

Vopat and colleagues[15] looked at NFL Scouting Combine data for navicular injury and its implications for prospective NFL career. They found that a previous navicular fracture results in a greater risk of developing posttraumatic osteoarthritis. Although only a low prevalence of navicular injury in prospective NFL players was noted, players with these injuries had a greater probability of going undrafted and not competing in at least 2 NFL seasons when compared with matched controls without an injury history.

The authors emphasize and commend the work invested in foot/cleat/playing surface research and its role in potential injury prevention. Much more work is on the horizon, which hopefully will translate to a further decrease in foot and ankle injuries.

Furthermore, the authors also agree with the significant consequences of midfoot injuries and liberally employ the use of multimodality advanced imaging (magnetic resonance imaging [MRI]/computed tomography [CT]/weight-bearing CT. and stress views) in the diagnosis of these injuries, many of which can be occult and difficult to see on static individual studies.

On the subject of Achilles tendon ruptures, the authors acknowledge what they believe is the superiority of minimally invasive surgical repair in achieving the highest-quality collagen repair and restoring resting motor unit tension and also reducing the relative risk profile of surgical treatment.

Aggressive surgical treatment of Jones fractures also is the preference of the authors, based on personal and literature support of lower rates of delayed union, nonunion and refracture, and quicker RTP.

The shoe and the playing surface, a complex relationship

This topic might hold the most promise for potential injury prevention to the foot and ankle and should be familiar to sports physicians and medical teams. Being in the early stages of discovery, there is much more to come.

Jastifer and colleagues[12] recently and fittingly have started to look closely at the relationship of the shoe and the surface, and the interaction of both, with injury to the foot and ankle. They suggest that the role of the cleat and the playing surface, in particular the interaction of the 2, is poorly understood and much more research is required.

They suggest there are several important factors to consider in terms of shoe design, including biomechanical compliance, cleat and turf interaction, and shoe sizing and fitting. They propose that the cleat should be considered a piece of protective equipment rather than an extension of the uniform, and this point is key.

Shoe plate stiffness has been implicated in turf toe and midfoot injuries by allowing excessive pathologic motion at these foot segments thus causing injury. Increasing plate stiffness, however, can decrease athletic ability; thus, there should be an attempt to match the stiffness to both an individual player's motion and athletic requirement. This subject area, however, is poorly understood, highlighted by the biomechanical literature surrounding this topic being complex and sometimes conflicting. What is understood is that quantifying and recording the stiffness of current cleats in relation to player statistics are important in establishing baseline data that will allow further analysis and hopefully meaningful data to impart improvements.

Current data support that the shoe plate may have a varying stiffness and should be designed with stiffness that allows a dorsiflexion angle of just shy of injury-level flexion angles and stiffness above performance levels to reduce injury risk.

Cleat design

This is a challenging area, with many variables and complex biomechanical literature. More recent literature, however, has shed some relatively simplistic light on this topic. Kent and colleagues[16] recently looked at the mechanical interaction of 19 different NFL cleats with natural and artificial turf. They discovered that all cleat designs failed by shear of the natural surface by either sliding across the surface in less aggressive cleat design or by generating a divot in the surface. In contrast, during testing on an artificial surface, only 1 cleat design released from the surface by way of sliding, with the rest enduring forces and torque to the limit of the testing device.

The investigators observed that when a cleat releases, either by sliding on the surface or creating a divot, the force-limiting factor is the interface between the cleat and playing surface. In the scenario where the cleat does not release, the force-limiting factor is the energy applied by the athlete, which, in extreme situations, can result in injury.

They suggest that an ideal scenario would be a cleat that releases from its interaction with the particular playing surface before the foot can experience an energy level known to cause particular injuries.

If an aggressive cleat is worn on artificial turf, the potential exists for an athlete's foot to experience high energy levels and thus potential injury, and they suggest this hypothesis might explain the higher level of foot, ankle, and knee injuries on synthetic turf compared with natural grass.

The NFL has published a ranking of cleats based on laboratory testing on synthetic turf, based on shoe safety and performance: https://www.playsmartplaysafe.com/resource/cleat-pattern-laboratory-testing-performance-results-synthetic-turf/.

Shoe sizing

It is proposed that poor shoe fit might contribute to foot and ankle injuries, in particular fifth metatarsal fractures, when the shoe is too narrow with the fifth metatarsal hanging over the edge of the sole of the shoe. Work in this area has shown there is significant variability in the measurement of any given size shoe between and even within manufacturers. It is suggested that there should be some form of standardization of sizing and fitting that might help prevent injury.[12]

Rugby

Whitehouse and colleagues[17] reviewed Australian Super Rugby teams during the 2014 season and found an injury incidence of 6.96 per 1000 hours, with a mean injury severity of 37.45 days lost from training and competition. Match play incidence was 66.07 per 1000 hours, with severity being 39.8 days lost. Injury rates were not significantly different between backs and forwards. The investigators compared this injury rate to reported rates for other sports; soccer, 32.8; ice hockey, 59.6; and Australian rules football, 25.7.

The ankle and foot accounted for 23% of these injuries. Approximately 80% of injuries were during contact, and being tackled as opposed to tackling or other contact was the most common event associated with injury.

Prior studies of South African rugby demonstrated an injury incidence of 83.3 per 1000 hours and of English rugby, 91 injuries per 1000 hours.

The author (CWH) has personal experience of collegiate-level participation in this traditionally winter sport, having grown up in the United Kingdom. The authors emphasize the importance of appropriate instruction regarding the tackle (being tackled and tackling) to prevent head and neck trauma.

The authors also emphasize the limited attention to the foot/cleat/playing surface relationship in injury prevention and expect the findings of the American football research work eventually to disseminate to other sports to help prevent injuries to the foot and ankle.

Running

van der Worp and colleagues[18] examined running associated injuries and found that men had a higher incidence of running-related injuries. A history of previous injury and use of orthotics was associated with higher risk of injury. Other risk factors that were identified included age, concrete surface running, marathon participation, weekly mileage of 30 m to 39 m, and running shoes older than 4 months to 6 months. Also, running experience of less than 2 years and restarting running after a period of downtime were associated with higher risk of injury. Acute injuries were rare, with 80% being overuse. The knee and lower leg were affected most commonly.

The authors acknowledge the invaluable contributions of running/shoe experts on advising running athletes on appropriate shoe wear.

Ice hockey
Crowley and colleagues[19] analyzed 10 years of NCAA ISS data looking at ice hockey foot and ankle injuries, in particular differences between male and female participation. They reported more injuries in men than women. The most common injury was a toe contusion, followed by ankle sprains. Low ankle sprains accounted for most moderate time-loss injuries (2–13 days) whereas high ankle sprains accounted for most severe time-loss injuries ($\geq$14 days).

Mixed martial arts
Jensen and colleagues[20] reviewed injury incidence in mixed martial arts sports. They identified that injury trends depended on the style of fighting employed. Most occurred in training, given the ratio of training to competition—approximately 23 to 29 injury incidence per 100 fights. Most injuries were to the head and face followed by hand/wrist. Lower extremity injuries primarily were secondary to strike and take down mechanisms.

Wrestling
Kay and colleagues[21] reviewed the incidence of severe injuries, defined as restricted participation greater than 21 days, in NCAA data over a 6-year period. Wrestling was found to have the highest incidence of severe injuries, with women's gymnastics coming second, ahead of football. The knee was affected most commonly (32.9%), followed by the lower leg/ankle/foot (22.5%).

Agel and colleagues[22] analyzed 16 years of NCAA wrestling injuries. Head and neck, musculoskeletal, and skin infections were most common. Musculoskeletal injuries predominantly were lower extremity injuries, with ankle injuries second most common (7%), behind the knee (23%). Injuries were significantly more common in the preseason; this might be due to early season attempts to drop body weight quickly, estimated to be a 10% change in body weight.

Snow sport
Mahmood and Duggal[23] examined lower extremity injuries in snowboarding. Although upper extremity injuries were more common, lower extremity injuries presented an issue, particularly for more inexperienced participants and those taking higher risks.

The ankle was the joint injured most frequently in the lower extremity, more likely on the leading side. Tall, stiffer boots have helped decrease the number of injuries.

The lateral process of the talus fracture, sometimes referred to as a snowboarding fracture, is the most common ankle fracture. The biomechanical etiology of this is not understood fully, but it has been suggested that it is an axial load on a dorsiflexed ankle that contributes with an external rotation moment.

Low readiness for speed, bad weather, snow conditions, and poor visibility all were associated with higher risk of injury.

Improved instruction (ie, on how to snowboard and how to fall) and equipment are responsible for a general decrease in injury. Proper ski bindings also have improved injury rates.

Epidemiologic Data Based on Injury

Achilles rupture

Achilles tendon rupture is one of the most common tendon injuries in the adult population, ranging between 7 to 40 per 100,000 person-years. Lemme and colleagues[24] performed a national surveillance study in the United States from 2012 to 2016 and found that men accounted for 77.1% of ruptures whereas women accounted for 22.9%, with a mean age at rupture of 37.5 years; 82% of these injuries occurred during sport or a recreational activity, with basketball (42.6%) the most common followed by soccer (9.9%), football (8.4%), tennis (6.9%), and running/hiking/stretching (5.8%).

Zellers and colleagues[25] performed a systematic review and meta-analysis and found that regardless of level of play, 80% of athletes were able to RTP after an Achilles tendon rupture, with a mean time to RTP of 6 months. Trofa and colleagues[26] identified NBA, NFL, Major League Baseball, and National Hockey League athletes who sustained a primary Achilles tendon rupture treated surgically between 1989 and 2013 and found that 30.6% of these professional athletes were unable to RTP. Those who did return played in fewer games, had less playing time, and performed at a lower level than their preinjury status. Basketball players appeared to be affected most in their postinjury careers. Lemme and colleagues[27] found that 37% of NBA players either did not RTP or started in fewer than 10 games the remainder of their career. They found the mean time to RTP was 10.5 months. Amin and colleagues[28] looked at data of 18 NBA players with an Achilles tendon repair over a 23-year period and found 39% of these players did not RTP and those who did performed at lower levels. Trofa and colleagues[29] went on to investigate Achilles ruptures in professional soccer players and found an RTP rate of 71%. At 2 years' postoperative, these athletes played 28.3% fewer minutes compared with their preoperative season. Finally, Jack and colleagues[30] examined RTP in the NFL and found 72.4% were able to return at a mean of approximately 11 months.

Again, the authors emphasize their personal experience and the support from recent literature showing the change in risk profile of minimally invasive surgical procedures for Achilles repair, which changes the much-debated conversation of surgical versus nonsurgical treatment of ruptures. The authors favor percutaneous (truly mini-incision) Percutaneous Achilles Repair System (Arthrex, Naples, Florida, USA) surgery for the majority of the ruptures in athletic patients.

Ankle sprain

Ankle sprains are one of the most common musculoskeletal injuries worldwide. More than 3 million ankle sprains presented to emergency departments in the United States during a 5-year period, and approximately half of these occurred during an athletic activity.[31] Surveillance studies from the NCAA showed lateral ankle sprains to be the most common, followed by high ankle sprains and then medial ankle sprains.[32–34]

Lateral ankle sprains occurred at the highest rates in men's and women's basketball and occurred more often during practice. In 44.4% of lateral ankle sprains, the athlete returned to play in less than 24 hours, whereas in 3.6%, athletes required more than 21 days before returning to play.[32]

In this same 5-year study period, high ankle sprains occurred at a rate of 1.00 per 10,000 athlete-exposures, with 57% occurring during competitions. Men's football, wrestling, and ice hockey had the highest rates of the 25 sports evaluated. Player contact was the most common injury mechanism; 69% of injuries resulted in greater than 1 days missed, 47% with greater than 7 days missed, and 16% with greater than 21 days of participation restriction.[33]

Deltoid ligament sprains occurred at a rate of 0.79 per 10,000 adverse events, with most happening during practice. These injuries were most common in women's gymnastics, men's and women's soccer, and men's football; 73% of these injuries required a restriction of less than 1 week from play.[34]

The authors reemphasize the NBA studies revealing the importance of proprioception training in reducing the incidence of ankle injuries and lost playing time.

Lisfranc injuries

Lisfranc injuries are relatively uncommon and account for approximately 0.2% of all fractures and, in the United States, the incidence has been reported to be 1 per 55,000 people annually.[35] Lisfranc injuries are increasingly common in athletes and it is reported that one-third occur in low energy sport trauma.

MacMahon and colleagues[36] followed their patients treated with primary partial arthrodesis and evaluated their ability to RTP. Most patients were able to return to their previous physical activities, many of which were high impact. Approximately 1 in 4 patients were unable to return to their preoperative activity levels; 97% of patients were satisfied with their surgical outcome.

Mora and colleagues[37] followed 31 patients treated with open reduction and internal fixation of their Lisfranc injuries and found 94% were able to return to some form of recreational sport, with 66% returning to their preinjury level. Interestingly, 33% of patients continued to have some degree of ongoing pain that limited their ability to RTP and physical activities.

Singh and colleagues[38] evaluated professional American football and rugby athletes with Lisfranc injuries. They identified 47 athletes, with 35 treated operatively; 83% of NFL players returned to play at a mean of 10 months at the cost of decreased participation and performance.

The authors re-emphasize the importance of multimodal static and dynamic imaging to evaluate midfoot injuries carefully and use MRI, CT, weight-bearing CT (bilateral), and stress views liberally to rule out detectable evidence of midfoot instability.

Fifth metatarsal fractures

The estimated incidence of proximal fifth metatarsal fractures is approximately 1.8 per 1000 person-years, although controversy exists regarding the classification of these injuries and collecting data on them.

Begly and colleagues[39] collected data on 26 NBA basketball players over 19 NBA seasons with Jones fractures, 24 of whom underwent operative fixation, 19% experienced a recurrence of their injury, and 12% underwent a second procedure. Return to previous level of competition was achieved by 85% of athletes, with no change in player efficiency rating.

O'Malley and colleagues[40] presented a case series of 10 NBA players who underwent operative fixation of their Jones fractures with the addition of either bone marrow aspirate concentrate or open bone grafting. They found average radiographic healing occurred at 7.5 weeks and RTP at 9.8 weeks, with 3 athletes experiencing refractures.

The authors acknowledge their preference for the aggressive surgical treatment of these injuries given the available data supporting the lower risks of delayed union, nonunion, and refracture and faster RTP.

Turf toe

Epidemiology of injuries to the plantar aspect of the hallux metatarsophalangeal joint continues to remain unknown due to most data arising from small case series. The incidence of turf toe was much higher in the 1970s when artificial playing surfaces first were introduced in the United States. The frequency of these injuries has declined over the years as more modern artificial turf designs have been implemented along with advancements in athletic shoe wear. RTP from turf toe injuries can range from a few days to upwards of 6 months, depending on injury severity.

The authors share the widely held opinion that these injuries can come in many different forms and are difficult injuries to diagnose and manage. They, therefore, evaluate them carefully using recorded footage of the injury, if available, and a careful history and physical examination. They also utilize MRI, weight-bearing bilateral CT scans, and dynamic stress and/or ultrasound imaging in the surgical decision-making process.

SUMMARY

Foot and ankle injuries are extremely common amongst all injuries sustained in sport and recreational activities. Incidence of sports-specific injuries, time lost due to injury, impact of future performance, and prevention measures all are of paramount importance to the sports medicine physician treating these athletes. Because of the paucity of evidence-based recommendations, it is imperative that, at minimum, understanding of the most common injuries is solidified to help take better care of patients.

DISCLOSURE

C.W. Hodgkins has a paid consultancy to disclose with Arthrex, Naples, Florida, USA. N.A. Wessling has nothing to disclose.

REFERENCES

1. Pfirrmann D, Herbst M, Ingelfinger P, et al. Analysis of Injury Incidences in Male Professional Adult and Elite Youth Soccer Players: A Systematic Review. J Athl Train 2016;51(5):410–24.
2. O'Connor A-M, James IT. Association of Lower Limb Injury with Boot Cleat Design and Playing Surface in Elite Soccer. Foot Ankle Clin 2013;18(2):369–80.
3. Ekstrand J, Nigg BM. Surface-related injuries in soccer. Sports Med 1989;8(1):56–62.
4. Williams S, Hume PA, Kara S. A review of football injuries on third and fourth generation artificial turfs compared with natural turf. Sports Med 2011;41(11):903–23.
5. Pardiwala DN, Rao NN, Varshney AV. Injuries in Cricket. Sports Health 2018;10(3):217–22.
6. Tummala SV, Hartigan DE, Makovicka JL, et al. 10-Year Epidemiology of Ankle Injuries in Men's and Women's Collegiate Basketball. Orthop J Sports Med 2018;6(11). 232596711880540.
7. Taylor JB, Ford KR, Nguyen A-D, et al. Prevention of Lower Extremity Injuries in Basketball: A Systematic Review and Meta-Analysis. Sports Health 2015;7(5):392–8.
8. Riva D, Bianchi R, Rocca F, et al. Proprioceptive Training and Injury Prevention in a Professional Men's Basketball Team: A Six-Year Prospective Study. J Strength Cond Res 2016;30(2):461–75.

9. Barboza SD, Joseph C, Nauta J, et al. Injuries in Field Hockey Players: A Systematic Review. Sports Med 2018;48(4):849–66.
10. Baugh CM, Weintraub GS, Gregory AJ, et al. Descriptive Epidemiology of Injuries Sustained in National Collegiate Athletic Association Men's and Women's Volleyball, 2013-2014 to 2014-2015. Sports Health 2018;10(1):60–9.
11. Dick R, Sauers EL, Agel J, et al. Descriptive epidemiology of collegiate men's baseball injuries: National Collegiate Athletic Association Injury Surveillance System, 1988-1989 through 2003-2004. J Athl Train 2007;42(2):183–93.
12. Jastifer J, Kent R, Crandall J, et al. The Athletic Shoe in Football: Apparel or Protective Equipment? Sports Health 2017;9(2):126–31.
13. Kluczynski MA, Kelly WH, Lashomb WM, et al. A Systematic Review of the Orthopaedic Literature Involving National Football League Players. Orthop J Sports Med 2019;7(8). https://doi.org/10.1177/2325967119864356.
14. Beaulieu-Jones BR, Rossy WH, Sanchez G, et al. Epidemiology of Injuries Identified at the NFL Scouting Combine and Their Impact on Performance in the National Football League: Evaluation of 2203 Athletes From 2009 to 2015. Orthop J Sports Med 2017;5(7). https://doi.org/10.1177/2325967117708744.
15. Vopat B, Beaulieu-Jones BR, Waryasz G, et al. Epidemiology of Navicular Injury at the NFL Combine and Their Impact on an Athlete's Prospective NFL Career. Orthop J Sports Med 2017;5(8). https://doi.org/10.1177/2325967117723285.
16. Kent R, Forman JL, Lessley D, et al. The mechanics of American football cleats on natural grass and infill-type artificial playing surfaces with loads relevant to elite athletes. Sports Biomech 2015;14(2):246–57.
17. Whitehouse T, Orr R, Fitzgerald E, et al. The Epidemiology of Injuries in Australian Professional Rugby Union 2014 Super Rugby Competition. Orthop J Sports Med 2016;4(3). https://doi.org/10.1177/2325967116634075.
18. van der Worp MP, ten Haaf DSM, van Cingel R, et al. Injuries in Runners; A Systematic Review on Risk Factors and Sex Differences. PLoS One 2015;10(2): e0114937.
19. Crowley SG, Trofa DP, Vosseller JT, et al. Epidemiology of Foot and Ankle Injuries in National Collegiate Athletic Association Men's and Women's Ice Hockey. Orthop J Sports Med 2019;7(8). https://doi.org/10.1177/2325967119865908.
20. Jensen AR, Maciel RC, Petrigliano FA, et al. Injuries Sustained by the Mixed Martial Arts Athlete. Sports Health 2017;9(1):64–9.
21. Kay MC, Register-Mihalik JK, Gray AD, et al. The Epidemiology of Severe Injuries Sustained by National Collegiate Athletic Association Student-Athletes, 2009–2010 Through 2014–2015. J Athl Train 2017;52(2):117–28.
22. Agel J, Ransone J, Dick R, et al. Descriptive epidemiology of collegiate men's wrestling injuries: National Collegiate Athletic Association Injury Surveillance System, 1988-1989 through 2003-2004. J Athl Train 2007;42(2):303–10.
23. Mahmood B, Duggal N. Lower extremity injuries in snowboarders. Am J Orthop (Belle Mead NJ) 2014;43(11):502–5.
24. Lemme NJ, Li NY, DeFroda SF, et al. Epidemiology of Achilles Tendon Ruptures in the United States: Athletic and Nonathletic Injuries From 2012 to 2016. Orthop J Sports Med 2018;6(11). https://doi.org/10.1177/2325967118808238.
25. Zellers JA, Carmont MR, Grävare Silbernagel K. Return to play post-Achilles tendon rupture: a systematic review and meta-analysis of rate and measures of return to play. Br J Sports Med 2016;50(21):1325–32.
26. Trofa DP, Miller JC, Jang ES, et al. Professional Athletes' Return to Play and Performance After Operative Repair of an Achilles Tendon Rupture. Am J Sports Med 2017;45(12):2864–71.

27. Lemme NJ, Li NY, Kleiner JE, et al. Epidemiology and Video Analysis of Achilles Tendon Ruptures in the National Basketball Association. Am J Sports Med 2019; 47(10):2360–6.
28. Amin NH, Old AB, Tabb LP, et al. Performance outcomes after repair of complete achilles tendon ruptures in national basketball association players. Am J Sports Med 2013;41(8):1864–8.
29. Trofa DP, Noback PC, Caldwell J-ME, et al. Professional Soccer Players' Return to Play and Performance After Operative Repair of Achilles Tendon Rupture. Orthop J Sports Med 2018;6(11). https://doi.org/10.1177/2325967118810772.
30. Jack RA, Sochacki KR, Gardner SS, et al. Performance and Return to Sport After Achilles Tendon Repair in National Football League Players. Foot Ankle Int 2017; 38(10):1092–9.
31. Waterman BR, Owens BD, Davey S, et al. The epidemiology of ankle sprains in the United States. J Bone Joint Surg Am 2010;92(13):2279–84.
32. Roos KG, Kerr ZY, Mauntel TC, et al. The Epidemiology of Lateral Ligament Complex Ankle Sprains in National Collegiate Athletic Association Sports. Am J Sports Med 2017;45(1):201–9.
33. Mauntel TC, Wikstrom EA, Roos KG, et al. The Epidemiology of High Ankle Sprains in National Collegiate Athletic Association Sports. Am J Sports Med 2017;45(9):2156–63.
34. Kopec TJ, Hibberd EE, Roos KG, et al. The Epidemiology of Deltoid Ligament Sprains in 25 National Collegiate Athletic Association Sports, 2009-2010 Through 2014-2015 Academic Years. J Athl Train 2017;52(4):350–9.
35. Desmond EA, Chou LB. Current concepts review: Lisfranc injuries. Foot Ankle Int 2006;27(8):653–60.
36. MacMahon A, Kim P, Levine DS, et al. Return to Sports and Physical Activities After Primary Partial Arthrodesis for Lisfranc Injuries in Young Patients. Foot Ankle Int 2016;37(4):355–62.
37. Mora AD, Kao M, Alfred T, et al. Return to Sports and Physical Activities After Open Reduction and Internal Fixation of Lisfranc Injuries in Recreational Athletes. Foot Ankle Int 2018;39(7):801–7.
38. Singh SK, George A, Kadakia AR, et al. Performance-Based Outcomes Following Lisfranc Injury Among Professional American Football and Rugby Athletes. Orthopedics 2018;41(4):e479–82.
39. Begly JP, Guss M, Ramme AJ, et al. Return to Play and Performance After Jones Fracture in National Basketball Association Athletes. Sports Health 2016;8(4): 342–6.
40. O'Malley M, DeSandis B, Allen A, et al. Operative Treatment of Fifth Metatarsal Jones Fractures (Zones II and III) in the NBA. Foot Ankle Int 2016;37(5):488–500.

In-Season Management of Acute and Subacute Sports Foot Injuries

William A. Davis III, MD[a],*, Gautam P. Yagnik, MD[b]

KEYWORDS

- Sports foot injuries • Turf toe • Plantar plate • Lisfranc • Jones fracture
- Fifth metatarsal base fracture • Navicular stress fracture • Plantar fasciitis

KEY POINTS

- Injuries of the foot are common in athletes during the season.
- Many foot injuries can be treated effectively nonoperatively.
- Understanding initial evaluation and workup is critical for choosing the appropriate management strategy.

INTRODUCTION

Injuries of the foot and ankle have a wide spectrum of mechanisms, acuteness, severity, and long-term disability in the athletic population. Many of these injuries can be managed during the season with nonoperative treatment. We review pertinent anatomy, presentation, workup, and management for common foot and ankle injuries. Although specific surgical technique is beyond the scope of this article, indications for operative and nonoperative treatment are reviewed.

TURF TOE

Turf toe describes a spectrum of injuries involving the structures associated with the first metatarsophalangeal joint. Injured structures can include the plantar plate and capsule, the plantar musculature, the sesamoid complex, and the articular surface of the metatarsal head. The injury was initially described by Bowers and Martin[1] in 1976 occurring in American football players, and following the introduction of artificial

---

[a] DuPage Medical Group, Team Physician – North Central College, 100 Spalding Drive, Suite 300, Naperville, IL 60540, USA; [b] Miami Orthopaedic and Sports Medicine Institute, Florida International University, Herbert Wertheim College of Medicine, Team Physician- NFL Miami Dolphins and NHL Florida Panthers, Baptist Health South Florida, 1150 Campo Sano Avenue, Coral Gables, FL 33146, USA
* Corresponding author.
E-mail address: William.davis@dupagemd.com

Foot Ankle Clin N Am 26 (2021) 187–203
https://doi.org/10.1016/j.fcl.2020.12.001
1083-7515/21/© 2020 Elsevier Inc. All rights reserved.

playing surfaces (Astroturf), the injury became more common. A 1990 study reported a 45% prevalence among active professional football players with the vast majority of those occurring on artificial turf.[2] More recent data suggest that the incidence of the injury is decreasing, presumably due to improvements in artificial turf designs.[3]

Anatomy

Turf toe describes a spectrum of injuries involving the structures associated with the first metatarsophalangeal joint. Injured structures can include the plantar plate and capsule, the plantar musculature, the sesamoid complex, and the articular surface of the metatarsal head. The injury was initially described by Bowers and Martin in 1976 occurring in American football players,[1] and following the introduction of artificial playing surfaces (Astroturf), the injury became more common. A 1990 study reported a 45 % prevalence among active professional football players with the vast majority of those occurring on artificial turf.[2] More recent data suggests that the incidence of the injury is decreasing, presumably due to improvements in artificial turf designs.[3]

Presentation

The injury most commonly presents following a hyperextension injury in which the first MTP joint experiences an axial load with the foot in equinus. This is commonly seen when the forefoot is fixed with the heel elevated and another player lands on the posterior aspect of the heel. It also can occur simply during active push-off. With such a mechanism, anything from a mild sprain of the plantar plate complex to a complete dorsal dislocation of the MTP joint can occur.[3] A valgus force vector at the time of injury may result in greater disruption to the medial sesamoid component, medial ligaments, and medial capsule, which can lead to a traumatic hallux valgus deformity over time.[4,5]

Sideline Management

If any instability is detected on physical examination, the player should be held out from participation for the rest of that practice or game. Initial clinical evaluation on the sideline or locker room should assess whether an obvious fracture is present, as exhibited by crepitus, and whether the first MTP joint is located, subluxed, or dislocated. If dislocation of the joint is obvious, a closed reduction can be attempted. If plain radiographs are available at the sports facility, then these should be obtained. Otherwise, a closed reduction of a dislocation may need to be performed before radiographs if gross deformity is noted to avoid delays in joint realignment. If a closed reduction is performed, the opportune time to assess stability is at that moment with a dorsal-plantar drawer sign, as this information may prove valuable to the player's injury management. A spectrum exists from grossly unstable with drawer (easily dislocated dorsally) to stable (resistance to dislocation provided by the joint anatomy and resting tension of the surround soft tissue structures).

Initial treatment should include rest, ice, elevation, and immobilization. A walking boot, cast shoe, or short leg cast with the hallux MTP joint in slight plantarflexion is recommended to allow for soft tissue rest.[5] Various modifications of durable medical equipment and injury-specific taping techniques can be used. A cut out under the hallux can be created within the foam of the boot insole or cast shoe surface to maintain the desired position of the hallux. Layered taping over the dorsal aspect of the first proximal phalanx provides a strong block so the hallux does not passively go beyond neutral while loaded on bearing weight. Plantarflexion positioning or creating a "dorsal block" at neutral can be achieved with taping techniques. Control of any varus, valgus, or rotational malalignment may be incorporated into taping technique to address specific components to the injury.

Workup

Appropriate imaging should be obtained to evaluate the extent of the injury, which will allow the team physician to formulate a treatment plan and return to play goals. Radiographs include weight-bearing anteroposterior (AP), lateral, and oblique views of the foot. In addition, an AP radiograph of the contralateral foot should be obtained for comparison of sesamoid position or other signs of significant asymmetry. Ideally the weight-bearing AP views should be performed with pressure on a single limb rather than shared, as with a bilateral AP view. If pain does not allow for this, a bilateral AP would suffice for demonstration of any obvious asymmetry. Radiographs may reveal sesamoid fractures, bony flecks indicating capsular avulsion, sesamoid diastasis, or sesamoid retraction. Proximal migration of one or both sesamoids is suggestive of a plantar plate rupture.[6]

MRI can delineate the pattern of injury and provide information on surrounding soft tissue disruption[1] (**Fig. 1**). MRI also may demonstrate bone marrow edema, osteochondral lesions, or an intra-articular loose body that may be impossible or difficult to visualize on plain radiographs. Depending on the circumstances and imaging findings, this additional information may provide useful information for injury management, particularly if surgical intervention is contemplated.

Classification and Treatment

A detailed injury classification was initially described by Clanton and Ford and later modified by McCormick and Anderson.[5,7] Grade I describes a capsular sprain without disruption. Grade II describes partial plantar plate tearing. Grade III describes a complete tear through the plantar plate.

Initial treatment is as described previously for sideline management. For grade I injuries, players will benefit from slight plantarflexion taping and the use of a stiff soled shoes or Morton extension orthotic. With a medial-sided injury, a toe spacer may be used to decrease the chance of developing posttraumatic hallux valgus. After the resolution of soft tissue swelling, generally in 3 to 5 days, athletes may return to low-impact activities as tolerated.[8] Taping or strapping to limit the degree of hallux dorsiflexion may be continued as the player initially returns to play.

For grade II injuries, initial treatment is the same as for grade I. The player will likely lose on average 2 weeks of playing time with this injury. Following the resolution of acute pain and swelling, low-impact activities may be initiated as tolerated, and toe

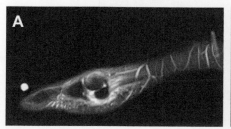
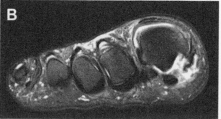

Fig. 1. Turf toe. T2-weighted MRI sagittal and axial images demonstrating rupture of the plantar plate from the distal aspect of the medial sesamoid (*A*) and disruption of the intersesamoid ligament (*B*).

protection is recommended. Once the athlete is tolerating low-impact activities, gradual advancement of running, jumping, and push-off activities may proceed.[1]

With grade III injuries, initial treatment remains the same; however, 8 weeks of immobilization may be required before returning to sports activities. In severe cases, complete resolution of symptoms may not occur for 6 months.[5]

Nonoperative treatment of grade III injuries is controversial, and most surgeons would advocate for surgery for a complete tear with instability. McCormick and Anderson[9] described indications for surgical repair to be large capsular avulsion with instability, diastasis of a bipartite sesamoid, diastasis of a sesamoid fracture, sesamoid retraction, traumatic hallux valgus deformity, vertical instability, loose body, chondral injury, and failed conservative treatment. Continued play on an unstable or inadequately rehabilitated high grade turf toe injury can predispose the player to developing late sequelae, including FHL tendon tears, hallux rigidus, and traumatic hallux valgus with cock-up or claw toe deformity. As such, we recommended to undergo surgical management once any operative indications are met.

Conclusion

Surgical treatment for turf toe injuries is rarely indicated and is beyond the scope of this article. It is typically reserved for severe grade III injuries, especially with concomitant injuries around the first MTP joint (**Fig. 2**). Regardless of treatment strategy, turf toe may be a significant injury to an athlete that can disrupt a season and cause significant pain and disability. Prompt diagnosis and appropriate treatment can allow most athletes to return to preinjury level of performance. Nevertheless, these injuries can lead to varying degrees of persistent pain, stiffness, posttraumatic arthritis, or deformity in the form of hallux rigidus or traumatic hallux valgus (traumatic bunion). Furthermore, athletic performance and career longevity can be negatively impacted.

LISFRANC INJURIES

The Lisfranc joint complex of the midfoot has a unique combination of osseous anatomy and stout ligamentous support that allows for effective force transfer from the

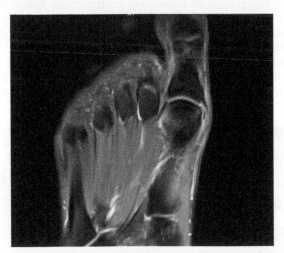

Fig. 2. Grade III turf toe. T2 MRI image demonstrating disruption of the medial collateral ligaments rand capsule. In addition, this high-grade injury results in the associated bone contusion seen in the metatarsal head, as well as surrounding soft tissue edema.

hindfoot to the forefoot during ambulation. It is, therefore, of critical importance in push-off activities in sports.

Lisfranc injuries are uncommon, and they present as a broad spectrum of injuries, ranging from low-energy sprains to high-energy fracture dislocations. Historically, the uncommon occurrence and potential for subtle presentation contributed to 20% to 40% of Lisfranc injuries being missed initially.[10] Recognition of this high rate of missed injury has led to improved early detection. If left untreated, players may develop posttraumatic arthritis and arch collapse.[11]

Anatomy

The Lisfranc joint complex receives osseous stability from the trapezoidal cuneiforms in a "Roman arch" configuration in combination with a proximally recessed second metatarsal base. Additionally, stout ligamentous support is conferred by the interosseous, as well as dorsal and plantar components, of the Lisfranc ligament, which runs obliquely from the plantar lateral base of the medial cuneiform to the plantar medial base of the second metatarsal.

Presentation

Injuries to the Lisfranc joint can occur through multiple mechanisms. Crush injuries can cause significant osseous and soft tissue damage. In sports, Lisfranc injuries can occur through 2 common mechanisms. One occurs when the hindfoot is anchored and a forceful rotation occurs about the midfoot, such as an equestrian who falls with the foot strapped. More commonly, a player with a plantarflexed forefoot and metatarsophalangeal joints in maximal dorsiflexion has an axial load applied to the hindfoot, such as when another player falls on the heel.[12]

Subtle Lisfranc injuries may be difficult to diagnose, particularly on the sideline. Players will typically have difficulty bearing weight following a Lisfranc injury. There may be swelling over the dorsomedial midfoot.[11] The presence of plantar ecchymosis is strongly associated with a Lisfranc injury although this finding is typically not present until 24-48 hours following injury.[13] The midfoot should be palpated for tenderness with particular attention to the metatarsal bases, tarsometatarsal joints, naviculocuneiform joint, and navicular tuberosity. Pain elicited with a passive pronation-abduction stress maneuver through the junction of the forefoot-midfoot is suggestive of injury. Dorsoplantar drawer testing of the individual first, second, and third TMT joints may reveal TMT instability or elicit pain on testing.

Sideline Management

If a Lisfranc injury is suspected due to swelling, tenderness, and difficulty bearing weight, the player should be made non–weight-bearing. Swelling can be significant; therefore, ice should be applied and the extremity elevated. Immobilization should be in a splint or controlled ankle motion (CAM) boot.

Workup

Imaging of a suspected Lisfranc injury begins with weight-bearing AP, lateral, and oblique views of the foot. On the AP view, the medial borders of the second metatarsal and the middle cuneiform should align. On the oblique view, the medial borders of the fourth metatarsal and cuboid should align. On the lateral view, there should be no dorsal or plantar subluxation of the metatarsals at the TMT joint. If there is a question of subtle irregularity, comparisons with the contralateral foot should be made. Greater than 2 mm of translation is diagnostic of injury[11] (**Fig. 3**). In addition, a "fleck

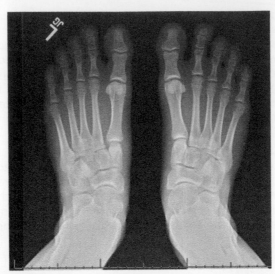

Fig. 3. Lisfranc injury. Bilateral weight-bearing AP radiographs demonstrating irregularity of the second metatarsal–middle cuneiform border and widening of the interval between the second metatarsal base and medial cuneiform.

sign," which is an avulsion of the base of the second metatarsal, is indicative of a Lisfranc ligament injury[14] (**Fig. 4**).

If plain radiographs are normal in a player with a suspected midfoot injury, stress radiographs or advanced imaging should be obtained. Stress radiographs are performed with an abduction-pronation stress maneuver but can be painful to the patient.[15] To perform this, an ankle block would likely be required to perform adequately or under intravenous sedation or general anesthesia. In our experience, however, this is rarely performed. Computed tomography (CT) scan may show bony abnormalities such as avulsion fractures and is useful for preoperative planning with injuries involving comminution. MRI can be useful for demonstrating ligamentous disruption, particularly in the setting of equivocal weight bearing radiographs and has been correlated with intraoperative instability.[16] MRI also may give findings consistent with injury pattern, such as disruption or partial tear of the Lisfranc ligament, signal intensity through the zones of the intercuneiform region, and bone contusions of the metatarsal bases or cuboid (**Fig. 5**).

Treatment

A mild Lisfranc injury can be treated successfully nonoperatively if subtle instability is ruled out. With appropriate plain radiographs and advanced imaging, if clinical findings are still suggestive of injury, an examination under anesthesia may have to be performed.[11]

For stable ligamentous injuries, nonoperative treatment consists of 4 to 6 weeks of non–weight-bearing immobilization. A short leg cast or CAM boot with arch support is recommended. After this period of immobilization, the player may benefit from a course of physical therapy to improve gait and balance. Return to play can occur after resolution of pain and swelling and may take 4 to 6 months or longer.[11] Simple Lisfranc fracture patterns can be treated successfully with nonoperative management as well. A recent study by Ponkilainen and colleagues[17] suggests that Lisfranc injuries involving avulsion fractures or simple non-displaced intra-articular fractures and less than 2 mm of medial

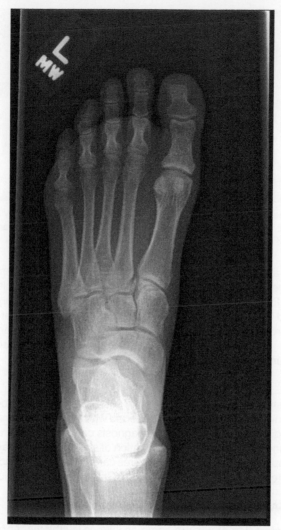

Fig. 4. "Fleck sign." AP radiograph demonstrating an avulsion of the second metatarsal base, indicating a Lisfranc injury.

cuneiform – second metatarsal displacement can be treated with 4-6 weeks of non-weightbearing cast immobilization with high functional outcomes.

For unstable or displaced injuries, surgical management is indicated. Definitive management is delayed until the soft tissue envelope can accommodate surgical incisions. The details of operative treatment are beyond the scope of this article but generally involve closed versus open reduction depending on the injury pattern, with rigid anatomic fixation of the medial and middle columns of the foot and possible flexible temporary fixation for the lateral column if necessary. An ongoing debate in the literature revolves around whether these injuries are best treated with open reduction and internal fixation (ORIF) or with primary arthrodesis. Future research is needed to delineate indications for each treatment option, particularly as it pertains to the athlete and ability to return to the same functional level.[11]

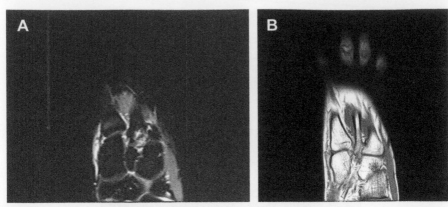

Fig. 5. T2-weighted (A) and T1-weighted (B) MRI scan of a Lisfranc injury demonstrating a tear of the Lisfranc ligament. Also present is associated soft tissue edema and a bone contusion of the base of the second metatarsal.

Posttraumatic arthritis can occur with both nonoperative and operative treatment, although it is generally accepted that anatomic fixation decreases this risk. However, the initial impact forces to the articular cartilage at the time of the injury must be taken into account, and the individual's biological cartilage response to that injury would be outside the control of the treating physician. Explaining these factors to the athlete may provide an understanding of some of the potential long-term implications following the trauma they sustained.

Conclusions

Lisfranc injuries, although uncommon, have the potential to be missed because of subtle presentations. A high index of suspicion is needed when a player suffers a midfoot injury with a corresponding mechanism. Missed diagnosis can lead to posttraumatic arthritis, persistent pain, and arch collapse. Determination of stability is necessary to guide operative versus nonoperative treatment and requires careful evaluation of advanced imaging and provocative testing if there is any question in the case of subtle injuries.

FIFTH METATARSAL BASE FRACTURES

Base of fifth metatarsal fractures are common injuries in athletes. Approximately 70% of metatarsal fractures are fifth metatarsal fractures, and 80% of these occur in the proximal end.[18,19] Basketball, American football, and soccer are among the 3 highest risk sports for fifth metatarsal base fractures.[20] Fractures may be acute fractures, stress fractures, or refracture through an incomplete union.

Anatomy

The fifth metatarsal is typically divided anatomically into the tuberosity, the metaphyseal-diaphyseal junction, and the proximal shaft. Lawrence and Botte[21] described them as Zones I, II, and III, respectively.

Zone I fractures are generally considered to be avulsion fractures by the lateral band of the plantar fascia or peroneus brevis tendon.

The metaphyseal-diaphyseal area, or Zone II, includes the fourth-fifth metatarsal articulation and is considered a vascular watershed. This area of relative hypovascularity predisposes fractures in this area, known as Jones fractures, to delayed union or nonunion[22] (**Fig. 6**).

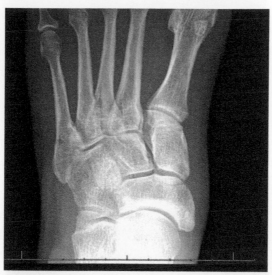

Fig. 6. Jones fracture (Zone II) of the fifth metatarsal. AP foot radiograph demonstrates an acute Jones fracture with the fracture line extending into the articulation of the fourth and fifth metatarsal bases.

The proximal diaphysis, or Zone III, is the area just distal to the fourth-fifth metatarsal articulation and is a common site of stress fractures in athletes[23] (**Fig. 7**).

Presentation

Fractures of the fifth metatarsal base may be either acute injuries or stress fractures. Players who sustain an acute fracture will usually present with pain, swelling, and difficulty bearing weight following a sudden inversion injury or pure adduction force on a loaded foot. Typically, there will be tenderness over the fracture site. The foot may exhibit erythema and bruising as well. Players who experience stress fractures will typically experience prodromal symptoms, such as activity-related pain over the lateral aspect of the foot followed by a sudden increase in symptoms once the cortical bone finally fails.[20]

Refracture may occasionally occur through a previous site of incompletely healed fracture or reveal that a nonunion had occurred through a relative biomechanically weak zone. If this does occur, both biologic and biomechanical sources should be reassessed. It would be prudent to investigate potential contributory factors that are intrinsic to the bone (eg, vitamin D deficiency or endocrine factors) and extrinsic to the bone (ie, varus hindfoot alignment contributing to lateral column overload).

Sideline Management

Following an acute injury, the ice, elevation, and pain control should be initiated. Immobilization in a CAM boot or splint will allow for soft tissue rest.

Workup

It is important to assess their overall foot and ankle alignment. This is easy to perform but often not done in the case of an acute fracture. Simply by having the player stand and viewing them front, side, and back may allow the treating physician to have a better understanding of predisposing factors, such as a varus hindfoot or cavovarus foot

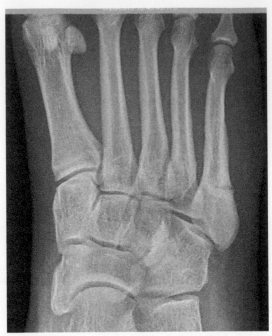

Fig. 7. Zone III fifth metatarsal fracture, immediately distal to the fourth-fifth metatarsal articulation.

shape, which may aid in the treatment of this condition and prevention of future issues with the contralateral foot.

Radiographic imaging should include weight-bearing AP, lateral, and oblique views of the foot. Contralateral comparison views are not typically needed, but may be helpful in a skeletally immature foot. Additional imaging, such as MRI or bone scan, may be helpful in the diagnosis of an early stress fracture. Bone scans have become less common over the years with the improvements that have occurred within the field of MRI. In addition, the MRI scan does not involve radiation to the patient. CT scan does expose the patient to radiation but can aid in the diagnosis of nonunion.[24]

Treatment

Zone II fractures, true Jones fractures, treated with ORIF have been shown to have higher union rates, earlier demonstration of radiographic healing, and, therefore, earlier return to baseline athletic activity. The typical form of ORIF has been intramedullary screw fixation. A systematic review from 2013[25] of 26 studies on treatment and return to sport following Jones fractures found a union rate of 76% for nonoperative treatment and 96% for screw fixation. Operative treatment allowed a return to sport between 4 and 18 weeks as compared with 9 to 22 weeks with nonoperative treatment. Gradual return to sport with stress protection of that zone will help with the transition. With full return to sport, it is recommended that adequate bony bridging is seen on plain radiographs and if in question, thin-slice CT scan confirmation can be obtained.

Use of a bone growth stimulator with immobilization has had mixed results as a treatment option for acute fracture, and no recommendations exist specifically for athletes. As such, the bone stimulator may be considered as an adjunctive therapy in combination with intramedullary screw fixation, although no specific literature has been presented to advocate its combined use.

Nonoperative treatment of Zone II fractures typically involves 6-8 weeks of non weight bearing cast immobilization; however, some surgeons advocate for early weight bearing. If nonoperative treatment is chosen, a slightly more frequent interval follow-up would be recommended. Four-week non–weight-bearing AP, lateral, and oblique foot radiographs could be obtained. Although fracture healing would not be anticipated at that time, certain radiographic signs, such as widening of the fracture line representing bone resorption, can be prognostic indicators of fracture healing and suggest potential development of delayed or nonunion. If this should occur, a CT scan can determine if callus formation is noted or absent and may help the treating physician in decision making of continued nonoperative management versus changing strategy to operative management. Assessment of patient compliance, reassessment of biological factors, and treatment plan alteration may be required.

Stress fractures of Zone III are at increased risk of nonunion in athletes, especially those with cavovarus deformities. Similar to Zone II fractures, these players should undergo intramedullary screw fixation, as there is a 33% risk of refracture of Zone III injuries with nonoperative treatment when the fracture is stress-related.[23] This high refracture rate may once again represent intrinsic or extrinsic predisposing factors. Therefore, the authors' recommendation would be for the treating physician to have a higher degree of suspicion when evaluating a player with a Zone III fracture; treat the acute fracture but also seek to determine why it occurred in this particular player.

A clinical challenge is the player who has been treated nonoperatively for a fifth metatarsal stress fracture, returns to play successfully, and then develops recurrence of symptoms. Many of these players can continue playing following a brief period of rest, boot immobilization, and management of symptoms. However, worsening of symptoms should raise suspicion for an acute on chronic injury and prompt new imaging. **Fig. 8** demonstrates such an injury in an 18 year old college football player. He underwent nonoperative management of a stress fracture as a high school senior. During his first collegiate season he experienced intermittent symptoms until experiencing a sudden acute injury. Radiographs demonstrated an acute fracture through a previous stress fracture, and he was treated with ORIF.

Given the significant risk of refracture, the treating physician should strongly consider ORIF in the player that continues to have symptoms after nonoperative management of a stress fracture. If symptoms permit, and if the player understands that there is a risk of refracture during continued play, this can be done following the season.

Conclusions

Proximal shaft fractures (Zone III) and refractures through a previous Jones (Zone 2) warrant higher level of investigation for biologic and biomechanical contributing factors. In the setting of acute Jones fractures (Zone II) and proximal shaft fractures (Zone III), operative treatment remains the preferred treatment in athletes. Operative treatment with an intramedullary screw yields higher union rates and an earlier return to sport than nonoperative treatment. Although successfully treated fractures may not be career threatening, missed time due to injury during the season can be significant.

NAVICULAR STRESS FRACTURES

Stress fracture of the navicular bone is not a common injury in the general population, but there is an increased prevalence in athletes. Those at particular risk include athletes engaging in explosive running or cutting sports.[26] One study found that up to

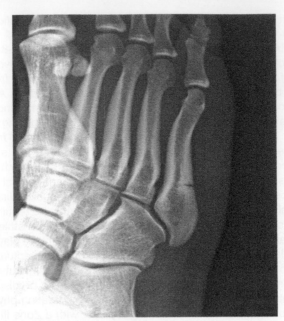

Fig. 8. Radiograph of an acute fifth metatarsal fracture through a previous Zone III stress fracture that had been treated nonoperatively.

73% of stress fractures in track athletes involved the navicular,[27] whereas the injury is uncommon in endurance runners.

Anatomy

The vascular anatomy of the navicular likely contributes to the development of stress fractures. The presence of dorsal and plantar blood supplies results in a watershed area with varying degrees of vascularity.[28]

Presentation

Athletes may have variable presentations. Initially, these fractures are often only painful during sports activity, but eventually this can progress to pain with daily activities or even pain at night. Tenderness over the dorsal navicular prominence is a common finding,[29] and has been referred to as the "N spot" (**Fig. 9**). Palpation of this region with maximal point of tenderness should raise suspicion for navicular stress fractures particularly in athletes with unexplained ongoing midfoot pain with activity. This is quite different from tenderness along the medial navicular tuberosity, which may represent either insertional posterior tibial tendon tendinitis or stress reaction through the synchondrosis bridge of an accessory navicular. Patients may have pain with single leg hop or doing a heel raise. Because of the insidious onset and vague symptoms, delay in diagnosis can range from 4 to 7 months from the onset of symptoms.[26]

Workup

Appropriate imaging begins with plain radiographs. A fracture line does not become apparent until late in the condition, however, and is therefore unlikely to be demonstrated on early plain radiographs. As few as 18% of stress fractures diagnosed on CT scan may be visible on plain radiographs.[30] CT scan is an excellent diagnostic tool for these fractures (**Fig. 10**). It is lower cost than MRI, has excellent sensitivity,

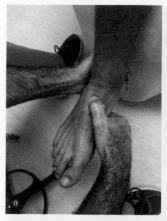
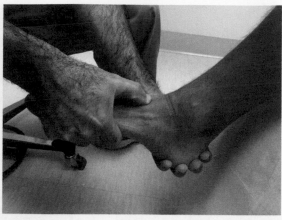

Fig. 9. "N spot." Clinical examination of the foot demonstrating palpation of the dorsal navicular prominence. Players with a navicular stress fracture will often exhibit a maximal point of tenderness at this specific location.

and provides detail of the fracture and surrounding bony involvement. MRI can be useful for identifying navicular stress reactions before the development of a fracture. Saxena and colleagues[31] developed a useful classification system based on coronal CT scan. Type 1 involves a dorsal cortical fracture. Type II involves a fracture line extending into the body of the navicular and type III is a complete fracture involving 2 cortices. Type 0.5 was subsequently added to describe stress reaction injuries visible only on MRI (**Fig. 11**).[32]

Treatment

Historically, nonoperative treatment has been favored except in cases in which a complete fracture line is noted on radiographs or CT scan. Identification of sclerotic edges at stress fracture zone, or any displaced fractures would mandate surgical repair. One meta-analysis found that non–weight-bearing immobilization in a cast for 6 weeks

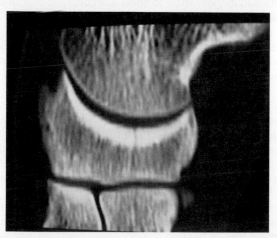

Fig. 10. Navicular stress fracture. CT image demonstrating fracture line in the mid portion of the navicular.

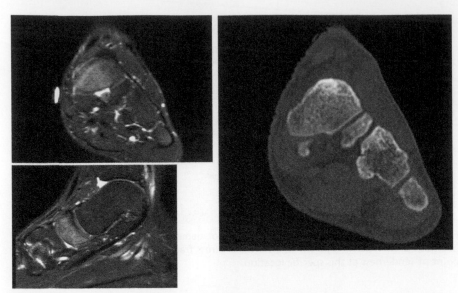

Fig. 11. Stress reaction of the navicular in a high school cross country runner visible on MRI. Coronal CT scan did not demonstrate and fracture line.

yielded a 96% success rate with return to sport of 4.9 months in patients with nondisplaced navicular stress fractures.[33] However, similar to Jones fractures, in the setting of a high-level athlete, operative treatment may be considered to minimize the time of immobility and improved the predictability of healing in a shorter timeframe. Recently, Saxena and colleagues[34] reported on outcomes of their treatment protocol in a large cohort of athletes, demonstrating a greater than 90% return to activity. They recommend ORIF of type II and III navicular stress fractures.

Early weight bearing and early surgical intervention have both been investigated as a means to speed up the return to sport. Early weight bearing has been shown to have worse results and longer return to sport than delayed weight-bearing immobilization.[30,33,35] Early surgical intervention has been shown to have similar return to sport times as 6 week cast immobilization.[33] One study, however, demonstrated a faster return to sport with early ORIF compared with nonoperative treatment for complete fractures.[36] Factors contributing to a faster recuperation with ORIF include less time immobilized in a cast, less muscle atrophy, and earlier range of motion.

Athletes with MRI-evident stress reactions (Type 0.5 injuries) can be treated well in a CAM boot with non or partial weightbearing restriction for several weeks until symptoms resolve, followed by progressive return to sport specific activity. Type I dorsal cortical fractures should undergo non-weight bearing cast immobilization for minimum of 6 weeks, followed by progressive weight bearing and physical therapy. To our knowledge, early fixation of type 0.5 or type I fractures has not been demonstrated to shorten return to play time.

For type II fractures, nonoperative management can be successful with non-weightbearing cast immobilization for 6 weeks, typically with an additional several weeks of progressive weight bearing in a boot until pain free. For high level athletes and those with recurrent fracture, ORIF should be considered. Players, coaches, and athletic trainers should understand that return to play time following ORIF may be 4-6 months. For Type III fractures, it is typically recommended that the player undergo ORIF.

Conclusions

Although navicular stress fractures are uncommon in the general population, physicians should maintain a high index of suspicion when dealing with nontraumatic midfoot pain in athletes, particularly track athletes or those doing explosive running and jumping. A delay in diagnosis is common, and combined with a significant return to sport time for all treatment strategies, players may be out of full participation for many months. Although larger, high-quality studies are needed to determine optimal treatments for navicular stress fractures, most of these fractures can be safely and effectively treated nonoperatively. In the high-level athlete, a lower threshold for operative treatment may exist due to the timeframe and desire for earlier return to sport.

DISCLOSURE

The authors have nothing to disclose.

REFERENCES

1. Bowers KD, Martin RB. Turf-toe: a shoe-surface related football injury. Med Sci Sports 1976;8:81-3.
2. Rodeo SA, O'Brien S, Warren RF, et al. Turf-toe: an analysis of metatarsophalangeal joint sprains in professional football players. Am J Sports Med 1990;18: 280-5.
3. Clough TM, Majeed H. Turf toe injury - current concepts and an updated review of literature. Foot Ankle Clin 2018;23:693-701.
4. George E, Harris AHS, Dragoo JL, et al. Incidence and risk factors for turf toe injuries in intercollegiate football: data from the National Collegiate Athletic Association injury surveillance system. Foot Ankle Int 2014;35:108-15.
5. Clanton TO, Ford JJ. Turf toe injury. Clin Sports Med 1994;13:731-41.
6. Prieskorn D, Graves SC, Smith RA. Morphometric analysis of the plantar plate apparatus of the first metatarsophalangeal joint. Foot Ankle 1993;14:204-7.
7. McCormick JJ, Anderson RB. Turf toe: anatomy, diagnosis, and treatment. Sports Health 2010;2:487-94.
8. McCormick JJ, Anderson RB. The great toe: failed turf toe, chronic turf toe, and complicated sesamoid injuries. Foot Ankle Clin 2009;14:135-50.
9. McCormick J, Anderson RB. The Great Toe: Failed Turf Toe, Chronic Turf Toe, and Complicated Sesamoid Injuries. Foot and Ankle Clinics 2009;14:135-50.
10. Aronow MS. Treatment of the missed Lisfranc injury. Foot Ankle Clin 2006;11: 127-142, ix.
11. Weatherford BM, Anderson JG, Bohay DR. Management of tarsometatarsal joint injuries. J Am Acad Orthop Surg 2017;25:469-79.
12. Eleftheriou KI, Rosenfeld PF. Lisfranc injury in the athlete: evidence supporting management from sprain to fracture dislocation. Foot Ankle Clin 2013;18:219-36.
13. Ross G, Cronin R, Hauzenblas J, et al. Plantar ecchymosis sign: a clinical aid to diagnosis of occult Lisfranc tarsometatarsal injuries. J Orthop Trauma 1996;10: 119-22.

14. Myerson MS, Fisher RT, Burgess AR, et al. Fracture dislocations of the tarsometatarsal joints: end results correlated with pathology and treatment. Foot Ankle 1986;6:225–42.
15. Coss HS, Manos RE, Buoncristiani A, et al. Abduction stress and AP weightbearing radiography of purely ligamentous injury in the tarsometatarsal joint. Foot Ankle Int 1998;19:537–41.
16. Raikin SM, Elias I, Dheer S, et al. Prediction of midfoot instability in the subtle Lisfranc injury. Comparison of magnetic resonance imaging with intraoperative findings. J Bone Joint Surg Am 2009;91:892–9.
17. Ponkilainen VT, Partio N, Salonen EE, et al. Outcomes after nonoperatively treated non-displaced Lisfranc injury: a retrospective case series of 55 patients. Arch Orthop Trauma Surg 2020.
18. Petrisor BA, Ekrol I, Court-Brown C. The epidemiology of metatarsal fractures. Foot Ankle Int 2006;27:172–4.
19. Hasselman CT, Vogt MT, Stone KL, et al. Foot and ankle fractures in elderly white women. Incidence and risk factors. J Bone Joint Surg Am 2003;85:820–4.
20. Hong CC, Pearce CJ, Ballal MS, et al. Management of sports injuries of the foot and ankle: An update. Bone Joint J 2016;98-B:1299–311.
21. Lawrence SJ, Botte MJ. Jones' fractures and related fractures of the proximal fifth metatarsal. Foot Ankle 1993;14:358–65.
22. Smith JW, Arnoczky SP, Hersh A. The intraosseous blood supply of the fifth metatarsal: implications for proximal fracture healing. Foot Ankle 1992;13:143–52.
23. Miller MD, Thompson SR, editors. Miller's review of orthopaedics. 7th edition. Philadelphia, PA: Elsevier; 2016.
24. Porter DA. Fifth metatarsal jones fractures in the athlete. Foot Ankle Int 2018;39:250–8.
25. Roche AJ, Calder JDF. Treatment and return to sport following a Jones fracture of the fifth metatarsal: a systematic review. Knee Surg Sports Traumatol Arthrosc 2013;21:1307–15.
26. Ramadorai MUE, Beuchel MW, Sangeorzan BJ. Fractures and dislocations of the tarsal navicular. J Am Acad Orthop Surg 2016;24:379–89.
27. Brukner P, Bradshaw C, Khan KM, et al. Stress fractures: a review of 180 cases. Clin J Sport Med 1996;6:85–9.
28. McKeon KE, McCormick JJ, Johnson JE, et al. Intraosseous and extraosseous arterial anatomy of the adult navicular. Foot Ankle Int 2012;33:857–61.
29. Burne SG, Mahoney CM, Forster BB, et al. Tarsal navicular stress injury: long-term outcome and clinicoradiological correlation using both computed tomography and magnetic resonance imaging. Am J Sports Med 2005;33:1875–81.
30. Khan KM, Fuller PJ, Brukner PD, et al. Outcome of conservative and surgical management of navicular stress fracture in athletes. Eighty-six cases proven with computerized tomography. Am J Sports Med 1992;20:657–66.
31. Saxena A, Fullem B. Comment on Torg et al, "management of tarsal navicular stress fractures: conservative versus surgical treatment". Am J Sports Med 2010;38:NP3–5.
32. Saxena A, Fullem B, Hannaford D. Results of treatment of 22 navicular stress fractures and a new proposed radiographic classification system. J Foot Ankle Surg 2000;39:96–103.
33. Torg JS, Moyer J, Gaughan JP, et al. Management of tarsal navicular stress fractures: conservative versus surgical treatment: a meta-analysis. Am J Sports Med 2010;38:1048–53.

34. Saxena A, Behan SA, Valerio DL, Frosch DL. Navicular Stress Fracture Outcomes in Athletes: Analysis of 62 Injuries. J Foot Ankle Surg 2017;56:943–8.
35. Potter NJ, Brukner PD, Makdissi M, et al. Navicular stress fractures: outcomes of surgical and conservative management. Br J Sports Med 2006;40:692–5 [discussion 695].
36. Saxena A, Fullem B. Navicular stress fractures: a prospective study on athletes. Foot Ankle Int 2006;27:917–21.

Imaging Techniques for Assessment of Dynamically Unstable Sports Related Foot and Ankle Injuries

Carolyn M. Sofka, MD

KEYWORDS

- Foot • Ankle • MRI • Radiographs • CT • Instability • Ligaments

KEY POINTS

- Dynamic information regarding both acute and chronic (or repetitive) foot and ankle sports injuries can be obtained from static imaging studies, including loading patterns in the setting of overuse injuries.
- Stress or loaded (weight-bearing) imaging studies provide an objective evaluation of the degree of instability.
- Absolute measurements and cutoff values for radiographic evaluation of a potentially unstable joint in the foot and ankle should be used with caution; comparison to the contralateral side is more reliable.
- Imaging findings always should be considered in conjunction with the clinical findings for the most accurate diagnosis in the setting of foot and ankle instability.

OVERUSE SYNDROMES

A diagnosis of osseous overuse syndromes on radiographs often is limited because it takes some time for bony turnover to result in endosteal callus or a visible fracture line. Depending on where the osseous abnormality is located, radiographic signs never may be seen if they are obscured by overlying osseous structures in the midfoot or hindfoot or do not frankly result in the creation of a discrete fracture. Radiographs are of benefit, however, in identifying potential biomechanical foot pathologies that may predispose to overuse injuries, such as pes planus, pes cavus, and hindfoot varus, with utilization of flexion and extension lateral views to demonstrate restricted ankle dorsiflexion.[1]

Magnetic resonance imaging (MRI) affords the ability to noninvasively diagnose repetitive stress injuries much earlier than radiographs, in the absence of a definable

Department of Radiology and Imaging, Hospital for Special Surgery, 535 East 70th Street, New York, NY 10021, USA
E-mail address: sofkac@hss.edu

Foot Ankle Clin N Am 26 (2021) 205–224
https://doi.org/10.1016/j.fcl.2020.10.003
1083-7515/21/© 2020 Elsevier Inc. All rights reserved.

fracture[2,3] (**Figs. 1** and **2**). High-resolution multiplanar imaging also helps diagnose less common stress injuries (and those more difficult to see on radiographs), including those of accessory ossicles of the foot and ankle (**Figs. 3** and **4**).

SYNDESMOSIS

Injuries to the supporting ligamentous structures of the lower leg and ankle can be devastating and a cause of chronic pain and instability, potentially resulting in severe posttraumatic ankle joint arthritis with the ultimate need for an ankle replacement or fusion. Defined measurements for the determination of a successfully reduced syndesmosis have been reported and historically utilized, which largely depend on the degree of overlap of the tibia and fibula as seen in the frontal (anteroposterior [AP] or mortise) projections.

The reliability and utility of these measurements recently have come into question, however. Statistically significant differences based on age and gender in the traditionally used tibiofibular overlap measurement have been reported.[4,5] A large review of the literature found that there was significant variability in the anatomic landmarks used for measurements in the determination of syndesmotic instability.[5] A subjective,

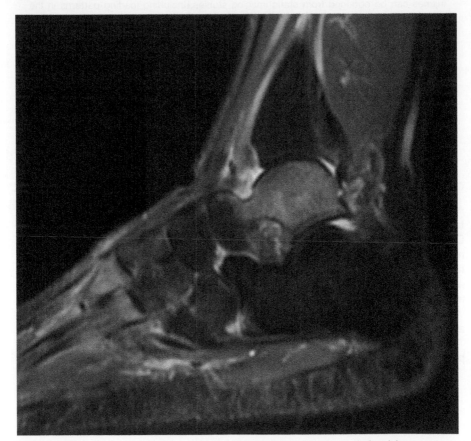

Fig. 1. Sagittal short tau inversion recovery image demonstrates multifocal bone marrow edema pattern, notably in the talus and imaged proximal metatarsals in this patient with overuse syndrome.

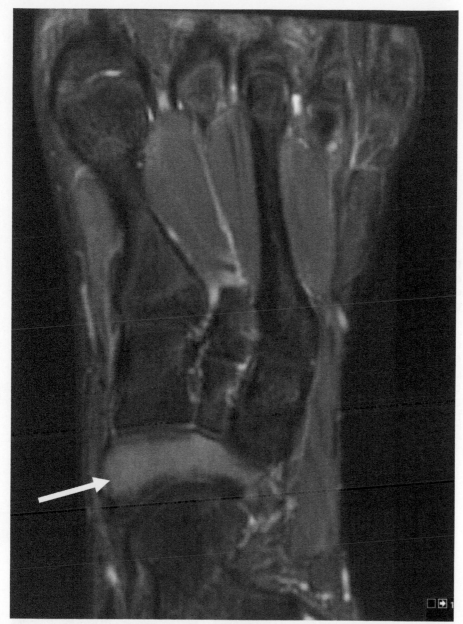

Fig. 2. Coronal inversion recovery image demonstrates marked navicular stress reaction (*arrow*) in the absence of a discrete fracture line either on MR or on radiographs.

thoughtful review and evaluation of ankle radiographs postreduction after a syndesmotic injury will reveal a wide range of appearances, with not all conforming to the strict measurement guidelines reported in the literature.

A tibiofibular clear space of more than 6 mm has been reported to be a normal variant, with many authors advocating for comparison with the contralateral side

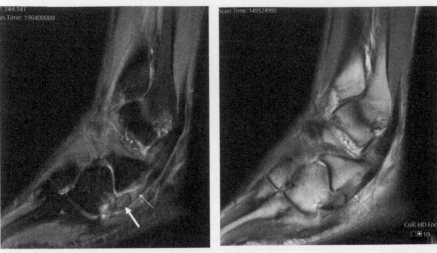

Fig. 3. Sagittal inversion recovery (*left*) and high-resolution fast spin-echo (*right*) images demonstrate high-grade stress reaction in the os peroneum (*thick arrow*), with additional edema in the adjacent cuboid in the setting of tendinopathy of the regional peroneus longus (*thin arrows*).

rather than relying on absolute numbers.[6–9] Exactly how great a difference is considered abnormal is uncertain, however, because the historically reported threshold of defining malreduction as a greater than 2 mm side-to-side difference also has been brought into question.[10–12] The incisura fibularis, a key landmark used in many syndesmotic measurements, has been demonstrated further to have variant anatomy based on age, gender, and location.[8,13]

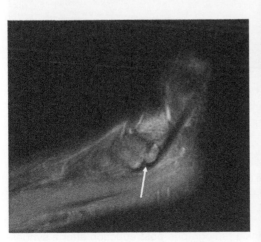
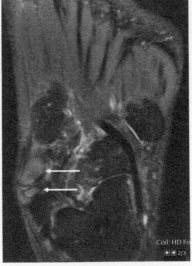

Fig. 4. Sagittal (*left*) and coronal (*right*) inversion recovery demonstrates marked reactive edema in an accessory navicular as well as the subjacent navicular (*arrows*) in this patient with an overuse syndrome.

Beyond the unreliability of commonly utilized and reported radiographic measurements for syndesmotic reduction, questions have been raised as to how precise a reduction needs to be. Warner and colleagues[10] studied 155 patients with either supination external rotation stage IV or pronation external rotation stage IV fractures with documented syndesmotic instability and, using standard radiographic measurements, found several patients malreduced yet experienced no adverse symptoms in clinical follow-up (median 15 months [range 12–120 months]). The investigators postulate that although a good syndesmotic reduction certainly is desirable, other factors, such as the quality of the articular reduction, may be more important.[10]

Although differences in age and gender may limit the utility of using strictly defined values when evaluating the quality of a reduced syndesmosis, other radiographic findings and, therefore, imaging techniques may prove more beneficial although certainly further renewed and reenergized research is required. As Warner and colleagues[10] postulated, the degree of articular malreduction may prove more clinically relevant, and observing lateral or anterior shift of the talus on weight-bearing radiographs likely is a more negative indicator for the development of future ankle joint arthritis. Computed tomography (CT) can identify anatomic landmarks precisely, thereby increasing reliability in determination of alignment although most standard CT scans are obtained non–weight bearing.

Determining the quality of a syndesmotic reduction at the time of surgery is ideal; however, it is also not without its limitations. Recent studies have described the advantages of using 3-dimensional intraoperative imaging, such as 3-dimensional fluoroscopy or cone-beam CT to judge the quality of the reduction though most surgeons do not have the luxury of such advanced imaging at their disposal.[14,15] Because standard frontal (AP and mortise) syndesmotic landmarks and measurements can be misleading, attempts have been made to use lateral fluoroscopy to evaluate syndesmotic reductions. Croft and colleagues[16] found that when approximately 40% of the anterior margin of the tibia was anterior to the fibular cortex at a location 1 cm superior to the plafond, this resulted in a satisfactory reduction. Other investigators have found the ratio of the anterior to posterior margins of the tibia helpful.[17] More recently, Cogan and colleagues[18] have reported that the posterior border of the fibula should intersect within 2 mm of the posterior extent of the tibial plafond to achieve a successful reduction and that greater differences, especially if displaced anteriorly, should raise concern for malreduction (**Fig. 5**).

Although its utilization of alignment is unreliable as it is non–weight bearing, MRI can directly visualize the supporting ligamentous structures of the syndesmotic complex. In a prospective review of grades III and IV supination external rotation ankle fractures without a posterior malleolar fracture, 97% of patients had abnormal posterior inferior tibiofibular ligaments on MRI, usually a delamination type tear from the posterior malleolus.[19] Because the syndesmosis is a complex structure, and it has a contribution to posttraumatic ankle arthritis and chronic instability, in conjunction with intraarticular pathology of the ankle joint proper, a complete evaluation, including weight-bearing CT with comparison to the contralateral normal ankle as well as MRI to directly visualize the morphology of the supporting soft tissue structures and potential intraarticular pathology is advocated because standard radiographs are unreliable for determination of an appropriate reduction for each individual patient.

ANKLE AND HINDFOOT

In the acute setting, tears of the anterior talofibular ligament (ATFL) are seen on MRI as diffuse increased signal intensity of the ligament, often with a wavy or lax appearance

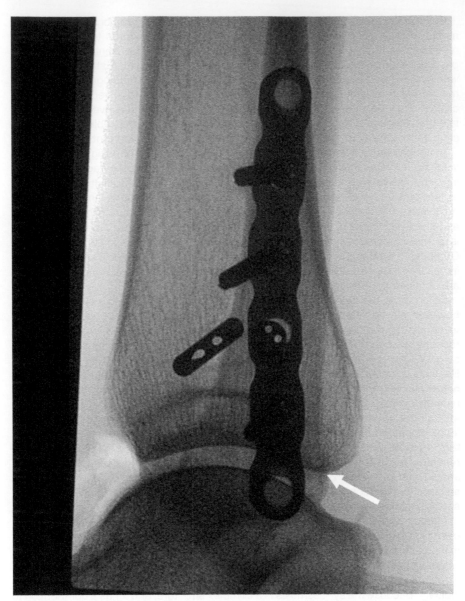

Fig. 5. Intraoperative lateral view of the ankle status post–distal fibular fracture reduction and syndesmotic fixation demonstrates a satisfactory reduction using the criteria of Cogan and colleagues[18] with the posterior cortex of the distal fibular just at the posterior margin of the plafond (*arrow*).

with remodeling of the ligament commencing usually about the fourth week after injury[20] (**Fig. 6**). Li and colleagues[21] reviewed changes in signal intensity of the ATFL in 70 patients with chronic ankle instability and found that those who had ATFLs that were of lower signal intensity had a higher rate of return to sport than those with a high signal intensity ATFL. This is in agreement with the general magnetic resonance

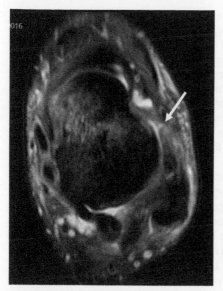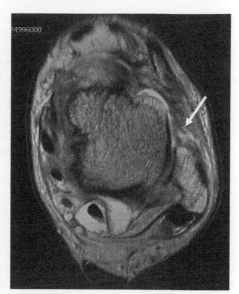

Fig. 6. Axial fast spin-echo inversion recovery (*left*) and proton density–weighted (*right*) images demonstrate complete disruption of the ATFL (*arrows*) in the setting of an acute ankle sprain.

(MR) principles of fluid imbibition and extracellular water within injured ligaments generating their MR appearance with remodeling over time resulting in a return to a more normal low signal intensity appearance.[22] Jung and colleagues[23] reviewed the MR findings in 132 ankles with chronic lateral ankle instability that underwent ligamentous reconstruction and found that, most commonly, chronically insufficient ATFLs or, less commonly, calcaneofibular ligaments, were attenuated or thinned, likely due to repetitive trauma and stretching. These same investigators also found a significant amount of abnormally thickened ligaments in their cohort attributed to a largely fibrotic response corresponding to previously described histologic examinations of abnormal ATFLs containing scar but lacking structurally sound type I collagen.[23,24] Ultrasound, particularly with anterior drawer and inversion stress, has been shown reliable in documenting alterations in ATFL morphology but is limited in its ability to provide a more global overview and potential associated lesions, such as intraarticular chondral injuries.[25–27]

Secondary and indirect findings of chronic lateral ankle instability can be observed on MRI, thus aiding in the diagnosis. Abnormal alignment can be appreciated even in the non–weight-bearing setting in cases of functionally incompetent ATFLs although the absence of abnormal alignment does not exclude it. Berkowitz and Kim[28] reported that the fibula was observed to be posteriorly displaced on axial MRI scans at the level of the ankle mortise in 65% of patients undergoing a lateral ankle stabilization procedure compared with 8% of controls. Associated injuries also are common in the setting of chronic lateral ankle instability, including peroneal tendon and peroneal retinacular injuries most commonly, although also osteochondral lesions, intraarticular loose bodies, and findings suggestive of anterolateral impingement, such as scarring and fibrosis in the anterolateral gutter can be seen.[29]

Although abnormalities of the ATFL are primarily implicated in the setting of chronic lateral ankle instability, deltoid ligament abnormalities can occur as well.[30] Both the superficial and deep portions of the deltoid are composed of multiple fascicles that, even at the time of this writing, are continuing to be explored anatomically.[31] In general, the superficial component of the deltoid is considered to be composed primarily of the tibiocalcaneal ligament (fascicle) with additional contributions of the anterior superficial tibiotalar fascicle, the tibionavicular fascicle, the tibioligamentous fascicle that blends with the superomedial fibers of the spring ligament, and the superficial posterior tibiotalar ligament.[32,33] The deep layer of the deltoid is largely composed of the deep anterior tibiotalar ligament, the deep posterior tibiotalar ligament, and the anterior tibiotalar fascicle.[32,33] It is rare to visualize every component of the deltoid on MRI; however, the major components of the deep fibers and the tibiocalcaneal fascicle can be identified consistently (**Figs. 7** and **8**).

It is recommended to view the deltoid in both the coronal and axial planes with high-resolution fast spin-echo proton density–weighted imaging. As with other ligaments, fibers normally should be seen as low signal intensity structures, although with some intervening fat, which should not be confused with a tear. If in doubt, correlate with inversion recovery or T2 fat-suppressed images, which should suppress out the fat. When abnormal, the ligament is hyperintense, ill defined, and often thickened. Visualizing a discrete cleft coursing through the ligament is rare; rather, a pattern of interstitial tearing is seen more frequently. Most tears of the deep fibers of the deltoid are midsubstance, whereas superficial tears usually are at its medial malleolar origin.[34,35]

The complex anatomy of the deltoid ligament renders it difficult to isolate specific fascicles on MRI. Crim and Longenecker[35] have proposed the concept of the "fascial sleeve of the medial malleolus" reflecting the broad fibrous covering of the medial malleolus consisting of the superficial deltoid origin, the periosteum, and the flexor retinaculum. When this complex is injured, diffuse high-signal intensity is seen along the medial malleolus with occasional identification of frank fluid insinuating between the fascial sleeve and the cortex of the medial malleolus (**Fig. 9**).

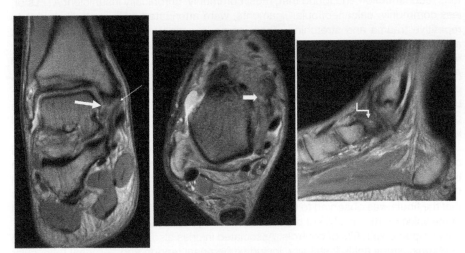

Fig. 7. Coronal (*left*), axial (*middle*) and sagittal (*right*) fast spin-echo high-resolution proton density–weighted images demonstrate tears of both the deep (*thick arrow*) and superficial components of the deltoid with involvement of the proximal fibers of the tibiocalcaneal ligament (*long thin arrow*), the tibioligamentous fascicle inserting on to the superomedial calcaneonavicular ligament (*short thick arrow*), and the tibionavicular fascicle (*wavy arrow*).

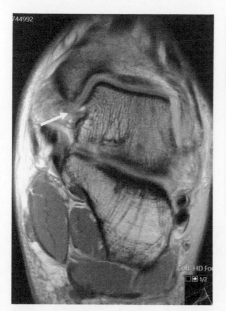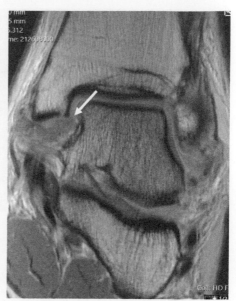

Fig. 8. Coronal fast spin-echo images of the ankle demonstrate complete disruption of the deep and superficial deltoid inclusive of the tibiotalar fascicle (*arrows*).

The deep fibers of the deltoid prevent eversion and lateral displacement of the talus.[29,30,36,37] The superficial fibers, however, also significantly stabilize against excessive external rotation and should be evaluated on all MRIs, notably in the setting of chronic lateral ankle instability.[36] Usually, the deep fibers more often are abnormal, but Crim and colleagues[38] found a significant number of patients in their series of surgically treated patient with lateral ankle instability had pathology of the anterior, superficial deltoid without involvement of the deep fibers. Ultrasound also can be used to identify isolated deltoid ligament tears given its relatively superficial location.[39]

In the acute setting, in addition to visualizing medial clear space widening, observing a cortical avulsion fracture from the medial malleolus can be a significant sign of potential ankle instability.[40] Nwosu and colleagues[40] studied a cohort of 166 rotational ankle injuries and found 1 out of 4 patients with a medial malleolar fleck sign had an unstable ankle. In the setting of chronic ankle instability, medial malleolar stress fractures also can be seen.[41]

Remodeling of ligament tears to a more uniform, low signal appearance on MRI does not guarantee, however, that they are functionally competent. Stress radiographs, although in and of themselves static images, taken in concert with the clinical and MRI findings can provide a functional assessment of the integrity of the supporting ligamentous structures[42–44] (**Fig. 10**). Stress radiographs usually are obtained with a standard amount of both talar tilt and anterior drawer force.[45–49] At the authors' institution, a force of 17 daN (Telos SD 900 Stress Device, TELOS Medical USA, Millersville, Maryland) is used in AP varus stress and anterior drawer in slight plantarflexion. A range of normal measurements has been reported but in general less than 10 mm tibiotalar joint translation with anterior drawer (or within 3–5 mm of the contralateral side) is considered normal, with less than 10° of talar tilt (or within 5° of the opposite side).[49] Nyska and colleagues[50] proposed using a modified method for performing the anterior drawer stress test with the patient supine with the knee

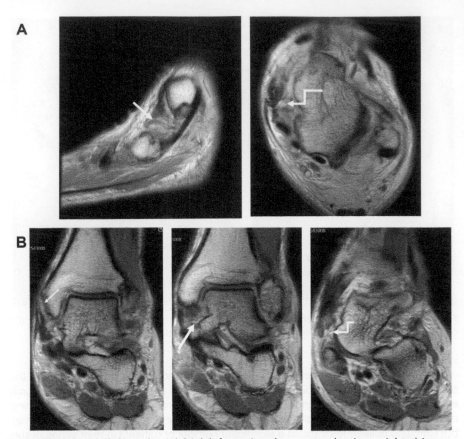

Fig. 9. (A) Sagittal (*left*) and axial (*right*) fast spin-echo proton density–weighted images demonstrate complete disruption of the deltoid ligament with essentially complete absence of ligament fibers as seen on the sagittal sequence (*arrow*). Axial fast spin-echo image demonstrates complete disruption of the tibioligamentous fascicle of the superficial deltoid (*wavy arrow*). (B) Oblique coronal fast spin-echo images in the same patient demonstrate avulsion of the proximal superficial fibers of the deltoid (the fascial sleeve of the medial malleolus) (*arrow*), complete tear of the deep fibers of the deltoid (*thick white arrow*), and complete disruption of the superomedial fibers of the spring ligament (*wavy arrow*).

flexed and the foot in 15° plantarflexion. In this way, the gastrocnemius is relaxed, providing the most maneuverability, and the ATFL the most elongated, therefore the tibiotalar joint the least stable.[50–52]

Stress radiographs can elucidate further between functional and mechanical ankle instability. Functional ankle instability is a subjective sense by the patient of the ankle being loose, unstable, or giving out.[53,54] Causes of functional instability can include nerve pathology or peroneal dysfunction.[54,55] Mechanical instability is the observation of the ankle translating outside of its normal physiologic range usually due to ligamentous laxity.[55] Stress radiographs can provide a quantitative evaluation and documentation of mechanical laxity, thus distinguishing between the 2 entities if a standard device, such as the TELOS stress device, is used.[43]

Sinus tarsi syndrome is a cause of instability that is somewhat more difficult to diagnose. It can be elusive clinically but there are some MRI findings that may assist

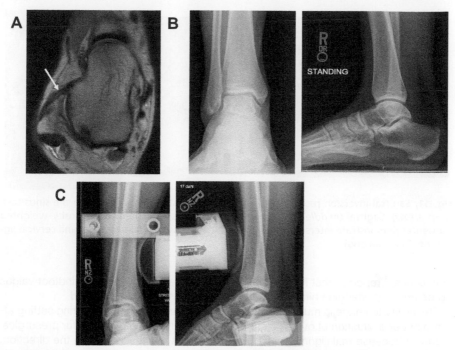

Fig. 10. (*A*) Axial fast spin-echo proton density–weighted MRI in a patient with chronic lateral ankle instability demonstrates a mildly thickened ATFL (*arrow*), although fibers appear largely in continuity and no focal defects or areas of ligamentous disruption are seen. (*B*) Standard AP (*left*) and lateral (*right*) weight-bearing radiographs in the same patient demonstrate normal alignment. (*C*) Stress radiographs in the same patient demonstrates marked anterior translation of the tibia with anterior drawer (*right*) and widening of the lateral gutter with application of forefoot stress (*left*) indicative of lateral ankle ligamentous laxity.

in directing the diagnosis, including increased signal intensity and abnormal talocalcaneal ligaments (**Fig. 11**). The sinus tarsi contains multiple ligaments that stabilize the ankle and prevent excessive eversion or inversion.[56] Patients may have a feeling of instability, notably on uneven surfaces.[57] Many causes have been postulated for the findings of sinus tarsi syndrome, but most investigators believe it is of a traumatic etiology with damage largely of the interosseous talocalcaneal and cervical ligaments[58,59] Isolated injuries to the talocalcaneal ligaments have been shown to be rare, however, with sinus tarsi syndrome only occurring after the lateral ligamentous stabilizers have failed.[60]

A reliable static imaging assessment of stability remains evasive, given variability in image acquisition techniques and absent standardization of the degree of loading to the affected ankle. Weight-bearing radiographs have been shown, however, to reliably predict stability in the setting of unstable ankle fractures.[61] Changes in medial clear space widening in the setting of supination external rotation ankle fractures have been shown significant in a cadaveric model compared with controls with weight-bearing CT.[62] Determination of alignment should be made cautiously with MRI because static images are obtained with the patient supine and with the foot generally largely fixed in a neutral position within a dedicated surface coil. Buber and

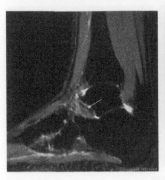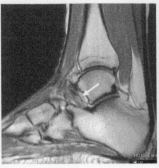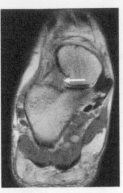

Fig. 11. Sagittal inversion recovery (*left*) image demonstrates high signal in the sinus tarsi (*thin arrow*). Sagittal (*middle*) and coronal (*right*) fast spin-echo proton density–weighted sequences demonstrate interstitial tearing of the interosseous talocalcaneal and cervical ligaments (*thick arrows*).

colleagues[63] reported that MRI tended to overestimate the degree of hindfoot valgus compared with standing hindfoot alignment views as the gold standard.

The ability to image in multiple orthogonal planes in a full weight-bearing setting affords better evaluation of overall alignment and significant information for presurgical planning because malalignment in 1 plane does not necessary dictate the direction, degree, or severity of malalignment in another. Nosewicz and colleagues[64] specifically found that talar tilt in the frontal projection did not correlate with talar sagittal alignment.

Weight-bearing CT has become more universally employed for evaluation of alignment and instability at some institutions and is in general perceived positively because it images the foot and ankle loaded in a weight-bearing position. Review of these images should be done with caution, however, as previously described, and universally used radiographic and clinical measurements may not be directly translatable to those obtained from weight bearing CT. Burssens and colleagues[65] have found that the largely universally accepted values of 2° to 6° of physiologic hindfoot valgus observed clinically and radiographically were not found in the general population with a cohort of 48 patients using weight-bearing CT; rather, a more neutral inferior calcaneal axis point was observed. Moreover, Colin and colleagues[66] found that the subtalar vertical angle changed depending on where the measurements were taken (anterior, middle, or posterior). It is further conceivable that measurements likely are different depending on how the coronal plane is prescribed (perpendicular to the floor vs perpendicular to the subtalar joint vs parallel to the talonavicular joint, and so forth).

Weight-bearing images are not infallible and care must be taken to ensure uniform consistent positioning not only of the ankle but also of the forefoot. Vuurberg and colleagues[67] found that significant changes in hindfoot alignment could be produced with greater than 10° changes in forefoot abduction or adduction.

Standard radiographs afford limited direct visualization of the subtalar joint, and subtle alterations in forefoot alignment can render this more difficult. Lenz and colleagues[68] have suggested that 20° of internal rotation of the foot provides the best positioning for visualizing the subtalar joint on an AP view of the ankle. Although less commonly utilized and difficult to reproduce, stress radiographs also can be used to evaluate and document potential subtalar instability.[59,69,70] Either direct measurements of the degree of separation of the posterior facet from the talus can be performed or evaluating the degree of the subtalar tilt angle.[69,71,72]

MIDFOOT

Isolated acute injuries to the spring ligament complex are rare and can be misdiagnosed initially as a medial ankle sprain although their ramifications can be significant, leading to classic components of adult-onset flatfoot deformity.[73,74] High-resolution MRIs can identify the components of the spring ligament and diagnose these injuries in the acute setting (**Figs. 12** and **13**).

Significant midfoot fracture dislocations are not a diagnostic dilemma on radiographs, but their true degree of severity can be underestimated. CT, either standard imaging or utilizing a weight-bearing cone-beam technique, is advocated for presurgical planning because radiographs may not demonstrate the relationships between the fracture fragments as well as the joint articulations accurately.

More subtle, low-grade and low-velocity midfoot sprains, such as those seen more commonly in the athletic population, however, are more challenging to diagnosis. The increased diagnostic accuracy of subtle midfoot injuries with weight-bearing has been advocated consistently. Shelton and colleagues[75] found that the talonavicular coverage angle and the talocalcaneal angle significantly increased with progressive weightbearing with loss of the cuboid-floor distance, suggesting progressive flattening of the arch with progressive weightbearing. These same investigators found, however, that other measurements, including the Lisfranc interval, did not change significantly between applying 25% and 100% of body weight, although there was an overall trend for these measurements to change between completely non–weight bearing and 25%

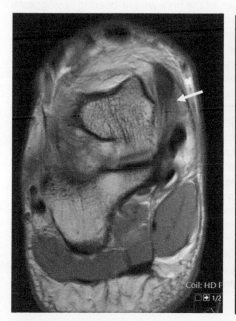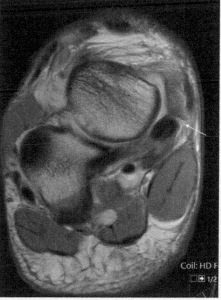

Fig. 12. Coronal fast spin-echo high-resolution proton density–weighted images of the ankle demonstrate high-grade interstitial tearing of the tibiocalcaneal fascicle of the deltoid ligament (*thick arrow*) as well as a discrete tear in the superomedial fibers of the spring ligament (*thin arrow*).

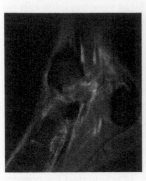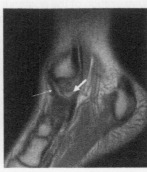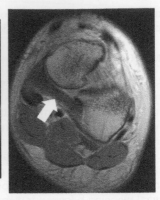

Fig. 13. Sagittal inversion recovery (*left*) and sagittal (*middle*) and oblique coronal (*right*) fast spin-echo proton density–weighted sequences demonstrate high-grade disruption of both the deep and superficial components of the deltoid inclusive of the tibiocalcaneal fascicle (*medium arrow*). The tibiotalar fascicle is markedly ill defined, wavy, and hyperintense (*thin arrow*). There is associated high-grade interstitial tearing of the superomedial fibers of the spring ligament, which are markedly thickened and hyperintense (*thick arrow*).

of full body weight, suggesting that as long as the patient is putting some weight on the foot, the measurements can be viewed as relatively reliable.[75]

Obtaining weight-bearing radiographs, including the opposite side for comparison, is ideal, but obtaining weight-bearing radiographs, especially in the acute setting, not always is possible, Most patients are in pain after an acute injury and cannot fully weight bear and images in the emergency room or clinic often are obtained non–weight bearing. A careful inspection; however, of the non–weight-bearing radiographs can provide useful information regarding a subtle Lisfranc injury with associated fractures reported in 39% of cases with Lisfranc injuries.[76] Seo and colleagues[77] further found that in most cases of Lisfranc injuries, some pathology at the first cuneiform–second metatarsal joint is present, such as a subtle avulsion fracture or diastasis. Stødle and colleagues[78] reported their series of 84 Lisfranc injuries, identifying intraarticular fractures in the second and third TMT joints and decreased height of the second TMT joint were predictive of instability.

Associated injuries sustained with low-energy athletic midfoot sprains can be identified on radiographs, thus elevating the clinical suspicion for potential midfoot instability. Cuboid fractures often occur with an abduction injury in equestrian sports and should heighten awareness for potential midfoot instability.[79] An additional, less common pattern of longitudinal instability can be diagnosed by observing diastasis of the first and second cuneiforms.[80] Pronation and abduction stress radiographs also can accentuate potential instability at the Lisfranc joint.[81]

Cuboid syndrome, usually occurring in gymnasts or ballet dancers, is an uncommon but limiting cause of lateral midfoot pain.[82] Chronic or repetitive injury with poor remodeling of the supporting ligamentous and capsular structures about the calcaneocuboid joint (the dorsolateral or lateral capsular ligaments) can be a significant cause of chronic lateral foot pain and instability.[82,83]

FOREFOOT

Plantar plate injuries, in the setting of not only first metatarsophalangeal (MTP) joint sprains (turf toe) but also the lesser toes, are a significant cause of pain and instability. Weight-bearing radiographs should be obtained, ideally with comparison with the contralateral side to identify subtle alterations in sesamoid alignment in the setting of acute first MTP joint sprains (**Fig. 14**). Dorsiflexion stress radiographs also can accentuate differences in alignment of the hallux sesamoids, thus identifying insufficiency of the first MTP plantar plate.[84]

Waldrop and colleagues[85] demonstrated a significant relationship between the severity of ligamentous injury at the first MTP joint in a cadaveric model with the distal of the sesamoids from the base of the first proximal phalanx using dorsiflexion stress radiographs with a greater than 3 mm distance indicative of significant injury to the plantar plate. Usually, the plantar plates of the lesser MTPs joints tear at the bases of the respective proximal phalanges.[86] Ultrasound of the lesser MTPs joints (specifically the second and third) can demonstrate the plantar plate reliably, although a grade 1 positive MTP drawer test may be present in asymptomatic individuals with a normal plantar plate on ultrasound.[87]

High-resolution MR imaging can be used to identify the structures of the plantar plate complex and associated injuries and thus help-grade MTP joint sprains by identifying where and how many structures are damaged. Bone marrow edema in the hallux sesamoids can be seen in the setting of injury to the first MTP joint (fractures), although it also is important to remember chronic stress reaction can be seen in the hallux sesamoids due to overuse injuries. Kulemann and colleagues[88] observed that isolated bone marrow edema pattern in the medial hallux sesamoid was more suggestive of pathology elsewhere in the forefoot other than at the first MTP joint proper,

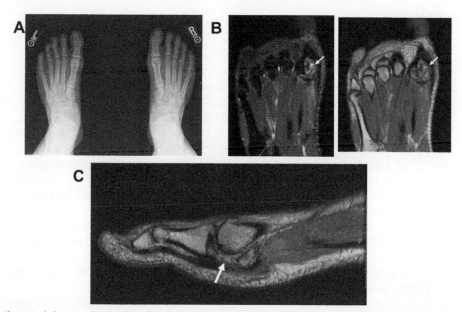

Fig. 14. (*A*) AP radiographs of both feet obtained with the patient weight bearing demonstrate asymmetric proximal retraction of the medial hallux sesamoid in the right foot in the setting of an acute first MTP joint sprain. (*B*) Coronal inversion recovery (*left*) and proton density (*right*) MR images demonstrate soft tissue hyperintensity about the plantar margin of the first MTP joint with a joint effusion, reactive edema in the medial hallux sesamoid and frank disruption of the medial sesamophalangeal ligament (*arrows*). (*C*) Sagittal high-resolution fast spin-echo MRI clearly demonstrates the disruption of the first MTP joint plantar plate (*arrow*) with associate retraction of the hallux sesamoid.

suggesting a mechanical overload at the hallux MTP joint, such as that seen with cavovarus deformities.

SUMMARY

In summary, although they are in and of themselves static images in time, radiographs and CT scans when performed with loading of the foot, in conjunction with the anatomic information provided by high-resolution MRIs, provide objective information to the clinician with regard to the potential presence and severity of instability, whether the supporting ligamentous structures of the distal leg, ankle, hindfoot, midfoot, or forefoot. Absolute numbers and measurement values historically reported in the literature should be used more as guidelines as opposed to dictating practice because significant age and gender discrepancies have been observed. Rather, comparison with a patient's normal internal control contralateral foot should be valued with more significance. Instability remains largely a clinical diagnosis and, although imaging can provide significant supportive information when performed properly, findings always should be taken in concert with the clinical presentation and findings in formulating a clinical treatment plan.

DISCLOSURES

Receives book royalties from Lippincott, Williams and Wilkins. Paid consultant—Ossio, Ltd.

REFERENCES

1. Kaufman KR, Brodine SK, Shaffer RA, et al. The effect of foot structure and range of motion on musculoskeletal overuse injuries. Am J Sports Med 1999;27(5): 585–93.
2. Niva MH, Sormaala MJ, Kiuru MJ, et al. Bone stress injuries of the ankle and foot: an 86 month magnetic resonance imaging-based study of physically active young adults. Am J Sports Med 2007;35(4):643–9.
3. Deutsch AL, Coel MN, Mink JH. Imaging of stress injuries to bone: radiography, scintigraphy and MR imaging. Clin Sports Med 1997;16(2):275–90.
4. Amin A, Janney C, Sheu C, et al. Weight-bearing radiographic analysis of the tibiofibular syndesmosis. Foot Ankle Spec 2019;12(3):211–7.
5. Prakash AA. Syndesmotic stability: is there a radiological normal? A systematic review. Foot Ankle Surg 2018;24:174–84.
6. Beumer A, van Hemert WL, Niesing R, et al. Radiographic measurement of the distal tibiofibular syndesmosis has limited use. Clin Orthop Relat Res 2004;423: 227–34.
7. Sclafani SJ. Ligamentous injury of the lower tibiofibular syndesmosis: radiographic evidence. Radiology 1985;156(1):21–7.
8. Shah AS, Kadakia AR, Tan GJ, et al. Radiographic evaluation of the normal distal tibiofibular syndesmosis. Foot Ankle Int 2012;33(10):870–6.
9. Prakash AA. Is incisura fibularis a reliable landmark for assessing syndesmotic stability? A systematic review of morphometric studies. Foot Ankle Spec 2016; 10(3):246–51.
10. Warner SJ, Fabricant PD, Garner MR, et al. The measurement and clinical importance of syndesmotic reduction after operative fixation of rotational ankle fractures. J Bone Joint Surg Am 2015;97(23):1935–44.

11. Cherney SM, Cosgrove CT, Spraggs-Hughes AG, et al. Functional outcomes of syndesmotic injuries based on objective reduction accuracy at a minimum of 1-year follow up. J Orthop Trauma 2018;32(1):43–51.

12. Laflamme M, Belzile EL, Bédard L, et al. A prospective randomized multicenter trial comparing clinical outcomes of patients treated surgically with a static or dynamic implant for acute ankle syndesmosis rupture. J Orthop Trauma 2015; 29(50):216–23.

13. Bozic KJ, Jaramillo D, DiCanzio J, et al. Radiographic appearance of the normal distal tibiofibular syndesmosis in children. J Pediatr Orthop 1999;19(1):14–21.

14. Cunningham BA, Warner S, Berkes M, et al. Effect of intraoperative multidimensional fluoroscopy versus conventional fluoroscopy on syndesmotic reduction. Foot Ankle Int 2020. https://doi.org/10.1177/1071100720959025.

15. Vetter SY, Euler J, Beisemann N, et al. Validation of radiological reduction criteria with intraoperative cone beam CT in unstable syndesmotic injuries. Eur J Trauma Emerg Surg 2020. https://doi.org/10.1007/s00068-020-01299-z.

16. Croft S, Furey A, Stone C, et al. Radiographic evaluation of the ankle syndesmosis. Can J Surg 2015;58(1):58–62.

17. Grenier S, Benoit B, Rouleau DM, et al. APTF: anteroposterior tibiofibular ratio, a new reliable measure to assess syndesmotic reduction. J Orthop Trauma 2013; 27(4):207–11.

18. Cogan C, Liu T, Toogood P. An assessment of normal tibiofibular anatomy on lateral fluoroscopy. Foot Ankle Int 2020;41(7):866–9.

19. Warner SJ, Garner MR, Schottel PC, et al. Analysis of PITFL injuries in rotationally unstable ankle fractures. Foot Ankle Int 2015;36(4):377–82.

20. Salat P, Le V, Velikovic A, et al. Imaging in foot and ankle instability. Foot Ankle Clin 2018;23(4):499–522.

21. Li H, Hua Y, Feng S, et al. Lower signal intensity of the anterior talofibular ligament is associated with a higher rate of return to sport after ATFL repair for chronic lateral ankle instability. Am J Sports Med 2019;47(10):2380–5.

22. Chu CR, Williams AA. Quantitative MRI UTE-T2* and T2* show progressive and continued graft maturation over 2 years in human patients after anterior cruciate ligament reconstruction. Orthop J Sports Med 2019;7(8):2325967119863056.

23. Jung HG, Kim NA, Kim TH, et al. Magnetic resonance imaging and stress radiography in chronic lateral ankle instability. Foot Ankle Int 2017;38(6):621–6.

24. Yasui Y, Takao M. Comparison of arthroscopic and histologic evaluation on the injured anterior talofibular ligament. American Academy of Orthopaedic Surgeons Annual Meeting. Chicago, March 19-23, 2013.

25. Kikumoto T, Akatsuka K, Nakamura E, et al. Quantitative evaluation method for clarifying ankle plantar flexion angles using anterior drawer and inversion stress tests: a cross-sectional study. J Foot Ankle Res 2019;12:27.

26. Abdeen R, Comfort P, Starbuck C, et al. Ultrasound characteristics of foot and ankle structures in healthy, coper, and chronically unstable ankles. J Ultrasound Med 2019;38(4):917–26.

27. Cho JH, Lee DH, Song HK, et al. Value of stress ultrasound for the diagnosis of chronic ankle instability compared to manual anterior drawer test, stress radiography, magnetic resonance imaging, and arthroscopy. Knee Surg Sports Traumatol Arthrosc 2016;24(4):1022–8.

28. Berkowitz MJ, Kim DH. Fibular position in relation to lateral ankle instability. Foot Ankle Int 2004;25(5):318–21.

29. DiGiovanni BF, Fraga CJ, Cohen BE, et al. Associated injuries found in chronic lateral ankle instability. Foot Ankle Int 2000;21(10):809–15.

30. Hintermann B, Boss A, Schäfer D. Arthroscopic findings in patients with chronic ankle instability. Am J Sports Med 2002;30(3):402–9.
31. Guerra-Pinto F, Fabian A, Mota T, et al. The tibiocalcaneal bundle of the deltoid ligament – prevalence and variations. Foot Ankle Surg 2020;S1268-7731(20): 30052-7.
32. Kelikian AS, editor. Sarrafin's anatomy of the foot and ankle: descriptive, topographic, functional. 3rd edition. New York (NY): Wolters Kluwer/Lippincott Williams and Wilkins; 2011. p. 176–82.
33. Lee S, Lin J, Hamid KS, et al. Deltoid ligament rupture in ankle fracture: diagnosis and management. J Am Acad Orthop Surg 2019;27:e648–58.
34. Jeong MS, Choi YS, Kim YJ, et al. Deltoid ligament in acute ankle injury: MR imaging analysis. Skeletal Radiol 2014;43(5):655–63.
35. Crim J, Longenecker LG. MRI and surgical findings in deltoid ligament tears. AJR Am J Roentgenol 2015;204:W63–9.
36. Rasmussen O, Kromann-Andersen C, Boe S. Deltoid ligament. Functional analysis of the medial collateral ligamentous apparatus of the ankle joint. Acta Orthop Scand 1983;54(1):36–44.
37. Ferkel RD, Chams RN. Chronic lateral instability: arthroscopic findings and long term results. Foot Ankle Int 2007;28(1):24–31.
38. Crim JR, Beals TC, Nickisch F, et al. Deltoid ligament abnormalities in chronic lateral ankle instability. Foot Ankle Int 2011;32(9):873–8.
39. Chen PY, Wang TG, Wang CL. Ultrasonographic examination of the deltoid ligament in bimalleolar equivalent fractures. Foot Ankle Int 2008;29(9):883–6.
40. Nwosu K, Schneiderman BA, Shymon SJ, et al. A medial malleolar "fleck" sign may predict ankle instability in ligamentous supination external rotation ankle fractures. Foot Ankle Spec 2018;11(3):246–51.
41. Lee HS, Lee YK, Kim HS, et al. Medial malleolar stress fracture resulting from repetitive stress caused by lateral ankle instability. Medicine (Baltimore) 2019; 98(5):e14311.
42. Jolman S, Robbins J, Lewis L, et al. Comparison of magnetic resonance imaging and stress radiographs in the evaluation of chronic lateral ankle instability. Foot Ankle Int 2017;38(4):397–404.
43. Hubbard TJ, Kaminski TW, Vander Griend RA, et al. Quantitative assessment of mechanical laxity in the functionally unstable ankle. Med Sci Sports Exerc 2004;36(5):760–6.
44. Phisitkul P, Chaichankul C, Sripongsai R, et al. Accuracy of anterolateral drawer test in lateral ankle instability: a cadaveric study. Foot Ankle Int 2009;30(7):690–5.
45. Martin DE, Kaplan PA, Kahler DM, et al. Retrospective evaluation of graded stress examination of the ankle. Clin Orthop Relat Res 1996;328:165–70.
46. Christensen JC, Dockery GL, Schuberth JM. Evaluation of ankle ligamentous insufficiency using the Telos ankle stress apparatus. J Am Podiatr Med Assoc 1986;76(9):527–31.
47. Rijke AM, Jones B, Vierhout PA. Stress examination of traumatized lateral ligaments of the ankle. Clin Orthop Relat Res 1986;210:143–51.
48. Beynnon BD, Webb G, Huber BM, et al. Radiographic measurement of anterior talar translation in the ankle: determination of the most reliable method. Clin Biomech 2005;20(3):301–6.
49. Shakked RJ, Sheskier S. Acute and chronic lateral ankle instability: diagnosis, management, and new concepts. Bull Hosp Jt Dis (2013) 2017;75(1):71–80.
50. Nyska M, Amir H, Porath A, et al. Radiological assessment of a modified anterior drawer test of the ankle. Foot Ankle 1992;13(7):400–3.

51. Nigg BM, Skarvan G, Frank CB, et al. Elongation and forces of ankle ligaments in a physiological range of motion. Foot Ankle 1990;11(1):30–40.
52. Kragh JF, Ward JA. Radiographic indicators of ankle instability: changes with plantarflexion. Foot Ankle Int 2006;27(1):23–8.
53. Smith RW, Reischl SF. Treatment of ankle sprains in young athletes. Am J Sports Med 1986;14(6):465–71.
54. Freeman MAR. Instability of the foot after injuries to the lateral ligament of the ankle. J Bone Joint Surg Br 1965;47(4):669–77.
55. Tropp H. Pronator muscle weakness in functional instability of the ankle joint. Int J Sports Med 1986;7(5):291–4.
56. Arshad Z, Bhatia M. Current concepts in sinus tarsi syndrome: a scoping review. Foot Ankle Surg 2020;S1268-7731(20):30183–91.
57. Aynardi M, Pedowitz PI, Raikin SM. Subtalar instability. Foot Ankle Clin N Am 2015;20:243–52.
58. Mittlmeier T, Rammelt S. Update on subtalar joint instability. Foot Ankle Clin 2018;23(3):397–413.
59. Kato T. The diagnosis and treatment of instability of the subtalar joint. J Bone Joint Surg Br 1995;77(3):400–6.
60. Frey C, Feder KS, DiGiovanni C. Arthroscopic evaluation of the subtalar joint: does sinus tarsi syndrome exist? Foot Ankle Int 1999;20(3):185–91.
61. Hastie GR, Akhtar S, Butt U, et al. Weightbearing radiographs facilitate functional treatment of ankle fractures of uncertain stability. J Foot Ankle Surg 2015;54(6):1042–6.
62. Lawlor MC, Kluczynski MA, Marzo JM. Weight bearing cone beam CT scan assessment of stability of supination external rotation ankle fractures in a cadaver model. Foot Ankle Int 2018;39(7):850–7.
63. Buber N, Zanetti M, Frigg A, et al. Assessment of hindfoot alignment using MRI and standing hindfoot alignment radiographs (Saltzman view). Skeletal Radiol 2018;47(1):19–24.
64. Nosewicz TL, Knupp M, Bollinger L, et al. Radiological morphology of peritalar instability in varus and valgus tilted ankles. Foot Ankle Int 2014;35(5):453–62.
65. Burssens A, van Herzele E, Leenders T, Clockaerts S, et al. Weight bearing CT in normal hindfoot alignment: presence of a constitutional valgus? Foot Ankle Surg 2018;24(3):213–8.
66. Colin F, Lang TH, Zwicky L, et al. Subtalar joint configuration on weightbearing CT scan. Foot Ankle Int 2014;35(10):1057–110.
67. Vuurberg G, Dahmen J, Dobbe JGG, et al. The effect of foot rotation on measuring ankle alignment using simulated radiographs: as safe zone for preoperative planning. Clin Radiol 2019;74(11):897.
68. Lenz AL, Krahenbuhl, Howell K, et al. Influence of the ankle position and xray beam angulation on the projection of the posterior facet of the subtalar joint. Skeletal Radiol 2019;48(10):1581–9.
69. Yamamoto H, Yagishita K, Ogiuchi T, et al. Subtalar instability following lateral ligament injuries of the ankle. Injury 1998;29(4):265–8.
70. Tourné Y, Besse JL, Mabit C, et al. Chronic ankle instability: which tests to assess the lesions? Which therapeutic options? Orthop Traumatol Surg Res 2010;96(4):433–46.
71. Heilman AE, Braly WG, Bishop JO, et al. An anatomic study of subtalar instability. Foot Ankle 1990;10(4):224–8.
72. Barg A, Tochigi Y, Amendola A, et al. Subtalar instabity: diagnosis and treatment. Foot Ankle Int 2012;33(2):151–60.

73. Bastias GF, Dalmau-Pastor M, Astudillo C, et al. Spring Ligament Instability. Foot Ankle Clin N Am 2018;23:659–78.
74. Masaragian HJ, Ricchetti HO, Testa C. Acute isolated rupture of the spring ligament: a case report and review of the literature. Foot Ankle Int 2013;34(1):150–4.
75. Shelton TJ, Singh S, Robinson EB, et al. The influence of percentage weight-bearing on foot radiographs. Foot Ankle Spec 2019;12(4):363–9.
76. Vuori JP, Aro HT. Lisfranc joint injuries: trauma mechanisms and associated injuries. J Trauma 1993;35(1):40–5.
77. Seo DK, Lee HS, Lee KW, et al. Nonweightbearing radiographs in patients with a subtle Lisfranc injury. Foot Ankle Int 2017;38(10):1120–5.
78. Stødle AH, Hvaal KH, Enger M, et al. Lisfrance injuries: incidence, mechanisms of injury and predictors of instability. Foot Ankle Surg 2019;26(5):535–40.
79. Hermel MB, Gershon-Cohen J. The nutcracker fracture of the cuboid by indirect violence. Radiology 1953;60(6):850–4.
80. Seybold JD, Coetzee JC. Lisfranc injuries: when to observe, fix or fuse. Clin Sports Med 2015;34(4):705–23.
81. Curtis MJ, Myerson M, Szura B. Tarsometatarsal joint injuries in the athlete. Am J Sports Med 1993;21(4):497–502.
82. Sullivan M, de Silva V, Panti JPL, et al. Operative technique for cuboid instability in an elite gymnast: a case report. Foot Ankle Int 2015;36(5):598–602.
83. Jennings J, Davies GJ. Treatment of cuboid syndrome secondary to lateral ankle sprains: a case series. J Orthop Sports Phys Ther 2005;35(7):409–15.
84. Rodeo SA, Warren RF, O'Brien SJ, et al. Diastasis of bipartite sesamoids of the first metatarsophalangeal joint. Foot Ankle 1993;14(8):425–34.
85. Waldrop NE, Zirker CA, Wijdicks CA, et al. Radiographic evaluation of plantar plate injury: an in vitro biomechanical study. Foot Ankle Int 2013;34(3):403–8.
86. Nery C, Coughlin MJ, Baumfeld D, et al. Lesser metatarsophalangeal joint instability: prospective evaluation and repair of plantar plate and capsular insufficiency. Foot Ankle Int 2012;33(4):301–11.
87. De Avila Fernandes E, Mann TS, Puchnick A, et al. Can ultrasound of plantar plate have normal appearance with a positive drawer test? Eur J Radiol 2015;84(3):443–9.
88. Kulemann V, Mayerhoefer M, Trnka HJ, et al. Abnormal findings in hallucal sesamoids on MR imaging: associated with different pathologies of the forefoot? An observational study. Eur J Radiol 2010;74(1):226–30.

Emerging Biological Treatment Methods for Ankle Joint and Soft Tissue Conditions

Clinical Applications as Alternative or Adjuvant

J. Nienke Altink, BSc[a,b,c], Gino M.M.J. Kerkhoffs, MD, PhD[a,b,c],*

KEYWORDS

- Biological treatment methods • Biologicals • Foot • Ankle • Achilles tendinopathy
- Osteochondral lesion • Ankle osteoarthritis • Current concepts

KEY POINTS

- Biological treatments are used widely in clinical practice despite limited understanding of working mechanisms, therapeutic effects, and contents.
- Current evidence is insufficient to support clinical use of platelet-rich plasma for ankle joint pathologies or Achilles tendinopathy.
- Current evidence is insufficient to support clinical use of minimally manipulated autologous cell preparations for ankle joint pathologies or Achilles tendinopathy.
- Current evidence is insufficient to support clinical use of culture-expanded connective tissue cells for ankle joint pathologies or Achilles tendinopathy.

INTRODUCTION

In the past 2 decades, there has been a rapid expansion of clinical studies investigating the safety and efficacy of biological treatment methods for a wide range of diseases, including diseases of the musculoskeletal system. These biological treatment methods have been explored as alternatives or adjuvants to conventional treatment options, with the aim of optimizing clinical outcomes by stimulating tissue

[a] Department of Orthopaedic Surgery, Amsterdam Movement Sciences, Amsterdam UMC, Location AMC, University of Amsterdam, K1-208, Meibergdreef 9, Amsterdam 1105 AZ, the Netherlands; [b] Academic Center for Evidence Based Sports Medicine (ACES); [c] Amsterdam Collaboration for Health and Safety in Sports (ACHSS), AMC/VUmc IOC Research Center
* Corresponding author. Department of Orthopaedic Surgery, Amsterdam Movement Sciences, Amsterdam UMC, Location AMC, University of Amsterdam, Meibergdreef 9, Amsterdam 1105 AZ, the Netherlands.
E-mail address: g.m.kerkhoffs@amsterdamumc.nl

Foot Ankle Clin N Am 26 (2021) 225–235
https://doi.org/10.1016/j.fcl.2020.11.001
1083-7515/21/© 2020 The Authors. Published by Elsevier Inc. This is an open access article under the CC BY license (http://creativecommons.org/licenses/by/4.0/).

regeneration.[1–3] Unlike conventional pharmaceuticals, where a known concentration of a bioactive substance is administered to achieve a certain therapeutic effect, the exact composition and working principles of biologicals often are unknown. Despite limited understanding of working mechanisms of biological treatment methods, they are used in widely clinical studies and clinical practice. Examples of biological substances that have been used to treat ankle joint and soft tissue conditions are platelet-rich plasma (PRP), bone marrow aspirate concentrate (BMAC), and mesenchymal stem cells (MSCs). High patient demand in combination with promising results in in vitro and animal studies have led to widespread clinical use of biologicals on the basis of minimal available evidence regarding the safety and efficacy of biological treatment methods. In order to provide evidence-based clinical care and to provide patients with accurate information, it is essential for health care providers to be familiar with the clinical evidence regarding biological treatment methods. Therefore, the aim of this article is to provide an overview of the existing evidence regarding emerging biological treatment methods for ankle joint and soft tissue conditions.

PLATELET-RICH PLASMA

PRP is an autologous blood-derived product with a platelet count higher than baseline autologous blood.[1] The rationale for the use of PRP is that platelets in PRP release growth factors and cytokines that may contribute to tissue regeneration by stimulating angiogenesis and progenitor cells and by dampening the local inflammatory response. PRP is a complex mixture containing a variable amount of plasma, platelets, leukocytes, and red blood cells. In this mixture, more than 300 cytokines and growth factors have been identified. The composition of PRP differs significantly between donors and preparation methods.[2,3] Despite limited understanding of its composition and working mechanism, there are more than 500 clinical trials registered that investigate the efficacy and safety of PRP in a broad spectrum of conditions, ranging from orthopedic conditions to erectile dysfunction, chronic obstructive pulmonary disease, and hair loss problems. Despite the high number of studies describing clinical outcomes of PRP, comparing outcomes is difficult due to incomplete reporting of factors that influence biologic activity and outcomes. A systematic review by Chahla and colleagues[4] showed that only 16% of the orthopedic studies reported quantitative metrics on the composition of the final PRP product. To address this concern, the American Academy of Orthopaedic Surgeons (AAOS) convened a symposium on biologicals and established a set of minimum reporting standards for studies regarding PRP.[1] The use of PRP is described in literature for the treatment of ankle osteoarthritis, osteochondral lesions of the talus (OLTs), and Achilles tendon pathology. The best available evidence for each indication is discussed in the following section.

Platelet-Rich Plasma for Ankle Osteoarthritis

High-quality clinical evidence on the efficacy of PRP on ankle osteoarthritis is lacking. No evidence is available of clinical trials comparing PRP with a placebo or other treatment modality to treat ankle osteoarthritis. Paget and colleagues,[5] however, recently published a protocol of a multicenter, randomized, double-blind placebo-controlled trial for the assessment of PRP for ankle osteoarthritis. Published results of studies investigating the safety and efficacy of PRP for ankle osteoarthritis currently consist only of case series and case reports. There is only 1 prospective study on the effect of PRP on ankle osteoarthritis. Fukawa and colleagues[6] reported no serious adverse effects and a significantly reduced visual analog scale (VAS) and improved Japanese Society for Surgery of the Foot scores after 2 injections of PRP in a cohort of 20 patients. Two other studies assessed the safety and efficacy of PRP for ankle osteo-arthritis. These are both retrospective case series and show conflicting results.[7,8]

Although evidence for PRP in the treatment of ankle osteoarthritis is lacking, there are numerous clinical trials investigating the safety and efficacy of PRP in knee osteo-arthritis. A systematic review by Shen and colleagues[9] included a total of 14 studies investigating the safety and efficacy of PRP for the treatment of knee osteoarthritis. Of the 14 included studies, 12 studies reported favorable outcomes in the PRP group compared with placebo or hyaluronic acid. However, 10 studies in this review had a high risk of bias and 4 studies had a moderate risk of bias according to Review Manager 5.3 (Cochrane Collaboration, Oxford, England).[10] Of the 4 studies with moderate risk of bias, only 2 studies reported favorable results of PRP compared with hyaluronic acid[11] or saline.[12] The other 2 studies reported no differences between PRP and hyaluronic acid.[13,14] Contradicting evidence regarding the efficacy might be due to differences in composition and preparation protocols. With regard to PRP composition, the use of leukocyte-poor PRP seems more beneficial than leukocyte-rich PRP in the treatment of knee osteoarthritis.[15]

No high-level clinical studies are available evaluating the efficacy of PRP for the treatment of ankle osteoarthritis. Results of clinical trials in the knee suggest that leukocyte-poor PRP seems more beneficial compared with leukocyte-rich PRP in the treatment of osteoarthritis. Further studies that report following the minimum reporting standards as established by the AAOS are needed before PRP should be used widely in clinical practice for ankle osteoarthritis. Conflicting evidence exists with regard to superiority of PRP compared with hyaluronic acid.

Platelet-Rich Plasma for Osteochondral Lesions of the Talus

PRP is described in the literature both as an injection therapy and as an adjuvant to surgical therapy for the treatment of OLTs. Mei-Dan and colleagues[16] compared the effect of intra-articular PRP injection with hyaluronic acid injection in 30 patients with an OLT. Significantly better VAS and ankle-hindfoot scale scores were found in the PRP group. These results, however, should be interpreted with care. In the study of Mei-Dan and colleagues, a 46% lost to follow-up rate was reported in the PRP group versus a 7% loss to follow-up rate in the hyaluronic acid group. In addition, only subjective outcome measures were studied in a nonblinded manner. Therefore, this study has a high risk of selection bias and observer bias.

Two randomized controlled trials (RCTs) have studied the effect of PRP as an adjuvant to surgical therapy for OLTs.[17–19] Guney and colleagues[20] compared the effect of microfracture surgery alone with microfracture surgery in combination with PRP in a total of 35 patients. They found improvement in both groups, but better AOFAS and VAS scores were found in the PRP group. In another study, Görmeli and colleagues[21] randomized 40 patients into 3 groups: 13 patients received microfracture surgery in combination with saline, 13 patients received microfracture surgery in combination with PRP, and 14 patients received microfracture surgery in combination with hyaluronic acid. Better AOFAS and VAS scores were found in the PRP group compared with the microfracture-only and hyaluronic acid groups. Additionally, 1 nonrandomized prospective comparative study is available that compared microfracture surgery, with and without PRP, with mosaicplasty. In this study, the mosaicplasty group showed significantly better results.

Although a positive effect is shown in all 3 studies that compared PRP with a control group, these results should be interpreted with care. In all 3 studies, both the participants and accessors were not blinded. This results in a significant risk of observer bias. Further studies are needed before PRP should be used widely in clinical practice for OLTs.

Platelet-Rich Plasma for Achilles Tendinopathies

Chronic Achilles tendinopathy

Multiple RCTs are available that have assessed the safety and efficacy of PRP in the treatment of chronic Achilles tendinopathy.[5,7,8,22,23] In these RCTs, PRP is administered both in combination with an eccentric training program or as an alternative to an eccentric loading program. de Vos and colleagues compared the effect eccentric training in combination with saline and in combination with PRP in 54 patients.[5,23] They found no effect of PRP compared with placebo with regard to tendon structure, neovascularization, pain, and function. Kearney and colleagues compared the effect of PRP injection with an eccentric loading program in a total of 20 patients.[7] Kearney and colleagues also found no significant differences between the PRP group and the eccentric loading group.[7] Krogh and colleagues compared the results of 1 PRP injection with 1 saline injection.[8] In this study, no significant difference in victorian institute of sports assessment - achilles questionnaire (visa-a) score was found between groups. An increased tendon thickness, however, was noticed in the PRP group compared with the saline group at 3 months after the injection.[8] Additionally, patients were informed that they could drop out 3 months after the injection if they were dissatisfied with the treatment, and this resulted in a 75% dropout rate in the PRP group, compared with a 33% dropout rate in the saline group.[8] This suggests that PRP injections result in inferior results compared with saline injections. These results should be interpreted with care, however, due to the small number of participants. The most recent randomized study comparing PRP with other treatments is the study of Boesen and colleagues in 2017.[23] They compared the effect of eccentric training in combination with subcutaneous saline, intra-articular PRP or a high-volume injection with steroids, saline, and a local anesthetic.[23] They found an improvement of VISA-A scores in all groups 6 weeks, 12 weeks, and 24 weeks after treatment. The high-volume injection group showed the best results with significantly better results at 6 weeks and 12 weeks compared with the saline and PRP group.[23] These results suggest that high-volume injection in combination with eccentric training is more effective at short term for the treatment of chronic Achilles tendinopathy compared with PRP.[23]

Evidence suggest that PRP is not an effective treatment strategy for the treatment of chronic Achilles tendinopathy. It is recommended that PRP is not used in clinical studies or clinical care, because better treatment options are available for patients with Achilles tendinopathy.

Achilles tendon rupture

In 2011, Schepull and colleagues[11] studied the effect of PRP on acute Achilles tendon ruptures in a randomized controlled trial of 30 patients. The effect of PRP as an adjuvant to surgical therapy was compared with surgical therapy alone.[11] The main outcome measures in this study were the heal raise index and Achilles tendon total rupture score. Due to the lower Achilles tendon rupture scores in the PRP group, Schepull and colleagues[11] concluded that PRP might have a detrimental effect and that PRP is not useful in the treatment of Achilles tendon ruptures. The results were assessed in a nonblinded manner, however, and only 16 patients were included in the PRP group. In 2019, the results of a larger randomized controlled study were published. Keene and colleagues[12] compared the effectiveness of PRP as a nonsurgical therapy with a placebo consisting of a dry needle for acute Achilles tendon ruptures in a randomized double blind multicenter trial. A total of 230 patients were randomized and included in either the PRP or the placebo group. No differences were found between groups with regard to pain, objective muscle tendon function, patient-reported function, or quality of life.[12]

Evidence suggests that PRP is not an effective treatment strategy for the treatment of Achilles tendon ruptures. It is recommended that further basic evidence and animal studies are conducted before PRP is used in clinical studies or clinical care, because better treatment options are available for patients with Achilles tendon ruptures.

CELL-BASED THERAPIES

Cell-based therapies increasingly are used to treat numerous orthopedic conditions.[13] These cell-based therapies include a wide range of products that often are marketed as stem cell therapy, despite poor characterization of these cells.[14] Additionally, unsubstantiated or incorrect information on the efficacy of cell therapies is marketed directly to consumers. A recent study showed that more than 95% of direct-to-consumer advertisements and Web sites regarding stem cell therapy in musculoskeletal diseases contain at least 1 statement of misinformation.[15] Direct-to-consumer marketing in combination with news articles in the general media about high-level athletes have led to high patient demand.[17,18] There is growing concern, however, that cell-based therapies are used in clinical practice based on minimal available evidence. To address this concern, the AAOS recently convened a symposium with the aim to optimize clinical use of biologicals in orthopedic surgery.[19] One of the main concerns of the AAOS was that misrepresentation of uncharacterized minimally manipulated products as stem cells would erode public trust and compromise development of legitimate cell therapies.[19] The term, *stem cell* (or MSCs), often is used for uncharacterized cell-based preparations with characteristics that do not meet the criteria for MSCs. Stem cells are unspecialized cells that can give rise to specialized cell types. Stem cells that can differentiate into musculoskeletal cells are called mesenchymal stem cells, or MSCs. These adult cells have the unique ability of division and self-renewal for long periods of time and differentiation into mesenchymal tissues, such as bone, cartilage, muscle, ligament, tendon, and fat.[24] Additionally, MSCs have shown to have anti-inflammatory and immunomodulatory effects.[25] Due to these characteristics, MSCs have therapeutic potential for tissue engineering and regenerative medicine for multiple musculoskeletal diseases and injuries. In the following section, the different types of cell-based treatments and indications of these cell types are discussed.

Minimally Manipulated Autologous Cell Preparations

Minimally manipulated autologous cell preparations are mixed cell populations from various sources with variable composition. Processing of these cells must not alter the biological characteristics of the cells or the tissues.[19] The biological attributes and function of this group of biologicals highly variates between donors and batches. Stem cells and progenitor cells may be present in this group of biologicals. MSCs, however, represent only approximately 0.001% to 0.01% of mononuclear cells.[26] Other biological attributes of minimally manipulated autologous cell preparations are highly dependent on the source of cells and the system used for centrifugation of the autologous cells. Types of minimally manipulated autologous cell preparations that are described in ankle joint and soft tissue treatment include BMAC and stromal vascular fraction (SVF).

Concentrated bone marrow aspirate

Bone marrow aspirate (BMA) is one of the most commonly used sources of MSCs. The contents of BMA are highly variable between donors, harvesting site, and harvesting method. Contents of BMAC include bone morphogenetic proteins, growth factors, and

MSCs.[27] Only a small minority of the cells within BMA, however, consists of MSCs.[19] The amount of red blood cells, granulocytes, and platelets can be reduced by density gradient centrifugation of the aspirate. Multiple commercial systems are available for the concentration of BMA. Hyer and colleagues[28] compared the amount of MSCs in different harvesting sites and found that the iliac crest contained many more MSCs compared with the calcaneus and distal tibia. Additionally, the posterior iliac crest might contain more MSCs compared with the anterior iliac crest.[29] BMAC is poorly characterized and results in inconsistent tissue formation compared with cultured MSCs, which most likely is due to contaminating cells with inhibitory effects on MSCs.[19]

Stromal vascular fraction

SVF is another source for MSCs. SVF is obtained after enzymatic digestion of adipose tissue. SVF can be suspended with PRP for intra-articular injection or delivered intraoperatively. When SVF is suspended with PRP, PRP acts as a source of platelets and growth factors, whereas SVF acts as a source of cells.

Minimally Manipulated Autologous Cell Preparations for Ankle Osteoarthritis

Concentrated bone marrow aspirate

Limited evidence is available to assess the safety and efficacy of BMAC for ankle osteoarthritis. There are, however, studies that assess the efficacy of BMAC in the knee. Hernigou and colleagues[30] compared the effect of BMAC injection with total knee arthroplasty in patients with bilateral osteoarthritis of the knee. They found a similar incidence of knee arthroplasty in patients after BMAC injection compared with the revision rate of patients who underwent a knee arthroplasty initially.[30] Shapiro and colleagues[31] compared the effect of BMAC in combination with leukocyte-poor PRP with saline. They found no significant differences between groups with regard to pain and function 12 months after injection.[31]

Stromal vascular fraction

No high-level clinical studies are available to assess the efficacy of SVF in the ankle joint. A recent randomized controlled trial, however, compared the use of SVF-injection with hyaluronic acid in the knee.[32] No differences were found between groups.[32] Because only 16 patients were enrolled in this study, however, further studies are indicated to determine if SVF is superior to hyaluronic acid.

Recommendation

No high-level clinical studies are available to evaluate the efficacy of BMAC for the treatment of ankle osteoarthritis. Results of clinical trials in the knee are conflicting. Further studies, reporting following the minimum reporting standards as established by the AAOS, are needed before BMAC should be used in clinical practice for ankle osteoarthritis. The additional value of SVF in the treatment of ankle osteoarthritis in unclear and needs to be studied further in RCTs following the minimum reporting standards as established by the AAOS.

Minimally Manipulated Autologous Cell Preparations for Osteochondral Lesions of the Talus

Concentrated bone marrow aspirate

No randomized trials are available to compare the effect of BMAC as injection therapy or as an adjuvant to surgical therapy for OLTs. Murphy and colleagues[33] compared the effect of BMAC as an adjuvant to microfracture surgery with microfracture surgery only in a prospective cohort study. They found similar patient reported outcomes in both groups. The revision rate was higher, however, in the microfracture-only group.

Hannon and colleagues[34] compared the effect of BMAC in combination with microfracture surgery with microfracture surgery only in a retrospective cohort study. In this study, they concluded that similar functional outcomes and improved border repair tissue integration with less evidence of fissuring and fibrillation on magnetic resonance imaging were observed in the patients treated with microfracture surgery in combination with BMAC.[34] Shimozono and colleagues[35] studied the additional effect of BMAC in patients treated with autologous osteochondral transplantation (AOT). They found similar patient-reported outcomes in patients treated with AOT in combination with BMAC compared with patients who received AOT only. Fewer postoperative cysts occurred, however, in patients treated with a combination of AOT and BMAC. Karnovsky and colleagues[36] also performed a retrospective study, in which they compared the results of juvenile allogenous articular cartilage with BMAC versus microfracture with and without BMAC. In this study, no differences were found between the microfracture group and the microfracture in combination with BMAC group. Another comparative study was the study of Richter and colleagues.[37] They compared the effects of matrix-associated stem cell transplantation (MAST) with autologous matrix-induced chondrogenesis plus peripheral blood concentrate (AMIC + PBC).[37] Both of these treatment use a collagen matrix with fibrin glue. The differences between the MAST technique versus the AMIC + PBC technique is the use of BMAC in MAST versus concentrated autologous blood in the AMIC + PBC group. In a matched cohort of 120 patients in total, both groups showed improvement of pain in the ankle and radiological outcomes.[37] No differences were found, however, between the group treated with autologous blood compared with the group treated with BMAC. These results suggest that there is no additional value of using BMAC compared with autologous blood as an adjuvant to autologous matrix induced chondrogenesis. These results should be interpreted with care, however, because only level III evidence is available.

Conflicting evidence exists to evaluate the efficacy of BMAC for the treatment of OLTs. Further randomized studies, reporting following the minimum reporting standards as established by the AAOS, are needed before BMAC should be used in clinical practice for ankle OLTs.

Minimally Manipulated Autologous Cell Preparations for Achilles Tendinopathy

Concentrated bone marrow aspirate
One retrospective cohort study showed good Achilles tendon rupture scores and a high return to sport rate of 92% after open repair of an Achilles tendon rupture in combination of BMAC injection.[38]

Stromal vascular fraction
Usuelli and colleagues[39] compared the effect of SVF for the treatment of Achilles tendinopathy. Both groups showed significant improvement of VAS, American Orthopaedic Foot & Ankle Society (AOFAS), and VISA-A scores. Comparing the 2 groups, VAS, AOFAS, and VISA-A scored significantly better at 15 days and 30 days in the SVF in comparison to PRP group.[39] After 60, 120 and 180 days from treatment, the scores were not significantly different between the 2 groups. No correlation has been found between clinical and radiological findings.[39]

Recommendation
Further studies are needed to access the safety and efficacy of BMAC and SVF for Achilles tendinopathies. Although SVF was superior to PRP in the study of Usuelli and colleagues[39] at early time points, it is unclear if SVF provides better results compared with exercise therapy.

Culture-Expanded Connective Tissue Cells

Culture-expanded connective tissue cells are defined as plastic adherent cells that tend to differentiate or undergo senescence with prolonged culture.[19] Biological attributes and function are dependent on the tissue source and culture conditions. Additionally, bioactivity varies between donors and batch. Culture-expanded connective tissue cells can be either autologous cells or allogeneic cells.[19] Autologous cells, however, generally raise fewer safety concerns compared with allogeneic cells. In contrast to minimally manipulated autologous cell preparations, culture-expanded connective tissue cells require prospective Food and Drug Administration (FDA) approval before they can be used in clinical trials. Matrix-associated autologous chondrocyte implantation (MACI) currently is the only treatment available with FDA approval. MACI uses autologous cultured chondrocytes on a porcine collagen membrane are transplanted for the repair of full-thickness cartilage of the knee.[40] In foot and ankle conditions, there currently (May 2020) are no treatments approved by the FDA that include culture-expanded connective tissue cells. Limited evidence is available for the use of culture-expanded connective tissue cells in the foot and ankle.

Mesenchymal stem cells for ankle joint pathology

A recent systematic review by McIntyre and colleagues[41] reviewed the safety and efficacy of MSC-based therapies in the human joint and concluded that that autologous intra-articular MSC therapy is safe, with generally positive clinical outcomes. Kim and Koh[42] assessed the outcomes of 49 patients with OLTs of the ankle treated with marrow stimulation in combination with lateral sliding calcaneal osteotomy; 26 of these patients received additional MSC injection. Second-look arthroscopy 1 year after surgery showed superior international cartilage repair society (ICRS) scores in patients treated with additional MSC injection.[42] Additionally, patients in the MSC-injection group showed superior clinical and radiological outcomes.[42] In a different cohort of 65 elderly patients with symptomatic OLTs, Kim and colleagues[43] found superior results in patients treated with marrow stimulation in combination MSCs compared with marrow stimulation only.

Although the initial results of MSCs in the ankle are promising, randomized studies with longer follow-up are needed to determine the additional effect of MSCs for ankle joint pathologies. Prospective clearance of the FDA is needed before the start of clinical trials.

Mesenchymal stem cells for Achilles tendinopathy

No clinical studies are available to assess the effect of MSCs for Achilles tendinopathy.

Amsterdam practice

In general, the authors only use PRP and stem cells as part of clinical research studies in Amsterdam and not as current practice.

In the authors' clinic, only PRP currently is used in a large, Amsterdam-based, multicenter clinical RCT on the effect of PRP injections as treatment of ankle joint osteoarthritis. The last patient has been included successfully and primary outcome analyses are expected in summer 2021.

The authors use concentrated BMA in a large, also Amsterdam-based, multicenter clinical RCT on the additional value of using BMAC in the treatment of small talar osteochondral lesions (diameter <15 mm) with bone marrow stimulation. This trial has just been started.

ACKNOWLEDGMENTS

The authors would like to thank Kaj Emanuel and Jari Dahmen for their valuable feedback at this work.

DISCLOSURE

No authors report receiving funding for this study or any other conflict of interest.

REFERENCES

1. Murray IR, Geeslin AG, Goudie EB, et al. Minimum Information for Studies Evaluating Biologics in Orthopaedics (MIBO): Platelet-Rich Plasma and Mesenchymal Stem Cells. J Bone Joint Surg Am 2017;99(10):809–19.
2. Castillo TN, Pouliot MA, Kim HJ, et al. Comparison of growth factor and platelet concentration from commercial platelet-rich plasma separation systems. Am J Sports Med 2011;39(2):266–71.
3. Mazzocca AD, McCarthy MB, Chowaniec DM, et al. Platelet-rich plasma differs according to preparation method and human variability. J Bone Joint Surg Am 2012;94(4):308–16.
4. Chahla J, Cinque ME, Piuzzi NS, et al. A Call for Standardization in Platelet-Rich Plasma Preparation Protocols and Composition Reporting: A Systematic Review of the Clinical Orthopaedic Literature. J Bone Joint Surg Am 2017;99(20): 1769–79.
5. Paget L, Bierma-Zeinstra S, Goedegebuure S, et al. Platelet-Rich plasma Injection Management for Ankle osteoarthritis study (PRIMA): protocol of a Dutch multicentre, stratified, block-randomised, double-blind, placebo-controlled trial. BMJ Open 2019;9(10):e030961.
6. Fukawa T, Yamaguchi S, Akatsu Y, et al. Safety and Efficacy of Intra-articular Injection of Platelet-Rich Plasma in Patients With Ankle Osteoarthritis. Foot Ankle Int 2017;38(6):596–604.
7. Kearney RS, Parsons N, Costa ML. Achilles tendinopathy management: A pilot randomised controlled trial comparing platelet-richplasma injection with an eccentric loading programme. Bone Joint Res 2013;2(10):227–32.
8. Krogh TP, Ellingsen T, Christensen R, et al. Ultrasound-Guided Injection Therapy of Achilles Tendinopathy With Platelet-Rich Plasma or Saline: A Randomized, Blinded, Placebo-Controlled Trial. Am J Sports Med 2016;44(8):1990–7.
9. Shen L, Yuan T, Chen S, et al. The temporal effect of platelet-rich plasma on pain and physical function in the treatment of knee osteoarthritis: systematic review and meta-analysis of randomized controlled trials. J Orthop Surg Res 2017; 12(1):16.
10. RevMan, V.5.3, Copenhagen: The Nordic Cochrane Centre, The Cochrane Collaboration, 2014.
11. Schepull T, Kvist J, Norrman H, et al. Autologous platelets have no effect on the healing of human achilles tendon ruptures: a randomized single-blind study. Am J Sports Med 2011;39(1):38–47.
12. Keene DJ, Alsousou J, Harrison P, et al. Platelet rich plasma injection for acute Achilles tendon rupture: PATH-2 randomised, placebo controlled, superiority trial. BMJ 2019;367:l6132.
13. Marks P, Gottlieb S. Balancing Safety and Innovation for Cell-Based Regenerative Medicine. N Engl J Med 2018;378(10):954–9.

14. Pean CA, Kingery MT, Strauss E, et al. Direct-to-Consumer Advertising of Stem Cell Clinics: Ethical Considerations and Recommendations for the Health-Care Community. J Bone Joint Surg Am 2019;101(19):e103.

15. Kingery MT, Schoof L, Strauss EJ, et al. Online Direct-to-Consumer Advertising of Stem Cell Therapy for Musculoskeletal Injury and Disease: Misinformation and Violation of Ethical and Legal Advertising Parameters. J Bone Joint Surg Am 2020;102(1):2–9.

16. Mei-Dan O, Carmont MR, Laver L, et al. Platelet-rich plasma or hyaluronate in the management of osteochondral lesions of the talus. Am J Sports Med 2012;40(3): 534–41.

17. Boren C. Kobe Bryant to have treatment on knee in Germany. Washington Post 2013. Available at: https://www.washingtonpost.com/news/early-lead/wp/2013/10/04/kobe-bryant-to-have-treatment-on-knee-in-germany/. Accessed May 2, 2020.

18. Cox L. Tiger Admits to Platelet-Rich Plasma Therapy, What's That?. 2010. Available at: https://abcnews.go.com/Health/Technology/tigerwoods-admits-platelet-rich-plasma-therapy/story?id=10303312. Accessed May 2, 2020.

19. Chu CR, Rodeo S, Bhutani N, et al. Optimizing Clinical Use of Biologics in Orthopaedic Surgery: Consensus Recommendations From the 2018 AAOS/NIH U-13 Conference. J Am Acad Orthop Surg 2019;27(2):e50–63.

20. Guney A, Akar M, Karaman I, et al. Clinical outcomes of platelet rich plasma (PRP) as an adjunct to microfracture surgery in osteochondral lesions of the talus. Knee Surg Sports Traumatol Arthrosc 2015;23(8):2384–9.

21. Görmeli G, Karakaplan M, Görmeli CA, et al. Clinical Effects of Platelet-Rich Plasma and Hyaluronic Acid as an Additional Therapy for Talar Osteochondral Lesions Treated with Microfracture Surgery: A Prospective Randomized Clinical Trial. Foot Ankle Int 2015;36(8):891–900.

22. Boesen AP, Hansen R, Boesen MI, et al. Effect of High-Volume Injection, Platelet-Rich Plasma, and Sham Treatment in Chronic Midportion Achilles Tendinopathy: A Randomized Double-Blinded Prospective Study. Am J Sports Med 2017;45(9): 2034–43.

23. de Vos RJ, Weir A, Tol JL, et al. No effects of PRP on ultrasonographic tendon structure and neovascularisation in chronic midportion Achilles tendinopathy. Br J Sports Med 2011;45(5):387–92.

24. Pittenger MF, Mackay AM, Beck SC, et al. Multilineage potential of adult human mesenchymal stem cells. Science 1999;284(5411):143–7.

25. Aggarwal S, Pittenger MF. Human mesenchymal stem cells modulate allogeneic immune cell responses. Blood 2005;105(4):1815–22.

26. Piuzzi NS, Chahla J, Jiandong H, et al. Analysis of Cell Therapies Used in Clinical Trials for the Treatment of Osteonecrosis of the Femoral Head: A Systematic Review of the Literature. J Arthroplasty 2017;32(8):2612–8.

27. Schafer R, DeBaun MR, Fleck E, et al. Quantitation of progenitor cell populations and growth factors after bone marrow aspirate concentration. J Transl Med 2019; 17(1):115.

28. Hyer CF, Berlet GC, Bussewitz BW, et al. Quantitative assessment of the yield of osteoblastic connective tissue progenitors in bone marrow aspirate from the iliac crest, tibia, and calcaneus. J Bone Joint Surg Am 2013;95(14):1312–6.

29. Pierini M, Di Bella C, Dozza B, et al. The posterior iliac crest outperforms the anterior iliac crest when obtaining mesenchymal stem cells from bone marrow. J Bone Joint Surg Am 2013;95(12):1101–7.

30. Hernigou P, Delambre J, Quiennec S, et al. Human bone marrow mesenchymal stem cell injection in subchondral lesions of knee osteoarthritis: a prospective randomized study versus contralateral arthroplasty at a mean fifteen year follow-up. Int Orthop 2020 [Online ahead of print].
31. Shapiro SA, Kazmerchak SE, Heckman MG, et al. A Prospective, Single-Blind, Placebo-Controlled Trial of Bone Marrow Aspirate Concentrate for Knee Osteoarthritis. Am J Sports Med 2017;45(1):82–90.
32. Hong Z, Chen J, Zhang S, et al. Intra-articular injection of autologous adipose-derived stromal vascular fractions for knee osteoarthritis: a double-blind randomized self-controlled trial. Int Orthop 2019;43(5):1123–34.
33. Murphy EP, McGoldrick NP, Curtin M, et al. A prospective evaluation of bone marrow aspirate concentrate and microfracture in the treatment of osteochondral lesions of the talus. Foot Ankle Surg 2019;25(4):441–8.
34. Hannon CP, Ross KA, Murawski CD, et al. Arthroscopic Bone Marrow Stimulation and Concentrated Bone Marrow Aspirate for Osteochondral Lesions of the Talus: A Case-Control Study of Functional and Magnetic Resonance Observation of Cartilage Repair Tissue Outcomes. Arthroscopy 2016;32(2):339–47.
35. Shimozono Y, Yasui Y, Hurley ET, et al. Concentrated Bone Marrow Aspirate May Decrease Postoperative Cyst Occurrence Rate in Autologous Osteochondral Transplantation for Osteochondral Lesions of the Talus. Arthroscopy 2019;35(1):99–105.
36. Karnovsky SC, DeSandis B, Haleem AM, et al. Comparison of Juvenile Allogenous Articular Cartilage and Bone Marrow Aspirate Concentrate Versus Microfracture With and Without Bone Marrow Aspirate Concentrate in Arthroscopic Treatment of Talar Osteochondral Lesions. Foot Ankle Int 2018;39(4):393–405.
37. Richter M, Zech S, Andreas Meissner S. Matrix-associated stem cell transplantation (MAST) in chondral defects of the ankle is safe and effective - 2-year-followup in 130 patients. Foot Ankle Surg 2017;23(4):236–42.
38. Stein BE, Stroh DA, Schon LC. Outcomes of acute Achilles tendon rupture repair with bone marrow aspirate concentrate augmentation. Int Orthop 2015;39(5):901–5.
39. Usuelli FG, Grassi M, Maccario C, et al. Intratendinous adipose-derived stromal vascular fraction (SVF) injection provides a safe, efficacious treatment for Achilles tendinopathy: results of a randomized controlled clinical trial at a 6-month follow-up. Knee Surg Sports Traumatol Arthrosc 2018;26(7):2000–10.
40. FDA. FDA approves first autologous cellularized scaffold for the repair of cartilage defects of the knee. 2016. Available at: https://www.fda.gov/news-events/press-announcements/fda-approves-first-autologous-cellularized-scaffold-repair-cartilage-defects-knee.
41. McIntyre JA, Jones IA, Han B, et al. Intra-articular Mesenchymal Stem Cell Therapy for the Human Joint: A Systematic Review. Am J Sports Med 2018;46(14):3550–63.
42. Kim YS, Koh YG. Injection of Mesenchymal Stem Cells as a Supplementary Strategy of Marrow Stimulation Improves Cartilage Regeneration After Lateral Sliding Calcaneal Osteotomy for Varus Ankle Osteoarthritis: Clinical and Second-Look Arthroscopic Results. Arthroscopy 2016;32(5):878–89.
43. Kim YS, Park EH, Kim YC, et al. Clinical outcomes of mesenchymal stem cell injection with arthroscopic treatment in older patients with osteochondral lesions of the talus. Am J Sports Med 2013;41(5):1090–9.

Moving?

Make sure your subscription moves with you!

To notify us of your new address, find your **Clinics Account Number** (located on your mailing label above your name), and contact customer service at:

Email: journalscustomerservice-usa@elsevier.com

800-654-2452 (subscribers in the U.S. & Canada)
314-447-8871 (subscribers outside of the U.S. & Canada)

Fax number: 314-447-8029

Elsevier Health Sciences Division
Subscription Customer Service
3251 Riverport Lane
Maryland Heights, MO 63043

*To ensure uninterrupted delivery of your subscription, please notify us at least 4 weeks in advance of move.